# Drug Resistance in Mammalian Cells

## Volume I
## Antimetabolite and Cytotoxic Analogs

Editor
**Radhey S. Gupta, Ph.D.**
Professor
Department of Biochemistry
McMaster University
Hamilton, Ontario, Canada

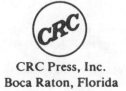

CRC Press, Inc.
Boca Raton, Florida

**Library of Congress Cataloging-in-Publication Data**

Drug resistance in mammalian cells / editor, Radhey S. Gupta
   p.   cm.
   Includes bibliographies and index.
   Contents: v. 1. Antimetabolite and cytotoxic analogs -- v. 2. Anticancer and other drugs.
   ISBN 0-8493-6921-5 (v. 1)
   ISBN 0-8493-6922-3 (v. 2)
   1. Antineoplasitc agents.  2. Drug resistance.
I. Gupta, Radhey S.
RC271.C5D776  1989         615'.7—dc19         89-466

Direct all inquires to CRC Press, Inc., 2000 Corporate Blvd., N.W., Boca Raton, Florida, 33431.

© 1989 by CRC Press, Inc.

International Standard Book Number 0-8493-6921-5 (v. 1)
International Standard Book Number 0-8493-6922-3 (v. 2)

Library of Congress Card Number 89-466
Printed in the United States

# PREFACE

During the past 15 to 20 years, extensive work has been carried out with mutants resistant to various cytotoxic drugs in mammalian cells. Such studies have had a major impact on research and development in a number of different areas including pharmacology, somatic cell genetics, cell biology, mutagenesis, etc. For example, analysis of the drug-resistant mutants have led to a detailed understanding of the cellular metabolism of drugs, molecular mechanisms of action of drugs, and of the different mechanisms by which resistance to various drugs develops in mammalian cells. Cross resistance studies with the mutants have yielded valuable information regarding similarities and/or differences in the mode of action of various drugs. Since development of drug resistance is one of the major causes for failure of chemotherapy, studies with the mutant cells should prove particularly useful in developing rational and more effective chemotherapeutic drug combinations.

The drug-resistant mutants have also played a dominant role in the fields of somatic and molecular cell genetics, which is reminiscent of the central role that the genetic approach had earlier played in providing a comprehensive understanding of prokaryotic systems. Mutants which are affected in specific components provide powerful probes to investigate the roles of the affected components in cell structure and function. They also facilitate molecular cloning as well as chromosomal mapping of the corresponding gene. The selection systems for the drug-resistant mutants also provide valuable genetic markers for quantitative mutagenesis and other genetic studies in mammalian cells. A number of these systems are now routinely employed for screening of agents which are potentially carcinogenic to mammals. In addition, some of the drug-resistant mutants are proving useful as in vitro models for human genetic diseases.

In view of the above, the main objective of these volumes is to provide a concise review of the work done with mutants resistant to different drugs in mammalian cells. The term "drug" is used here in a broad sense to include various cytotoxic agents and inhibitors of cellular processes. Each chapter provides an overview of the mechanism of action of a particular drug or group of drugs and covers the various mechanisms by which resistance to these drugs have been found to develop in mammalian cells. The available information regarding cross resistance/collateral sensitivity patterns of the mutants to other drugs and inhibitors is also included. The information regarding cell structure and function that studies of such mutants have provided, as well as application of the mutants to other types of studies, is also covered. Further, the chemical structures of different drugs/inhibitors are included in various chapters and in some chapters information regarding structure-activity relationship, which has emerged from studies with the mutant cells, is also provided.

Currently, no book which covers all these aspects for mammalian cell mutants resistant to different drugs is available. It is hoped that these volumes will serve as resource and reference books to specialists (e.g., researchers, graduate students, clinicians) in the fields of pharmacology, mammalian cell genetics, and cell biology. In addition, these volumes should also prove useful to researchers, students, and nonspecialists in various allied fields who are using these drugs and inhibitors as probes in their studies and are interested in understanding and learning about the mechanisms of action of these compounds. The first of these volumes covers mainly the antimetabolites and analogs of nucleosides and amino acids while the second volume is devoted to other inhibitors of cellular processes.

I am grateful to many of my colleagues, particularly Dr. K. B. Freeman, who have provided valuable comments and criticisms on many of my own chapters in these volumes. I also wish to express my thanks and appreciation to Barbara Sweet for her highly skilled and efficient secretarial assistance during the course of preparing these volumes. The editorial assistance of the CRC staff deserves special mention. Finally, I would also like to thank my family for their encouragement, understanding, and continued support during this work.

# THE EDITOR

**Radhey S. Gupta, Ph.D.,** is Professor of Biochemistry at McMaster University in Hamilton, Ontario, Canada. Dr. Gupta received undergraduate education at Delhi and Agra and an M.Sc. degree in Chemistry/Biochemistry from the Indian Institute of Technology, New Delhi in 1968. After obtaining his Ph.D. degree in Molecular Biology from the Tata Institute of Fundamental Research (University of Bombay) in 1973, Dr. Gupta pursued postdoctoral work at the Washington University School of Medicine, St. Louis and at the University of Toronto, Canada. His stay in Toronto in Dr. Louis Siminovitch's laboratory had a major influence on his current research interests in the areas of somatic cell genetics and drug resistance in mammalian cells. In 1978 he joined McMaster University as an Assistant Professor and moved through the ranks to his present position in 1986.

Dr. Gupta is a member of the American Association for Cancer Research, New York Academy of Sciences, American Society of Microbiology, Tissue Culture Association of America, Environmental Mutagen Society, Genetic Society of Canada, Canadian Biochemical Society, and Canadian Society for Cell Biology. He has been on several research grant panels and task forces and is currently Associate Editor (for North America) for the journal *Mutagenesis* (IRL Press).

Dr. Gupta, at present, is a recipient of the prestigious "MRC Scientist" award of the Medical Research Council of Canada. From 1979—1984 he also received the "MRC Scholarship" award. The research work in Dr. Gupta's laboratory has been generously supported by grants and personnel support from the Medical Research Council of Canada, Heart and Stroke Foundation of Ontario, Canadian Heart Foundation, National Cancer Institute of Canada, and the Arthritis Society. Dr. Gupta has published over 100 papers, most of which involve studies with drug-resistant mutant cells. The main focus of his current research is on understanding the mechanisms of action of antimitotic drugs, several anticancer drugs, and cardiac glycosides.

# CONTRIBUTORS

**Irene L. Andrulis, Ph.D.**
Assistant Professor
Department of Medical Biophysics
University of Toronto
Toronto, Ontario, Canada

**Gérard Buttin, Ph.D.**
Professor
Department of Immunology
Institut Pasteur
Paris, France

**Elizabeth Cairney, M.D.**
Research Fellow
Department of Research
Mount Sinai Hospital Research Institute
Toronto, Ontario, Canada

**Carol E. Cass, Ph.D.**
Professor
McEachern Laboratory
Department of Biochemistry
University of Alberta
Edmonton, Alberta, Canada

**Chia-Cheng Chang, Ph.D.**
Associate Professor
Department of Pediatrics and Human
  Development
Michigan State University
East Lansing, Michigan

**Michelle Debatisse, Ph.D.**
Maitre de Conférences
Department of Genetics
Institut Pasteur
Paris, France

**Anil K. Dudani, Ph.D.**
Post Doctoral Fellow
Department of Biochemistry
McMaster University
Hamilton, Ontario, Canada

**Wayne F. Flintoff, Ph.D.**
Associate Professor
Department of Microbiology and
  Immunology
University of Western Ontario
London, Ontario, Canada

**Radhey S. Gupta, Ph.D.**
Professor
Department of Biochemistry
McMaster University
Hamilton, Ontario, Canada

**Satish Jindal, Ph.D.**
Post Doctoral Fellow
Department of Biochemistry
McMaster University
Hamilton, Ontario, Canada

**Elliot R. Kaufman, Ph.D.**
Associate Professor
Department of Genetics
University of Illinois College of Medicine
Chicago, Illinois

**William H. Lewis, Ph.D. (Deceased)**
Associate Professor
Department of Microbiology
University of Toronto
Toronto, Ontario, Canada

**Grant A. McClarty, Ph.D.**
Post Doctoral Fellow
Department of Biochemistry
Manitoba Insitiue of Cell Biology
Winnipeg, Manitoba, Canada

**K. John Morrow, Jr., Ph.D.**
Professor
Department of Biochemistry
Texas Tech University Health Sciences
  Center
Lubbock, Texas

**David A. Rintoul, Ph.D.**
Assistant Professor
Biology Division
Kansas State University
Manhattan, Kansas

**Amrik Sahota, Ph.D.**
Research Associate
Department of Medical Genetics
Indiana University School of Medicine
Indianapolis, Indiana

**B. Robert de Saint Vincent, Ph.D.**
Charge de Recherche
Department of Immunology
C.N.R.S.
Paris, France

**Immo E. Scheffler, Ph.D.**
Professor
Department of Biology
University of California at San Diego
LaJolla, California

**Bernard P. Schimmer, Ph.D.**
Professor
Banting and Best Department of Medical
 Research
University of Toronto
Toronto, Ontario, Canada

**P. R. Srinivasan, Ph.D.**
Professor
Department of Biochemistry and Molecular
 Biophysics
Columbia University
New York, New York

**Brian G. Talbot, Ph.D.**
Professor
Department of Biology
University of Sherbrooke
Sherbrooke, Quebec, Canada

**Milton W. Taylor, Ph.D.**
Professor
Department of Biology
Indiana University
Bloomington, Indiana

**Jean-Paul Thirion, Ph.D.**
Professor
Department of Microbiology
University of Sherbrooke
Sherbrooke, Quebec, Canada

**James E. Trosko, Ph.D.**
Professor
Department of Pediatrics and Human
 Development
Michigan State University
East Lansing, Michigan

**Buddy Ullman, Ph.D.**
Associate Professor
Department of Biochemistry
Oregon Health Sciences University
Portland, Oregon

**Jim A. Wright, Ph.D.**
Professor
Departments of Biochemistry and
 Microbiology
Mantioba Institute of Cell Biology
University of Manitoba
Winnipeg, Manitoba, Canada

# TABLE OF CONTENTS

Chapter 1
Methotrexate ...................................................................................................................... 1
**W. F. Flintoff**

Chapter 2
Hydroxyurea and Related Compounds ........................................................................... 15
**J. A. Wright, G. A. McClarty, W. H. Lewis, and P. R. Srinivasan**

Chapter 3
Aphidicolin ...................................................................................................................... 29
**C. C. Chang and J. E. Trosko**

Chapter 4
Ornithine Analogs ........................................................................................................... 45
**I. E. Scheffler**

Chapter 5
Mycophenolic Acid .......................................................................................................... 59
**B. Ullman**

Chapter 6
Adenosine, Deoxyadenosine, and Deoxyguanosine ....................................................... 69
**B. Ullman**

Chapter 7
Purine Nucleoside Analogs .............................................................................................. 89
**R. S. Gupta**

Chapter 8
Adenine Analogs .............................................................................................................. 111
**M. W. Taylor**

Chapter 9
9-β-D-Arabinofuranosyladenine and 9-β-D-Arabinofuranosyl-2-Fluoroadenine ............... 125
**C. E. Cass**

Chapter 10
Guanine and Hypoxanthine Analogs ............................................................................... 145
**K. J. Morrow, Jr. and D. A. Rintoul**

Chapter 11
Halogenated and Other 5-Position Substituted Pyrimidines ........................................... 159
**E. R. Kaufman**

Chapter 12
Cytosine Arabinoside, Deoxycoformycin, and Coformycin .............................................. 171
**G. Buttin, M. Debatisse, and B. Robert de Saint Vincent**

Chapter 13
Cyclic AMP and Other Effectors of Cyclic AMP-Dependent Pathways ............................ 185
**B. P. Schimmer**

Chapter 14
Amino Acid Analogs .................................................................................................... 211
**A. E. L. Cairney and I. L. Andrulis**

Chapter 15
Carbohydrate Analogs ................................................................................................. 233
**J.-P. Thirion and B. Talbot**

Chapter 16
Miscellaneous Drugs — I .............................................................................................. 247
**A. K. Dudani, S. Jindal, and R. S. Gupta**

Index ........................................................................................................................... 259

Chapter 1

# METHOTREXATE

**Wayne F. Flintoff**

## TABLE OF CONTENTS

I.      Introduction ................................................................... 2

II.     Structural Features ............................................................ 2

III.    Cytotoxicity ................................................................... 2

IV.     Structural Changes in DHFR ..................................................... 3

V.      Alterations in the Transport of Mtx ............................................ 4

VI.     Quantitative Changes in DHFR .................................................. 6

VII.    Defects in Polyglutamation .................................................... 7

VIII.   Other Resistant Phenotypes .................................................... 7

IX.     Genetics of Mtx Resistance .................................................... 7

X.      Summary and Perspectives ...................................................... 10

Acknowledgments ................................................................... 10

References ........................................................................ 10

# I. INTRODUCTION

The use of the first rationally designed cancer chemotherapeutic agent, aminopterin, in clinical trials[1] some 38 years ago has stimulated considerable interest in the antifolate compounds not only for their therapeutic value but also as important agents to probe several aspects of the basic biology of the cell. Since aminopterin is no longer used clinically, interest has shifted more recently to methotrexate (Mtx), which is still used in the treatment of certain types of malignancies.[2] The main research interests of several laboratories are to understand the mechanisms of its cytotoxic action and the basis for cellular resistance. This latter goal is stimulated by the observation that resistance does develop in vivo and as a result model in vitro systems have been developed to gain insights into this process. It is anticipated that knowledge gained from such systems may lead to the rationale design of other drugs and protocols to aid in overcoming the resistance in addition to providing important basic information about the eukaryotic cell. It is the purpose of this article to review the current knowledge on the mechanisms of resistance to Mtx in model systems.

There have been several recent reviews on antifolates and their resistances. Readers are referred to these articles which deal in greater depth with certain aspects of this subject.[2-6] Because of the extensive literature in this area this article will not be an exhaustive review, but rather will concentrate on the more significant findings related to the biochemical, genetic, and phenotypic features of Mtx resistance.

# II. STRUCTURAL FEATURES

Methotrexate or amethopterin is the $N^{10}$-methyl-4-aminopteroglutamic derivative of folic acid (Figure 1). These alterations in the structure of folic acid lead to a wide variety of effects on the cell mainly through an interaction and inhibition of the enzyme dihydrofolate reductase (DHFR), which is responsible for the conversion of dihydrofolate (DHF) to tetrahydrofolate (THF).[7] Methotrexate has a higher affinity than folic acid for DHFR which is attributed to the substitution of the 4 amino group for the 4 hydroxyl group.

# III. CYTOTOXICITY

The cytotoxic effect of Mtx is a complex set of interactions occurring at the level of transport and intracellular metabolism.[8] The drug is transported across the cell membrane by the same carrier-mediated, energy requiring system used by the naturally occurring folates.[9] Once inside the cell, it is rapidly polyglutamated[10] which contributes to a longer intracellular retention thus prolonging its exposure to intracellular targets.[11] Methotrexate or its polyglutamated form exerts its most profound effect on the cell by inhibiting DHFR thus blocking the synthesis of THF. During the synthesis of thymidylate there is a rapid conversion of L5,10 methylene THF to DHF.[8] Thus, during treatment with Mtx the THF cofactor is depleted resulting in a subsequent inhibition of both DNA and RNA synthesis. For cellular death to occur from thymidylate starvation, the intracellular levels of Mtx exceed the level of DHFR.[12] This implies that a site other than DHFR is of importance, or that a low affinity form of DHFR that does not bind Mtx tightly exists in the cell, or that DHF is not the rate limiting step in dUMP utilization. Although Mtx does bind to thymidylate synthetase (Kd $10^{-6}$)[13,14] it does so at several orders of magnitude lower than it binds to DHFR (Kd $10^{-11}$)[14] and thus may not contribute significantly to cell death. Current information indicates that cytotoxicity involves both starvation for thymidine and for purines. The extent to which each contributes to cell death is not clearly understood and may depend upon the nature of the folate interconversions within the cell types that have been studied.

Because Mtx affects several aspects of cellular metabolism, various mechanisms of ac-

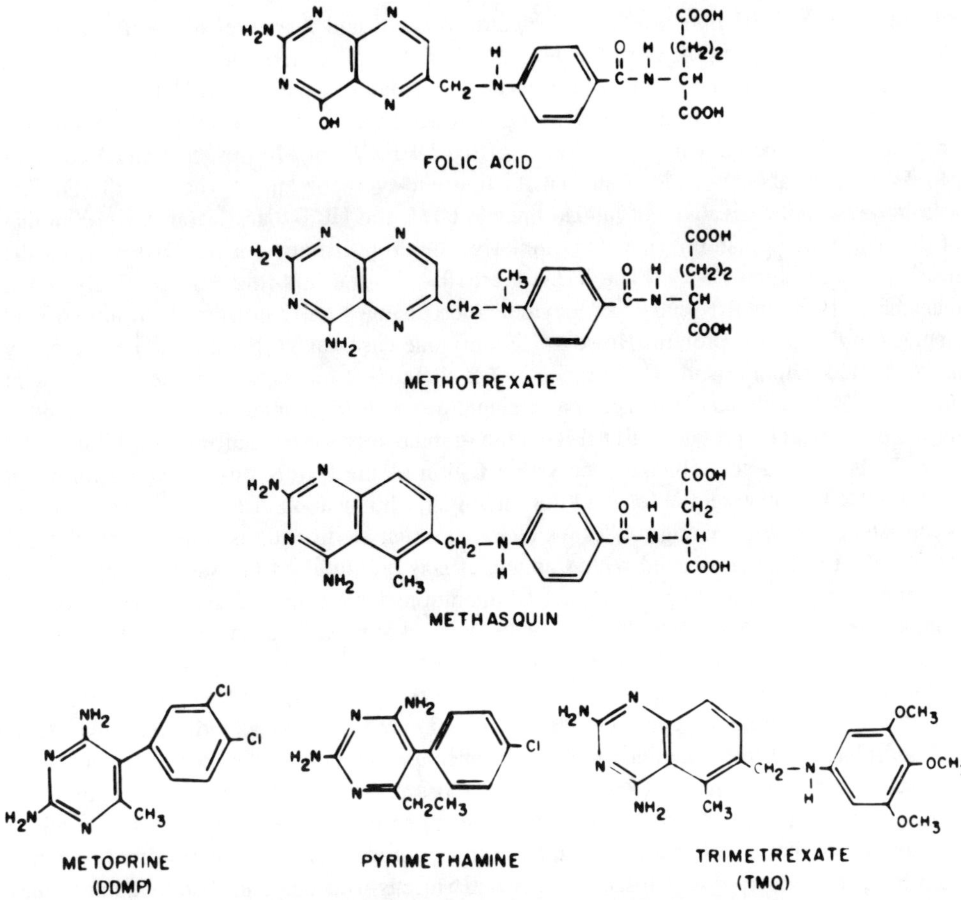

FIGURE 1.    Structures of folic acid and folic acid antagonists.

quired resistance might be expected. To date resistant mechanisms have been associated with alterations both qualitatively and quantitatively in DHFR, in antifolate transport, in polyglutamation, and in thymidylate synthetase. These mechanisms are not mutually exclusive since multiple mechanisms can occur in the same cell. This in part may be a reflection of the multi-step or continuous selection schemes employed to isolate resistant cells.

## IV. STRUCTURAL CHANGES IN DHFR

Since the major intracellular target for Mtx is DHFR, it is not surprising that alterations in this function are detected in Mtx-resistant cells, although this type of change appears not to be the most frequent. Qualitative changes in the DHFR from Mtx-resistant derivatives of murine (L5178Y,[15] L1210,[16] 3T6,[17] L4946[18]), hamster (Chinese hamster ovary [CHO]),[19] Chinese hamster lung, (CHL),[20] and human (lymphoid W1-L2,[21] colon HCT-8[2]) cell lines have been documented. A majority of these isolates have been selected in multistep selection protocols and the phenotype is complex. Not only do these isolates contain an altered DHFR but they may also contain an alteration in the transport of the drug and an overproduction of the DHFR. In some cases the selections have been done in single steps[19] and the only mechanism of resistance can be attributed to the structural change in the DHFR.

Biochemical studies comparing the properties of these altered DHFRs to the corresponding wild type enzyme indicate that a wide spectrum of functional changes can occur. These changes include alterations in substrate binding parameters,[2,15,17,19-22] Vmax,[15,17] susceptibility to heat,[21,22] pH optima,[15,17,21] isoelectric point,[17] and response to modifying agents such as p-chloromercuriphenylsulfonate (pCMS).[15] Not all of the altered DHFRs show all of these changes. The common feature in all the isolates is the altered DHFRs decreased sensitivity to inhibition by the drug, which is reflected in a lower affinity for binding the drug than wild type enzyme. The affinity of the DHFR from Mtx-resistant CHO cells for Mtx is lowered about sixfold from that for the wild-type enzyme,[23] whereas, the DHFRs from the resistant derivatives of human lines W1-L2, and HCT-8 are 1/50th to 1/100th that of the wild-type human enzyme.[21,22] Similarly, the drug affinities of the DHFRs from the resistant murine lines L5178Y and 3T6400 are $10^5$-$10^{15}$ and 300-fold,[17] respectively, lower than the affinity for the wild-type enzyme. Such changes are consistent with amino acid changes in the DHFR protein. However, in only one case has such a change been directly demonstrated. Cloning and DNA sequencing of the DHFR message from the Mtx-resistant murine 3T6400 cells has indicated that a single amino acid change of an arginine residue for a leucine residue produces a DHFR with a dramatically lowered affinity for binding the drug.[24] This amino acid change occurs in a region of the DHFR protein which forms an hydrophobic pocket essential for inhibitor binding.[25] The location of this amino acid change is consistent with drug analog studies which indicate that modifications of the p-aminobenzyl moiety of Mtx were associated with dramatic effects on binding to this altered DHFR.[17]

Indirect support indicating that structural alterations have occurred in the DHFRs comes from studies with structural analogs of folate. Mtx-resistant cells carrying an altered DHFR are cross resistant to both classical (aminopterin)[19] and so called "non-classical"[26] (diaminopyrimidines, triazines, 2,4-diaminoquinazolines) folate analogs. Antifolates with the 2,4-diamino-structure and with the glutamate moiety are the classical antifolates. Nonclassical antifolates lack the glutamate moiety. In one case the cross resistance is not absolute. A Mtx-resistant CHL line, DC-3F/A3, is not cross resistant to the quinazoline antifolate methasquin (Figure 1).[20] This implies that the alteration in the DHFR is at a binding/interaction site that is not shared by the two drugs. Various studies using purified enzymes from both the wild type and resistant cells and various triazines and diaminoquinazolines have indicated that some of these drugs are more effective in inhibiting the wild type enzyme, while others are more effective against the altered DHFR.[27] This is probably a reflection of differences in the binding affinities and sites of interactions which are related to the structural changes in the DHFR proteins.

From various studies, it has been shown that 13 amino acids in the DHFR protein are involved in Mtx binding.[25,28] It is possible that a mutation in any one of these binding/interaction sites would produce a DHFR with altered properties. In the various systems described above it will be of interest to determine where the amino acid changes map in relation to the known sites of interaction of the enzyme with the drug.

## V. ALTERATIONS IN THE TRANSPORT OF MTX

A more common mechanism of resistance to Mtx are changes affecting the ability of the drug to be taken up or transported by the resistant cell. This was first demonstrated by Fisher in 1968 for Mtx-resistant cells from the mouse L5178Y line.[29] A similar phenotype has been shown for resistant cells isolated from the murine lines L1210,[16,30,31] and S180,[32] for lines derived from CHO cells,[19] for lines obtained from rat cells (Yoshida sarcoma,[33] H35[34]), human lines derived from the lines W1-L2,[35] CCRF-CEM (leukemia),[2] HCT-8,[2] MOLT-3 (T-cell),[36] and SAOS-2 (osteosarcoma).[37]

Since the process of Mtx transport is complex involving cell membrane binding, translocation across the membrane, release intracellularly, and efflux from the cell,[9] a wide spectrum of alterations could yield a defective drug uptake phenotype. Sorting out whether the defective drug uptake results from a single lesion or multiple lesions is further complicated since most isolates have been generated in multistep selection schemes where it is possible that multiple events could occur. Furthermore, often these isolates have complex phenotypes with more than a single mechanism of resistance operative. Some isolates, however, have been selected in a single step[19] making an understanding of the mechanism of resistance somewhat simpler. A common feature of a majority of the resistant isolates in this category is a higher Km for drug uptake.[30,31,35,36,38] This is reflected in some cases in a decreased binding of the drug to the surface of the resistant cell in comparison to its binding to the wild type cell.[38] In one resistant isolate from the mouse L1210 line the Km for the transport of Mtx is altered with no change in this parameter for the L5-formyl and L5-methyl derivatives of folate implying a specific alteration in the protein binding domain unique to Mtx.[39] In some cases the Km change is coupled with an alteration in the Vmax of transport. In others no alteration in the Km of transport is evident but the Vmax is decreased suggesting that in these cells the number of membrane binding sites or their turnover rate is reduced. In a Mtx-resistant CHO cell, selected in a single step, the resistant phenotype was correlated directly with the inability of the cells to transport the drug because of an inability to bind the drug at the cell surface.[38] Such a mutant has been useful in demonstrating that both folate and the reduced forms of folate share a common transport system, since this isolate is also defective in the ability to transport folate and 5-methyl THF. This shared transport system has been recently confirmed by kinetic data.[40] Lines showing alterations in the Km for drug transport show cross resistance to folate analogs such as aminopterin[19] and dichloro-Mtx[36] as would be expected for compounds that share the same transport system.

A second class of resistant cells altered in drug transport is represented by a resistant isolate from the L1210 line.[31] These cells may be defective in the ability to permit the translocation of the drug across the cell membrane since they show some influx of drug although this occurs with an altered Km and Vmax when compared to wild type cells. It would be of interest to determine whether this is a single mutational event. To date no isolates have been identified that are defective in the efflux of the drug.

In some of the earlier work it was demonstrated that some resistant cells took up radiolabeled Mtx but to a lesser degree than the corresponding wild-type cells. It would be of importance to reevaluate these observations in light of the demonstration of impurities in the radiolabeled Mtx that are transported via different routes and at a faster rate than Mtx.[41]

Not only have resistant cell defective in Mtx transport been isolated in vitro, but similar such isolates have been selected in vivo.[39] A series of mouse L1210 variants have been isolated by exposure of mice carrying such cells to Mtx. The alterations identified fall into three categories (1) cells with an altered Km for taking up the drug, (2) cells with a lower Vmax for transporting the drug, and (3) cells which contain both a higher Km and a lower Vmax for drug transport. As with the in vitro systems employing continuous selection schemes, it is difficult to determine whether these alterations result from single or multiple genetic events.

An interesting feature of the altered transport phenotype is collateral sensitivity of the cells to lipophilic inhibitors of DHFR. These compounds, which are not actively transported by the cell nor polyglutamated once inside the cell, include such agents as 2,4-diamino-5-(3′,4′ dicholorphenyl)-6-methyl pyrmidine (DDMP, metroprine), pyrimethamine, and 2,4-diamino-6-[(3,4,5,-trimethoxyanilino) methyl] quinazoline (trimetrexate, TMQ) (Figure 1). This increased sensitivity has been demonstrated for resistant CHO cells[42] which are unable to bind the drug at the cell surface, and for both resistant cells derived from mouse L1210[43] and human lines CEM and SAOS-2.[37,44] These resistant isolates possess increased Km parameters for transport when compared to the wild type cells. The mechanism for the increased sensitivity to lipophilic inhibitors is not known. It is speculated that cells defective in Mtx transport will also have a diminished uptake of the natural folates and thus may have a reduced level of the folates intracellularly.[43] This would make the cells sensitive to agents, such as these lipophilic DHFR inhibitors, that affect folate metabolism but enter the cell via different routes than Mtx.

At present the molecular basis of the defects affecting the ability of Mtx to be transported across the cell membrane are lacking as is information of this process in the wild type cells. Part of this results from the limited number of drug binding sites on the surface of the cell. The availability of a cell line which has upregulated the rate of synthesis of the carrier/ binding protein[45] may be useful in the analysis of the transport process at a biochemical/ molecular level and aid in an understanding of the mutational basis of this class of resistant cells.

## VI. QUANTITATIVE CHANGES IN DHFR

The most frequently isolated Mtx-resistant phenotype occurring after a multistep or continuous selection scheme is the overproduction of the DHFR protein. Isolates have been obtained from mouse lines (S180,[46] L1210,[31] L5178Y,[47] EL4,[48,49] PG19[49]), hamster lines (BHK,[50] CHL,[20,51,52] CHO[53]), human lines (HeLa,[54] CEM-CCRF,[2] K562,[2,55] HCT-8,[2] TE 85,[37] MG-63,[37] W1-42,[37] W1L2,[35] RA51[37]), and rat lines (HTC).[56] In most cases examined except one, the overproduction correlates with an overproduction of the DHFR message as a result of an amplification of its gene. This was first demonstrated by Alt et al.[57] for the resistant S180 cells isolated by Hakala et al.[46] and has been subsequently shown for the other systems using specific cloned cDNAs. In one case however, a resistant isolate from the human line HL60 has been shown to overproduce the DHFR protein with no corresponding increase in the abundance of the message nor the gene sequences.[58] Presumably, an alteration in the structural gene for DHFR has occurred and the resulting protein has an enhanced activity.

At low levels of gene amplification there is a good correlation among the levels of resistance, DHFR protein overproduction, mRNA abundance, and gene copy number. At higher levels of amplification, the correlation appears to fall off perhaps due to supplementary mechanisms including decreased affinities of the DHFR for Mtx, altered transport of the drug, or decreased activity of thymidylate synthetase.[59] The DHFR protein overproduced by these resistant cells is either indistinguishable from the wild type enzyme[60,61] or is altered in such a manner as to affect its kinetic parameters.[15,17,23] These latter changes can occur as early[19] or late events[17] in the development of the resistant phenotype. In the latter case, presumably a mutational event occurs in one of the copies of the amplified genes producing the gene product with altered properties. The overproduction of the DHFR protein appears to be specific to this folate enzyme since no other folate utilizing enzymes show any types of changes relative to similar such enzymes from wild type cells.[2,21] The functions examined include folyl glutamate synthetase, thymidine synthetase, serine hydroxymethyl transferase, 10-formyltetrahydrofolate synthetase, and 5,10-methylene tetrahydrofolate synthetase.

At present, the mechanism whereby the additional copies of the DHFR gene are made in the highly amplified lines is unknown. Based on the study of the strucure of the amplified DNA,[49,62] what is apparent is that more DNA than the DHFR gene is amplified. These amplified sequences are of variable lengths in clonal isolates and may undergo changes in what may be a complex process associated with DNA replication, recombination, and genomic rearrangements. In one system there is evidence to indicate that the structure of the amplified unit is constant with little indication of major changes in the DNA sequence arrangement through many fold amplification.[63] For further discussions of the mechanisms of the amplification process, readers are referred to the articles by Schimke,[4] Stark and Wahl,[64] and Hamlin et al.[65]

Since more DHFR protein is synthesized and present in the lines with amplified copies of the DHFR gene than the corresponding wild-type cell, one might expect such isolates to be cross resistant to compounds which have as their target the DHFR protein. These DHFR amplified lines are cross resistant to varying degrees to analogs such as aminopterin,[19] DDMP,[42] pyrimethamine,[42] triazinate,[66] and trimetrexate (TMQ).[66] The level of resistance is in good agreement with the DHFR gene copy number.

The availability of cell lines overproducing the DHFR protein, message, and gene have been invaluable in gaining insights into the structure of this gene, its mRNA, and its regulation.[67]

## VII. DEFECTS IN POLYGLUTAMATION

A less common mechanism of resistance is the lack of detectable polyglutamation of Mtx once it has entered the cell. This has been demonstrated for a human breast cell line with a complex phenotype.[68] These cells, Mtx[R]ZR-75, are about 1000-fold more resistant than wild type cells to the cytotoxic action of Mtx, have a 3-fold lower influx of Mtx than the wild-type cells, a 3-fold decrease in thymidylate synthetase activity, and no detectable polyglutamation of Mtx. However, no changes were detected in the folyl glutmate synthetase enzyme which is responsible for the polyglutamation event. Recently, a human small cell carcinoma has been shown to have a 1.5 to 4-fold lower ability than wild type cells to form polyglutamated derivatives of Mtx with no apparent changes in the synthetase enzyme.[69] In both these cases described, the nature of the alteration(s) yielding low levels of polyglutamation is unknown.

These cells with the complex phenotype including defects in polyglutamation are cross resistant to compounds such as aminopterin, but show little cross resistance to agents such as DDMP, triaznide, and trimetrexate.[68] This may be related to differences in the structures of Mtx and these compounds. These latter compounds lack the end terminal glutamyl residues and thus cannot be converted to polyglutamated forms.

## VIII. OTHER RESISTANT PHENOTYPES

Since Mtx has been shown to have an affinity for thymidylate synthetase[13] and also to affect purine metabolism,[70] one might expect that with a large number of mutants that alterations in some of these functions might be found. In the latter case, there is no direct evidence that such mutants exist, however, there are some reports indicating alterations in thymidylate synthetase.[59,68] These occur as part of complex phenotypes and it appears that the nature of these alterations have not been pursued.

## IX. GENETICS OF MTX RESISTANCE

The frequency to Mtx resistance is dependent upon the cell type, the stringency of selection, and the dose of the drug. Because of the nature of the selection schemes, a majority of the resistant isolates obtained have multiple phenotypes which make it difficult to ascertain the frequency of any single event yielding a mutant phenotype. This is further complicated by the demonstration that certain phenotypes may be lost when the selection pressure is increased.[35] In one study using single step selections the spontaneous frequency to Mtx resistance at a drug dose of $10^{-7} M$ was $10^{-6}$ for the CHO system.[19] Approximately one half of these were stable and all of these displayed qualitative changes in the DHFR protein. The mutational rate for the stable phenotype was $2 \times 10^9$/cell/generation.[71] The other half of the isolates were unstable and may have represented a low level of gene amplification. At this stringency of selection (i.e., $10^{-7} M$ Mtx) no stable isolates were obtained that had amplified DHFR genes and none were defective in Mtx transport. In mutagenized cultures of CHO the frequency to Mtx resistance at this selection pressure was increased five- to tenfold above the spontaneous frequency.[19] In this case all the isolates were stable; about one half displayed qualitative changes in DHFR while the remainder were defective in Mtx uptake. None were shown to contain amplified genes. A second step selection to higher resistance on those isolates displaying an altered DHFR produced isolates which contain stable amplifications of the DHFR gene at a frequency of $10^{-4}$ to $10^{-5}$.[19] More recent work in this system has indicated that a similar frequency of DHFR amplification can be obtained in a single step if the stringency of the selection pressure is reduced to a drug concentration of $5 \times 10^{-8} M$.[96]

These frequencies for DHFR amplification in the CHO system are similar to other systems where resistant colonies with from 5 to 10 copies of the DHFR gene occur at a frequency of $10^{-4}$ to $10^{-6}$ after some 2 to 3 weeks exposure to the drug.[72] This, however, may not be a true reflection of the frequency of gene amplification events, particularly if such genes are highly unstable and are lost within the growth period or if the selection conditions are such that extensive amplification must occur to support growth. The frequency to gene amplification may be greater than this. Recent studies with a fluorescent conjugate of Mtx and a fluorescent activated cell sorter to identify cells with increased levels of the DHFR protein indicate that the spontaneous frequency to DHFR gene amplification in the absence of selection is in the order of $10^{-3}$/cell/generation.[73]

As indicated above, the frequency to Mtx resistance in CHO cells can be increased by treatment with mutagens,[19] however, in general there is a paucity of information on the effects of mutagens on the generation of Mtx-resistant cells. Some interesting observations, however, have been made on the effect of various agents on the frequency of DHFR gene amplification. Agents that reversibly inhibit DNA synthesis, such as Mtx,[74] hydroxyurea,[72] ultraviolet light, and a carcinogen (*N*-acetoxy *N*-acetylaminofluorene)[75] increase the frequency of gene amplification 10- to 100-fold. It is at present not clear as to the mechanism of this increased frequency but it may be related to the mechanism of the gene amplification process. Recent work indicates that treatment of cells with these agents results in the increased synthesis of the DHFR protein due to alterations in the transcriptional patterns which subsequently lead to an increase in the DNA content of the cells.[76]

The phenotypic changes of an altered DHFR protein or defects in the ability of the cells to take up Mtx are stable maintaining their properties in the absence of selection pressure.[19] In contrast, the gene amplification phenotype can be either stable or unstable.[4,64,65] These stability properties appear to correlate to some extent with the arrangement of the amplified genes in the resistant cells. Highly stable lines have the amplified genes located on chromosomes with homogeneously staining regions (HSRs),[77] whereas, unstable lines have the amplified genes present on small, paired, acentric, extrachromosomal bodies called double minutes (DMs).[78-80] This correlation between stability and chromosomal location of amplified genes is not absolute since there have been reports of cell lines containing HSR chromosomes in which the amplified sequences are lost in the absence of selection pressure.[3,81] The HSR type chromosomes were initially observed in hamster cells by Biedler and Spendler[82] and have been subsequently observed in several systems.[80] If present in a cell the HSRs may be on more than a single chromosome,[53] often one of these is the chromosome to which the native DHFR gene maps. For Chinese hamster this is chromosome 2[83-85] and for human it is chromosome 5.[86] Not all chromosome regions containing the amplified DHFR genes are as homogeneously staining as the HSRs originally described.[80] Some HSRs may be banded and in low level amplification the chromosomes containing the amplified gene sequences may have deranged band patterns with small homogeneously staining regions.[3,51] This HSR type chromosome and the abnormally banded chromosomes appear to confer a greater short-term stability or an apparently irreversible altered phenotype on the resistant cell in the absence of selective pressure. In contrast the double minute chromosomes, which contain amplified sequences, are associated with an unstable phenotype when selection pressure is removed. This presumably results from unequal partitioning of the double minutes to the daughter cells at mitosis since these chromosome structures lack centromeres.[87] Coupled to this is the observation that cells which contain fewer double minutes have a selective growth advantage over those with large numbers of these chromosomal structures. Thus the stability of the DHFR amplified genes is dictated in part by the chromosomal structure containing the amplified genes and in part by the species. In general, Mtx-resistant Chinese hamster lines tend to have chromosomally located amplified genes, whereas, mouse and human lines have either HSRs or DMs.

HSR and DM chromosomes are not the only type of chromosomal changes that have been identified in Mtx-resistant lines carrying the amplified genes. Chromosomal rearrangements have been detected both in low[85] and high level[53] amplification of the DHFR gene, but their relationship to the amplification process is at present unclear.

Reversions of the various Mtx-resistant phenotypes to wild type levels of drug sensitivity have not been extensively examined. This is in part due to lack of simple back selection reversion schemes. Revertants of unstably amplified genes to low level gene copy number are readily selected by removal of the selection pressure. Over a period of time there is a concomitant loss of the resistant phenotype and the amplified genes presumably by unequal segregation of the amplified genes during mitosis, at least for the cases where these genes are present on DMs. To date there has been a single report of the reversion of a stable low level DHFR amplified CHO cell line.[88] This was obtained by treatment of the cells with irradiation and subsequent suicide treatment with $^3$H-dUMP. Reversion results from deletions of all or part of the amplified genes. Also in the CHO system revertant schemes for wild type phenotypes have been described for cells containing either an altered DHFR or a defect in the ability to bind the drug at the cell surface. In the former case, a suicide selection scheme using $^3$H-dUMP was employed to isolate revertants.[89] These revertants were shown to have a wild-type sensitivity to Mtx and to contain a DHFR with similar properties as the enzyme from wild type cells. These are presumably point mutations, but it is not known whether the reversion occurred at the same site as the initial mutation or at a secondary site. Wild type revertants from cells with defective Mtx membrane binding were selected by exposure of the resistant cells to pyrimethamine.[42] The resistant cells show an increased sensitivity to this drug and isolates were obtained that could grow in wild type levels of the drug. Some of these showed wild type sensitivities to Mtx and were able to transport the drug in a similar manner as the wild-type cell. Others, however, were able to grow in wild type levels of pyrimethamine but retained the resistance to Mtx and the inability to transport this drug. The nature of the reversion process and the generation of the pyrimethanine resistant cells are unknown.

Somatic cell hybrid analyses have been carried out with the Mtx-resistant cells in combination with wild type cells to examine the genetic behavior of the resistant phenotypes. In such a combination, in systems that have been examined, both the resistant phenotype characterized by an altered DHFR and the overproduction of DHFR behave as co-dominant traits.[50,71] The hybrids show a resistance to Mtx that is intermediate between that of the wild type and resistant diploid parents. As well, the biochemical parameters of the DHFR present in such hybrids is indicative of the expression from both parental cell genomes. In contrast, the alteration in the CHO system resulting in a decreased binding of Mtx to the cell surface and thus a defect in drug transport behaves as a genetically recessive trait.[71] The hybrids between the wild-type cells and the resistant cells have a similar sensitivity to Mtx and transport the drug in a similar manner as the wild-type parental cells. Hybrid studies have not been carried out on the various other types of alterations that can give rise to the defective or altered drug transport phenotypes.

## X. SUMMARY AND PERSPECTIVES

The studies of model systems have provided important information on the mechanisms of resistance to Mtx. It is apparent that this process is complex both biochemically and genetically. Clearly, this analysis is far from complete. The further application of recombinant DNA techniques to the study of Mtx resistance should extend our knowledge on the molecular details of the various phenotypes. Such studies should aid in defining sites on the DHFR protein that are important for drug interaction, in characterizing the membrane binding/transport protein and to defining sites on it which are important for drug binding, and in identifying genomic changes that can occur as a consequence or part of the gene amplification process. Such studies are underway in several laboratories and may lead to the rationale design of drugs to overcome the resistance.

The study of the Mtx-resistant cells has indicated that this drug has several sites of action and it is conceivable that others may exist but mutations in these have not been detected because they occur at low frequencies. Since one of the major sites is the DHFR protein, it might be informative to examine the development of resistance in cells that lack this function.[90] This may be complicated since for growth such cells require the addition of both purines and pyrimidines to the media. However, by a judicial control of these components it might be possible to develop resistance to Mtx in this line that does not involve the DHFR gene.

Reversion analysis in this system has not been explored to any great extent and it might be useful to exploit this approach not only to more completely define the phenotypes but also to identify primary and secondary sites that are used to overcome resistance.

The studies outlined above have been carried out on model systems but it is clear that similar such mechanisms arise clinically in treatments with this drug.[2,5,91-94] Furthermore, the genomic changes, such as HSR chromosomes and DMs, associated with gene amplification have been observed in several malignancies.[80,95] Thus, understanding the biochemical and genetic aspects of the development of resistance to Mtx in model systems may lead to important applications at the clinical level.

## ACKNOWLEDGMENTS

The author wishes to thank Drs. J. Bertino, J. Freisham, J. Goldie, R. Schimke, and F. Sirotnak for providing reprints and preprints of articles prior to their publication. Work in the author's laboratory was supported by a grant from the Medical Research Council of Canada. The author wishes to thank Wendy Dodds for valuable assistance in the typing and preparation of this article.

## REFERENCES

1. **Farber, S., Diamond, L. K., Mercer, R. D., Sylvester, R. F., Jr., and Wolff, J. A.,** Temporary remissions in acute leukemia in children produced by a folic anatagonist, 4-aminopteroylglutamic acid (aminopterin), *New Engl. J. Med.,* 238, 787, 1948.
2. **Bertino, J. R., Srimatkandada, S. Carman, M. D., Mini, E., Jastreboff, M., Moroson, B. A., and Dube, S. K.,** Mechanisms of drug resistance in human leukemia, *Haematology Blood Transfusion,* 29, 90, 1985.
3. **Albrecht, A. M. and Biedler, J. I.,** Acquired resistance of tumor cells to folate antagonists, in *Folate Antagonists as Theurapeutic Agents,* Vol. 1, Sirotnak, F. M., Ed., Academic Press, New York, 1984, 317.
4. **Schimke, R. T.,** Gene Amplification in cultured cells, *Cell,* 37, 705, 1984.

5. **Bertino, J. R. and Rodenhuis, S.,** Methotrexate and drug resistance, in *Advances in Cancer Chemotherapy. Bladder Cancer: Future Directions for Treatment,* Yagoda, A., Ed., John Wiley and Sons, New York, 1986, in press.
6. **Sirotnak, F. M.,** Determinants of resistance to antifolates: biochemical phenotypes, their frequency of occurrence and circumvention, *Cancer Treatment Symposia,* 1986, in press.
7. **Blakley, R. L.,** *The Biochemistry of Folic Acid and Related Pteridines,* North Holland, Amsterdam, 1969, 188.
8. **Jackson, R. C. and Grindey, G. B.,** The biochemical basis for methotrexate cytotoxity, in *Folate Antagonists as Therapeutic Agents,* Vol. 1, Sirotnak, F. M., Ed., Academic Press, New York, 1984, 289.
9. **Dembo, M. and Sirotnak, F. M.,** Membrane transport of folate compounds in mammalian cells, in, *Folate Antagonists as Therapeutic Agents,* Sirotnak, F. M., Ed., Academic Press, New York, 1984, 113.
10. **Whitehead, V. M.,** Synthesis of methotrexate polyglutamates in L1210 murine leukemia cells, *Cancer Res.,* 37, 408, 1977.
11. **Balinska, M., Nimec, Z., and Galivan, J.,** Characteristics of methotrexate polyglutamate formation in cultured hepatic cells, *Arch. Biochem. Biophys.,* 216, 466, 1982.
12. **Goldman, I. D.,** Membrane transport considerations in high-dose methotrexate regimins with leucovorin rescue, *Cancer Treat. Rep. Suppl.,* 65, 13, 1981.
13. **Borsa, J. and Whitmore, G. F.,** Cell killing studies on the mode of action of methotrexate on L-cells *in vitro, Cancer Res.,* 29, 737, 1969.
14. **Jackson, R. C.,** Biological effects of folic acid antagonists with antineoplastic activity, *Pharmacol. Ther.,* 25, 61, 1984.
15. **Goldie, J. H., Dedhar, S., and Krystal, G.,** Properties of a methotrexate-insensitive variant of dihydrofolate reductase derived from methotrexate-resistant L5178Y cells, *J. Biol. Chem.,* 256, 11629, 1981.
16. **Jackson, R. C., Niethammer, D., and Huennekens, F. M.,** Enzymic and transport mechanisms of amethopterin resistance in L1210 mouse leukemia cells, *Cancer Biochem. Biophys.,* 1, 151, 1975.
17. **Haber, D. A., Beverley, S. M., Kiely, M. L., and Schimke, R. T.,** Properties of an altered dihydrofolate reductase encoded by amplified genes in cultured mouse fibroblasts, *J. Biol. Chem.,* 256, 9501, 1981.
18. **Blumenthal, G. and Greenberg, D. M.,** Evidence for two molecular species of dihydrofolate reductase in amethopterin resistant and sensitive cells of the mouse leukemia L4946, *Oncology,* 24, 223, 1970.
19. **Flintoff, W. F., Davidson, S. V., and Siminovitch, L.,** Isolation and partial characterization of three methotrexate-resistant phenotypes from Chinese hamster ovary cells, *Somat. Cell Genet.,* 2, 245, 1976.
20. **Albrecht, A., Biedler, J. L., and Hutchison, D. J.,** Two different forms of dihydrofolate reductase in mammalian cells differentially resistant to amethopterin and methasquin, *Cancer Res.,* 32, 1539, 1972.
21. **Jackson, R. C. and Niethammer, D.,** Acquired methotrexate resistance in lymphoblasts resulting from altered kinetic properties of dihydrofolate reductase, *Eur. J. Cancer,* 13, 567, 1977.
22. **Gupta, R. S., Flintoff, W. F., and Siminovitch, L.,** Purification and properties of dihydrofolate reductase from methotrexate-sensitive and methotrexate-resistant Chinese hamster ovary cells, *Can. J. Biochem.,* 55, 445, 1977.
23. **Flintoff, W. F. and Essani, K.,** Methotrexate-resistant Chinese hamster ovary cells contain a dihydrofolate reductase with an altered affinity for methotrexate, *Biochemistry,* 19, 4321, 1980.
24. **Simonsen, C. C. and Levinson, A. D.,** Isolation and expression of an altered mouse dihydrofolate reductase cDNA, *Proc. Natl. Acad. Sci. U.S.A.,* 80, 2495, 1983.
25. **Voltz, K. W., Matthews, D. A., Alden, R. A., Freer, S. T., Hansch, C., Kaufman, B. T., and Kraut, J.,** Crystal structure of avian dihydrofolate reductase containing phenyltriazine and NADPH, *J. Biol. Chem.,* 257, 2528, 1982.
26. **Hamrell, M. R.,** Inhibition of dihydrofolate reductase and cell growth by antifolates in a methotrexate-resistant cell line, *Oncology,* 41, 343, 1984.
27. **Dedhar, S., Freisham, J. H., Hynes, J. B., and Goldie, J. H.,** Further studies on substituted quinazolines and triazines as inhibitors of a methotrexate-insensitive murine dihydrofolate reductase, *Biochem. Pharmacol.,* 35, 1143, 1986.
28. **Matthews, D. A., Alden, R. A., Bolin, J. T., Freer, S. T., Hamlin, R., Xuong, N., Kraut, J., Poe, M., Williams, M., and Hoogsteen, K.,** Dihydrofolate reductase: x-ray structure of the binary complex with methotrexate, *Science,* 197, 452, 1977.
29. **Fischer, G. A.,** Defective transport of amethopterin (methotrexate) as a mechanism of resistance to the antimetabolite in L5178Y leukemic cells, *Biochem. Pharamacol.,* 11, 1233, 1962.
30. **Sirotnak, F. M., Kurita, S., and Hutchison, D. J.,** On the nature of a transport alteration determining resistance to amethopterin in the L1210 leukemia, *Cancer Res.,* 28, 75, 1968.
31. **McCormick, J. I., Susten, S. S., and Freisheim, J. J.,** Characterization of the methotrexate transport defect in a resistant L1210 lymphoma cell line, *Arch. Biochem. Biophys.,* 212, 311, 1981.
32. **Hakala, M. T.,** On the role of drug penetration in amethopterin resistance of sarcoma 180 cells *in vitro, Biochem. Biophys. Acta.,* 102, 198, 1965.

33. **Braganca, B. M., Diverar, A. Y., and Vaidya, N. R.,** Defective transport of aminopterin in relation to development of resistance in Yoshida sarcoma cells, *Biochem. Biophys. Acta.,* 135, 937, 1967.

34. **Galivan, J.,** Transport and metabolism of methotrexate in normal and resistant cultured rat hepatoma cells, *Cancer Res.,* 39, 735, 1979.

35. **Niethammer, D. and Jackson, R. C.,** Changes of molecular properties associated with the development of resistance in human lymphoblastoid cells, *Eur. J. Cancer,* 11, 845, 1975.

36. **Ohnoshi, T., Ohnuma, T., Takahashi, I., Scanlon, K., Kamen, B. A., and Holland, J. F.,** Establishment of methotrexate-resistant human acute lymphoblastic leukemia cells in culture and effects of folate antagonists, *Cancer Res.,* 42, 1655, 1982.

37. **Diddens, H., Niethammer, D., and Jackson, R. C.,** Patterns of cross-resistance to the antifolate drugs trimetrexate, metoprine, homofolate, and CB3717 in human lymphoma and osteosarcoma cells resistant to methotrexate, *Cancer Res.,* 43, 5286, 1983.

38. **Flintoff, W. F. and Nagainis, C. R.,** Transport of methotrexate in Chinese hamster ovary cells: a mutant defective in methotrexate uptake and cell binding, *Arch. Biochem. Biophys.,* 223, 433, 1983.

39. **Sirotnak, F. M., Moccio, D. M., Kelleher, L. E., and Goutas, L. J.,** Relative frequency and kinetic properties of transport-defective phenotypes among methotrexate-resistant L1210 clonal cell lines derived *in vivo, Cancer Res.,* 41, 4447, 1981.

40. **Henderson, G. B., Suresh, M. R., Vitols, K. S., and Huennekens, F. M.,** Transport of folate compounds in L1210 cells: kinetic evidence that folate influx proceeds via the high-affinity transport system for 5-methyltetrahydrofolate and methotrexate, *Cancer Res.,* 46, 1639, 1986.

41. **Kamen, B. A., Cashmore, A. R., Dreyer, R. N., Moroson, B. A., Hsieh, P., and Bertino, J. R.,** Effect of [3H] methotrexate impurities on apparent transport of methotrexate by a sensitive and resistant L1210 cell line, *J. Biol. Chem.,* 255, 3254, 1980.

42. **Flintoff, W. and Saya, L.,** The selection of wild-type revertants from methotrexate permeability mutants, *Somat. Cell Genet.,* 4, 143, 1978.

43. **Sirotnak, F. M., Moccio, D. M., Goutas, L. J., Kelleher, L. E., and Montgomery, J. A.** Biochemical correlates of responsiveness and collateral sensitivity of some methotrexate-resistant murine tumors to the lipophilic antifolate, metoprine, *Cancer Res.,* 42, 924, 1982.

44. **Schornagel, J. H., Chang, P. K., Sciarini, L. J., Moroson, B. A., Mini, E., Cashmore, A. R., and Bertino, J. R.,** Synthesis and evaluation of 2,4-diaminoquinazoline antifolates with activity against methotrexate-resistant human tumor cells, *Biochem. Pharmacol.,* 33, 3251, 1984.

45. **Sirotnak, F. M., Moccio, D. M., and Yang, C. H.,** A novel class of genetic variants of the L1210 cell up-regulated for folate analogue transport inward, *J. Biol. Chem.,* 259, 13139, 1984.

46. **Hakala, M. T., Zakrzewski, S. F., and Nichol, C. A.,** Relation of folic acid reductase to amethopterin resistance in cultured mammalian cells, *J. Biol. Chem.,* 236, 952, 1961.

47. **Dedhar, S. and Goldie, J. H.,** Overproduction of two antigenically distinct forms of dihydrofolate reductase in a highly methotrexate-resistant mouse leukemia cell line, *Cancer Res.,* 43, 4863, 1983.

48. **Tyler-Smith, C. and Alderson, T.,** Gene amplification in methotrexate-resistant mouse cells. I. DNA rearrangement accompanies dihydrofolate reductase gene amplification in a T-cell lymphoma, *J. Mol. Biol.,* 153, 203, 1981.

49. **Bostock, C. J. and Tyler-Smith, C.,** Gene amplification in methotrexate-resistant mouse cells. II. Rearrangement and amplification of non-dihydrofolate reductase gene sequences accompany chromosomal changes, *J. Mol. Biol.,* 153, 219, 1981.

50. **Littlefield, J. W.,** Hybridization of hamster cells with high and low folate reductase activity, *Proc. Natl. Acad. Sci. U.S.A.,* 62, 88, 1969.

51. **Lewis, J. A., Biedler, J. L., and Melera, P. W.,** Gene amplification accompanies low level increases in the activity of dihydrofolate reductase in antifolate-resistant Chinese hamster lung cells containing abnormally banding chromosomes, *J. Cell Biol.,* 94, 418, 1982.

52. **Melera, P. W., Lewis, J. A., Biedler, J. L., and Hession, C.,** Antifolate-resistant Chinese hamster cells. Evidence for dihydrofolate reductase gene amplification among independently derived sublines overproducing different dihydrofolate reductases, *J. Biol. Chem.,* 255, 7024, 1980.

53. **Flintoff, W. F., Weber, M. K., Nagainis, C. R., Essani, A. K., Robertson, D., and Salser, W.,** Overproduction of dihydrofolate reductase and gene amplification in methotrexate-resistant Chinese hamster ovary cells, *Mol. Cell. Biol.,* 2, 275, 1982.

54. **Morandi, C. and Attardi, G.,** Isolation and characterization of dihydrofolate reductase from methotrexate-sensitive and -resistant human cell lines, *J. Biol. Chem.,* 256, 10169, 1981.

55. **Srimatkandada, S., Medina, W. D., Cashmore, A. R., Whyte, W., Engel, D., Moroson, B. A., Franco, C. T., Dube, S. K., and Bertino, J. R.,** Amplification and organization of dihydrofolate genes in a human leukemia cell line, K-562, resistant to methotrexate, *Biochemistry,* 22, 5774, 1983.

56. **Fougere-Deschatrette, C., Schimke, R. T., Weil, D., and Weiss, M. C.,** A study of chromosomal changes associated with amplified dihydrofolate reductase genes in rat hepatoma cells and their dedifferentiated variants, *J. Cell Biol.,* 99, 497, 1984.

57. **Alt, F. W., Kellems, R. D., Bertino, J. R., and Schimke, R. T.,** Selective multiplication of dihydrofolate reductase genes in methotrexate-resistant variants of cultured murine cells, *J. Biol. Chem.,* 253, 1357, 1978.

58. **Dedhar, S., Hartlet, D., and Goldie, J. H.,** Increased dihydrofolate reductase activity in methotrexate-resistant human promyelocytic-leukemia (HL-60) cells, *Biochem. J.,* 225, 609, 1985.

59. **White, J. C. and Goldman, I. D.,** Methotrexate resistance in an L1210 cell line resulting from increased dihydrofolate reductase, decreased thymidylate synthetase activity and normal membrane transport, *J. Biol. Chem.,* 256, 5722, 1981.

60. **Nakamura, H. and Littlefield, J. W.,** Purification, properties, and synthesis of dihydrofolate reductase from wild type and methotrexate-resistant hamster cells, *J. Biol. Chem.,* 247, 179, 1972.

61. **Alt, F. W., Kellems, R. E., and Schimke, R. T.,** Synthesis and degradation of folate reductase in sensitive and methotrexate-resistant lines of S-180 cells, *J. Biol. Chem.,* 251, 3063, 1976.

62. **Federspiel, N. A., Beverley, S. M., Schilling, J. W., and Schimke, R. T.,** Novel DNA rearrangements are associated with dihydrofolate reductase amplification, *J. Biol. Chem.,* 259, 9127, 1984.

63. **Montoya-Zavala, M. and Hamlin, J.,** Similar 150-kilobase DNA sequences are amplified in independently derived methotrexate-resistant Chinese hamster cells, *Mol. Cell Biol.,* 5, 619, 1985.

64. **Stark, G. R. and Wahl, G. M.,** Gene amplification, *Ann. Rev. Biochem.,* 53, 447, 1984.

65. **Hamlin, J. L., Milbrandt, J. D., Heintz, N. H., and Azizkhan, J. C.,** DNA sequence amplification in mammalian cells, *Int. Rev. Cytology,* 90, 31, 1984.

66. **Mini, E., Moroson, B. A., Franco, C. T., and Bertino, J. R.,** Cytotoxic effects of folate anatagonists against methotrexate-resistant human leukemic lymphoblast CCRF-CEM cell lines, *Cancer Res.,* 45, 325, 1985.

67. **Chasin, L.,** The dihydrofolate reductase locus, in *Molecular Cell Genetics,* Gottesman, M. M., Ed., John Wiley and Sons, New York, 1985, 449.

68. **Cowan, K. H. and Jolivet, J.,** A methotrexate-resistant human breast cancer cell line with multiple defects, including diminished formation of methotrexate polyglutamates, *J. Biol. Chem.,* 259, 10793, 1984.

69. **Curt, G., Carney, D., and Jolivet, J.,** Defective methotrexate (MtxG1) polyglutamation: a mechanism of drug resistance in human small cell cancer (SCLC), *Proc. Am. Assoc. Cancer Res.,* 24, 283, 1983.

70. **Allegra, C. J., Fine, R. L., Drake, J. C., and Chabner, B. A.,** The effect of methotrexate on intracellular folate pools in human MCF-7 breast cancer cells. Evidence for direct inhibition of purine synthesis, *J. Biol. Chem.,* 261, 6478, 1986.

71. **Flintoff, W. F., Spindler, S. M., and Siminovitch, L.,** Genetic characterization of methotrexate-resistant Chinese hamster ovary cells, *In Vitro,* 12, 749, 1976.

72. **Brown, P. C., Tlsty, T. D., and Schimke, R. T.,** Enhancement of methotrexate resistance and dihydrofolate reductase gene amplification by treatment of mouse 3T6 cells with hydroxyurea, *Mol. Cell Biol.,* 3, 1097, 1983.

73. **Johnston, R. N., Beverley, S. M., and Schimke, R. T.,** Rapid spontaneous dihydrofolate reductase gene amplification shown by fluorescent activated cell sorting, *Proc. Natl. Acad. Sci. U.S.A.,* 80, 3711, 1983.

74. **Varshavsky, A.,** Phorbol ester dramatically increases incidence of methotrexate-resistant mouse cells: possible mechanisms and relevance to tumor promotion, *Cell,* 25, 561, 1981.

75. **Tlsty, T. D., Brown, P. C., and Schimke, R. T.,** UV radiation facilitates methotrexate resistance and amplification of the dihydrofolate reductase gene in cultured 3T6 mouse cells, *Mol. Cell Biol.,* 4, 1050, 1984.

76. **Johnson, R. N., Feder, J., Hill, A. B., Sherwood, S. W., and Schimke, R. T.,** Transient inhibition of DNA synthesis results in increased dihydrofolate reductase enzyme synthesis and subsequent increased DNA content per cell, *Mol. Cell Biol.,* 6, 3373, 1986.

77. **Nunberg, J. H., Kaufman, R. F., Schimke, R. T., Urlaub, G., and Chasin, L.,** Amplified dihydrofolate genes are localized to a homogeneously staining region of a single chromosome in a methotrexate-resistant Chinese hamster ovary cell line, *Proc. Natl. Acad. Sci. U.S.A.,* 75, 5553, 1978.

78. **Kaufman, R. J., Brown, P. C., and Schimke, R. T.,** Amplified dihydrofolate reductase genes in unstably methotrexate-resistance cells are associated with double minute chromosomes, *Proc. Natl. Acad. Sci. U.S.A.,* 76, 5669, 1979.

79. **Haber, D. A. and Schimke, R. T.,** Unstable amplification of an altered dihydrofolate reductase gene associated with double minute chromosomes, *Cell,* 26, 355, 1981.

80. **Cowell, J. K.,** Double minutes and homogeneously staining regions: gene amplification in mammalian cells, *Annu. Rev. Genet.,* 16, 21, 1982.

81. **Biedler, J. L., Melera, P. W., and Spengler, B. A.,** Specifically altered metaphase chromosomes in antifolate-resistant Chinese hamster cells that overproduce dihydrofolate reductase, *Cancer Genet. Cytogenet.,* 2, 47, 1980.

82. **Biedler, J. L. and Spengler, B. A.,** Metaphase chromosome anomaly: association with drug resistance and cell-specific products, *Science,* 191, 185, 1976.

83. **Worton, R., Duff, C., and Flintoff, W.,** Microcell mediated cotransfer of genes specifying methotrexate resistance, emetine sensitivity and chromate sensitivity with Chinese hamster chromosome 2, *Mol. Cell Biol.,* 1, 330, 1981.
84. **Roberts, M., Melera, P. W., Davide, J. P., Hart, J. T., and Ruddle, F. H.,** Assignment of the native Chinese hamster dihydrofolate reductase gene to chromosome 2, *Cytogenet. Cell Genet.,* 36, 599, 1983.
85. **Flintoff, W. F., Livingston, E., Duff, C., and Worton, R. G.,** Moderate-level amplification in methotrexate-resistant Chinese hamster ovary cells is accompanied by chromosomal translocations at or near the site of the amplified DHFR gene, *Mol. Cell Biol.,* 4, 69, 1984.
86. **Anagnou, N. P., O'Brien, S. J., Shimada, T., Nash, W. G., Chen, M. J., and Nienhuis, A. W.,** Chromosomal organization of the human dihydrofolate reductase genes: dispersion, selective amplification, and a novel form of polymorphism, *Proc. Natl. Acad. Sci. U.S.A.,* 81, 5170, 1984.
87. **Barker, P. E., Drwinga, H. L., Hittelman, W. N., and Maddox, A. M.,** Double minutes replicate once during S phase of the cell cycle, *Exp. Cell Res.,* 130, 353, 1980.
88. **Urlaub, G., Kas, E., Carothers, A. M., and Chasin, L.,** Deletion of the diploid dihydrofolate reductase locus from cultured mammalian cells, *Cell,* 33, 405, 1983.
89. **Flintoff, W. F. and Weber, M.,** Selection of wild-type revertants from methotrexate-resistant cells containing an altered dihydrofolate reductase, *Somat. Cell Genet.,* 6, 517, 1980.
90. **Urlaub, G. and Chasin, L. A.,** Isolation of Chinese hamster cell mutants deficient in dihydrofolate reductase activity, *Proc. Natl. Acad. Sci. U.S.A.,* 77, 4216, 1980.
91. **Curt, G. A., Carney, D. N., Cowan, K. H., Jolivet, J., Bailey, B. D., Drake, J. C., Kao-Shan, C. S., Minna, J. D., and Chabner, B. A.,** Unstable methotrexate resistance in human small-cell carcinoma associated with double minute chromosomes, *N. Engl. J. Med.,* 208, 199, 1983.
92. **Horns, R. C., Dower, W. J., and Schimke, R. T.,** Gene amplification in a leukemic patient treated with methotrexate, *J. Clin. Oncol.,* 2, 2, 1984.
93. **Trent, J. M., Buick, R. N., Olson, S., Horns, R. C., and Schimke, R. T.,** Cytologic evidence for gene amplification in methotrexate resistant cells obtained from a patient with ovarian adenocarcinoma, *J. Clin. Oncol.,* 2, 8, 1984.
94. **Carmen, M. D., Schornagel, J. H., Rivest, R. S., Srimatkamdada, S., Portlock, C. S., Duffy, T., and Bertino, J. R.,** Resistance to methotrexate due to gene amplification in a patient with acute leukemia, *J. Clin. Oncol.,* 2, 16, 1984.
95. **Barker, P. E.,** Double minutes in human tumor cells, *Cancer Genet. Cytogenet.,* 5, 81, 1982.
96. **Flintoff, W. F.,** unpublished observations.

Chapter 2

# HYDROXYUREA AND RELATED COMPOUNDS

**Jim A. Wright, Grant A. McClarty, William H. Lewis, and P. R. Srinivasan**

## TABLE OF CONTENTS

I. Introduction to Hydroxyurea and Ribonucleotide Reductase ..................... 16

II. Cellular Properties of Drug Resistant Cells ..................................... 16
   A. Ribonucleotide Reductase Inhibitors..................................... 16
   B. Hydroxyurea Resistance and Cross Resistance to Other Drugs ........... 18
   C. Bleomycin Collateral Sensitivity and Ribonucleotide Reductase
      Hypersensitivity ....................................................... 20
   D. Hydroxyurea Resistance and Modifications in Cell Proliferation ......... 20

III. Altered Expression of Ribonucleotide Reductase and the Role of Gene
   Amplification in Drug Resistant Cells ........................................ 23
   A. Protein Elevations ...................................................... 23
   B. Analysis of M1 and M2 mRNA and DNA .............................. 24

IV. Summary ................................................................... 24

Acknowledgments................................................................ 25

References...................................................................... 25

# I. INTRODUCTION TO HYDROXYUREA AND RIBONUCLEOTIDE REDUCTASE

Hydroxyurea was first synthesized in 1869 by Dresler and Stein,[1] but very little interest was shown in the drug until 1960, when it was reported to have antitumor activity in animal screening tests,[2] and in 1964, when it was shown to produce responses in patients with neoplastic disease.[3] In general, hydroxyurea has been used clinically in the treatment of a wide range of solid tumors as well as acute and chronic leukemia,[3-5] and it has shown promise as a radiation potentiator,[6] as a myelosuppressive agent in treating polycythemia vera,[7] and in controlling proliferation of the epidermis in psoriasis.[8] Furthermore, in many cell biology studies, the drug has been used as a cell synchronizing tool because it is a specific and reversible inhibitor of DNA synthesis.[9] Hydroxyurea enters mammalian cells by a diffusion mechanism and rapidly inhibits DNA synthesis upon addition of cytotoxic concentrations to cultured cells,[10,11] making the drug a convenient selective agent for isolating drug resistant cell lines.[12-14]

The major site of action for hydroxyurea is at the highly regulated enzyme, ribonucleotide reductase.[14-17] DNA synthesis requires a continuous and balanced supply of the four deoxyribonucleoside triphosphates that originate from the direct reduction of the 2′-carbon atom on the ribose moiety of ribonucleotides. In mammalian cells, this reduction occurs at the diphosphate level in the presence of ribonucleotide reductase, which occupies a critical rate-limiting position in the synthesis of DNA (Figure 1). In keeping with the importance of this enzyme in the physiology of the cell, substrate specificity and activity is strictly regulated in a complex manner by nucleotide effectors. For example, the reduction of CDP to dCDP and UDP to dUDP occurs in the presence of an ATP activated enzyme. The reduction of GDP to dGDP and ADP to dADP takes place in the presence of dTTP and dGTP, respectively. Further controls are exerted by various nucleotides acting as inhibitors of the reductions of one or more of the enzyme substrates. For example, dATP acts as a general regulator of activity by inhibiting the reduction of all four ribonucleotides, and dTTP and dGTP are potent inhibitors of pyrimidine reductions. The control of ribonucleotide reductase occurs by one of the most interesting and complex allosteric mechanisms in the cell. Structural properties of the enzyme are also interesting. The mammalian enzyme has been separated into two nonidentical components,[18] often called M1 and M2[14,17] (Figure 2). Effectors and substrates bind to protein M1, a dimer of molecular weight 170,000. The M2 protein is a dimer of molecular weight 88,000 containing stoichiometric amounts of nonheme iron and a unique tyrosine free radical required for activity.[19] Hydroxyurea inhibits ribonucleotide reduction by specifically inactivating the M2 tyrosine free radical (Figure 2). Although both M1 and M2 are required for enzyme activity, different mechanisms regulate the levels of the two components during cell growth; the regulation of M2 is particularly interesting since it varies significantly during the cell cycle and closely correlates with S-phase.[17,20,21] Clearly, hydroxyurea resistant cell lines altered in ribonucleotide reductase activity would be useful for studying both mammalian drug resistance characteristics, and the regulation of an exceptionally interesting enzyme playing a central role in DNA synthesis, and therefore, cell proliferation.

# II. CELLULAR PROPERTIES OF DRUG RESISTANT CELLS

## A. Ribonucleotide Reductase Inhibitors

A variety of drugs are available which inhibit ribonucleotide reductase in vivo, by acting at the M1 or M2 proteins of the enzyme. As outlined in a previous review,[14] these compounds can be placed into three different classes. The first group contains drugs which interact with the M2 protein and interfere with tyrosine free radical formation, which is essential for the

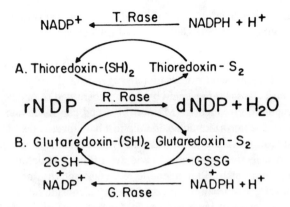

FIGURE 1.   Reduction of ribonucleotides (rNDP) to deoxy-ribonucleotides (dNDP) by ribonucleotide reductase (R.R ase) (EC 1.17.4. 1).[14] Two small proteins, thioredoxin through the thioredoxin reductase (T.Rase) system (A) and glutaredoxin via the glutathione (GSH) and glutathione reductase (G.Rase) system (B) can function as hydrogen carriers in the reaction

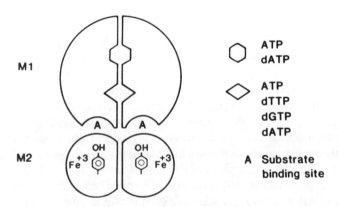

FIGURE 2.   A subunit structure model for ribonucleotide reductase.[14] There are two independent regulatory domains on the M1 protein dimer. One is responsible for regulating overall activity through binding of ATP (activator) or dATP (inhibitor), and the other regulates substrate specificity through the binding of ATP, dTTP, and dGTP. Apparently, dATP can also bind to the substrate specificity site of M1 and mimic the effects observed with ATP. Protein M2 also forms a dimer containing nonheme iron which is involved in stabilizing the tyrosine-free radical. Hydroxyurea acts by destroying the tyrosine-free radical required for enzyme activity.

reduction process. Included in this group are the hydroxamic acids like hydroxyurea, thiosemicarbazones such as MAIQ (4-methyl-5-amino-1-formylisoquinoline thiosemicarbazone), diazoles like IMPY (2,3-dihydro-1-H-pyrazole 2,3-A imidazole), the triazole guanazole (3,5-diamino-1,2,4-triazole), hydroxy- and amino-substituted benzohydroxamic acids, *N*-carbamoyloxyurea, and the glycopeptide antibiotic bleomycin. The second group of compounds inhibit the substrate and effector binding protein, M1. These include natural metabolites like deoxyguanosine, deoxyadenosine, and deoxythymidine, which are converted by the cell to natural allosteric effectors of ribonucleotide reductase, and unnatural drugs such as bromodeoxyuridine which inhibit enzyme activity when converted to the triphosphate level by cellular activities. The periodate oxidized dialdehyde derivatives such as oxidized inosine (Inox) and 5'-inosinic acid (PI-IMP) are also included in this group. The polyphenolic compound gossypol also inhibits ribonucleotide reductase,[22] but does not inactivate the M2 tyrosine free radical (unpublished observations) suggesting that the target for gossypol is the M1 protein. A third class is represented by the 2' substituted ribonucleoside diphosphates which require a functioning reductase (M1 and M2) and can inactivate either component. For example, 2'deoxy-2-chlororibonucleoside diphosphate inactivates M1 whereas 2'deoxy-2-azidoribonucleoside diphosphate is an M2 inactivator. Clearly, there are a large number of potentially useful selective agents with widely different structures for isolating drug resistant lines with alterations in ribonucleotide reductase activity, and some of them (e.g., hydroxyurea, guanazole, *N*-carbamoyloxyurea, deoxyadenosine, deoxythymidine, deoxyguanosine, bromodeoxyuridine) have been used for that purpose.[14] Furthermore, the antibiotic aphidicolin which inhibits DNA polymerase but not ribonucleotide reductase, and the arabinofuranosyl nucleoside analogs (Ara-A and Ara-C), which are much better inhibitors of DNA polymerase than the reductase, have also been good selective agents for isolating drug resistant cell lines with alterations in ribonucleotide reductase activity.[14] We have initiated the study of cell lines selected for resistance to hydroxyurea and related drugs such as guanazole and *N*-carbamoyloxyurea.[12-14] Single and multiple step procedures for isolating cell lines and strains resistant to the cytotoxic effects of these drugs have been described elsewhere.[23-28]

## B. Hydroxyurea Resistance and Cross Resistance to Other Drugs

Earlier work from our laboratory suggested that hydroyxurea and guanazole shared a common site of action.[21] Electron paramagnetic resonance (EPR) spectroscopy studies have now shown that hydroxyurea and guanazole inactivate the M2 tyrosine free radical (Figure 2) of ribonucleotide reductase.[19,29] Also, drug resistance and enzyme inhibition studies have led to the proposal that *N*-carbamoyloxyurea acts by a similar mechanism.[26] The chemical structures of these three compounds are shown in Figure 3. These drugs have been effective selective agents for the isolation of resistant lines from rapidly proliferating cells. As an example, the drug resistance properties of a Chinese hamster ovary (CHO) cell line selected for the ability to grow in normally cytotoxic concentrations of hydroxyurea is shown in Figure 4. Cells resistant to hydroxyurea have been shown to be cross resistant to hydroxyurethane and formamidoxime.[24] In addition, a common feature of hydroxyurea resistant cell lines is the ability to form colonies in the presence of very high concentrations of guanazole and *N*-carbamoyloxyurea as well as the selective agent, when compared to parental wild-type cells. Similarly, cell lines selected for resistance to guanazole or *N*-carbamoyloxyurea are highly cross resistant to the other two nonselective agents.[23,26] These results support the view that the three drugs share at least one major site of action, presumably the M2 component of ribonucleotide reductase. Enzyme studies support this point as well since cell lines resistant to these drugs exhibit alterations in ribonucleotide reductase.[12-14]

Cell lines selected for resistance to hydroxyurea frequently contain increased levels of ribonucleotide reductase activity, which is accompanied by an elevation in M2 activity, or by an elevation in both the M1 and M2 components.[14,27] This suggests that some hydroxyurea resistant lines, especially those showing an increase in both components, may be cross resistant to compounds that act at enzyme sites other than the M2 tyrosine free radical. We have recently found that gossypol (Figure 3), a DNA synthesis inhibitor and antifertility agent, is a potent inhibitor of ribonucleotide reductase.[22] As noted earlier, EPR studies indicate that, unlike hydroxyurea, gossypol does not destroy the tyrosine free radical of M2 (unpublished observations), suggesting that gossypol is an M1 inhibitor. Hydroxyurea resistant cells that overproduce ribonucleotide reductase activity can show cross resistance to

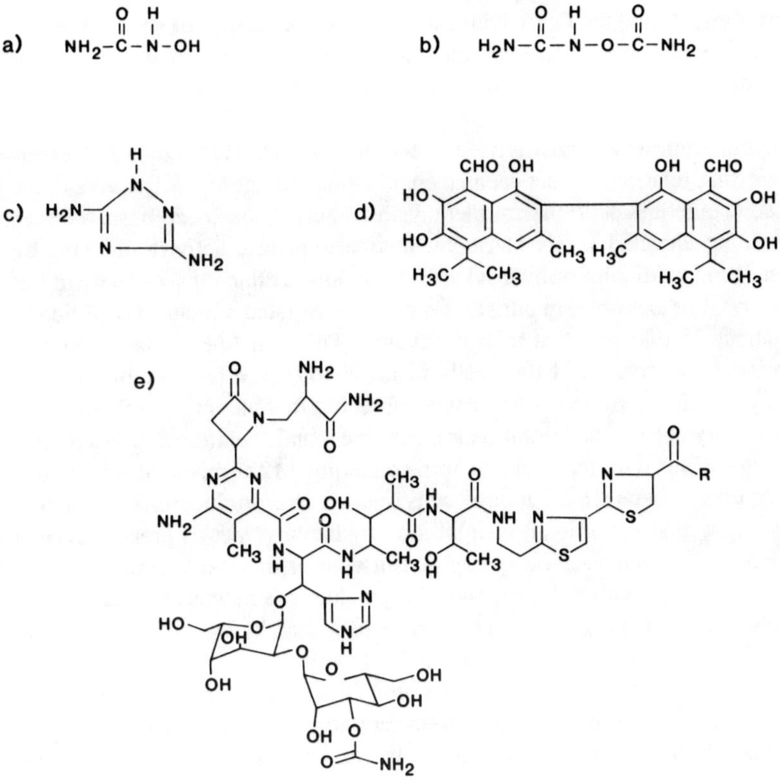

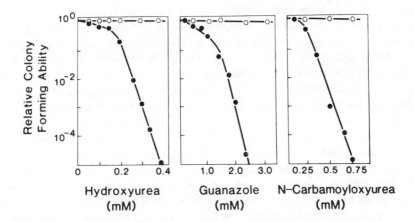

FIGURE 3. Chemical structures of some inhibitors of ribonucleotide reductase: (a) hydroxyurea, (b) *N*-carbamoyloxyurea, (c) guanazole, (d) gossypol, (e) bleomycin (various forms exist which are different from each other only in the terminal cation moiety, R, which consists of an amine or polyamine).[45]

FIGURE 4. Relative colony forming ability of wild type Chinese hamster ovary cells (○) and a cell line selected for resistance to hydroxyurea (●) in the presence of increasing concentrations of drugs.[14]

the cytotoxic effects and the DNA synthesis inhibitory properties of gossypol.[22] These results are in keeping with the biochemical alterations in the drug resistant cells, and the finding that gossypol is a ribonucleotide reductase inhibitor.

## C. Bleomycin Collateral Sensitivity and Ribonucleotide Reductase Hypersensitivity

An interesting relationship between ribonucleotide reductase, hydroxyurea, and the commonly used chemotherapeutic agent bleomycin (Figure 3) has been observed recently. Cell lines containing elevated levels of ribonucleotide reductase activity obtained by selection for resistance to aphidicolin or hydroxyurea can exhibit collateral sensitivity to the antibiotic bleomycin.[30,31] For example, in our studies we have isolated a mouse L cell line called SC2, which is about 35-fold resistant to hydroxyurea. This cell line is also approximately 8.5-fold more sensitive than wild-type cells to the cytotoxic effects of bleomycin in colony forming experiments.[31] In addition, we have observed that bleomycin inhibits ribonucleotide reductase activity.[31] Enzyme inhibition is due to the metal chelating abilities of this antitumor agent, which enables it to inactivate the iron containing M2 component (see Figure 2). Using the hydroxyurea resistant SC2 mouse cells, which overproduce enzyme activity, it was possible to show that the amount of inhibition by bleomycin was greatly enhanced if ribonucleotide reductase was previously exposed in vivo or in vitro to drugs like hydroxyurea, guanazole, or MAIQ, which destroy the M2 tyrosine free radical. For example, when SC2 cells were cultured in the presence or absence of 5 m$M$ hydroxyurea, and CDP reductase activity was measured in the presence of 8$\mu$ $M$ bleomycin, we observed 70% inhibition with enzyme from hydroxyurea treated cells and only 20% inhibition with enzyme prepared from nontreated cells. This conversion of ribonucleotide reductase to a form hypersensitive to bleomycin occurs rapidly in vivo (within 15 min) and in vitro (within 20 min). The increased sensitivity to bleomycin is likely due to a decrease in the stability of the iron center of protein M2 following exposure to hydroxyurea and related drugs. These observations may have important implications for the use of bleomycin as an anticancer agent, especially in combination chemotherapy where it can be used with other drugs whose target is ribonucleotide reductase.

## D. Hydroxyurea Resistance and Modifications in Cell Proliferation

Since the main site of action of hydroxyurea is ribonucleotide reductase, a key rate-limiting step in DNA synthesis, drug-resistant cells altered in this activity may exhibit significant differences in proliferation-related characteristics, and therefore be useful model systems for investigating the role of ribonucleotide reduction and DNA synthesis in this process. Several model systems in which proliferation is strictly regulated in a normal or near-normal fashion were chosen to test this hypothesis. The first model was the normal human diploid fibroblast culture which exhibits a limited lifespan in vitro and is often used to investigate problems in senescence.[25,32] Three independent clones of human diploid fibroblasts resistant to hydroxyurea were isolated from young (low passage) cell cultures. The drug resistance properties of these human strains appeared to be entirely due to elevated ribonucleotide reductase activity, which was accompanied by alterations in deoxyribonucleotide pools, especially in the dCTP pool size. Interestingly, the three variant human strains exhibited substantial reductions in their replicative abilities (between 20 and 40%) when compared to cultures of normal human diploid fibroblasts.[25] In a second approach, our laboratory has used the rat $L_6$ and $L_8$ myoblast cell lines.[33-34] Cell proliferation and the induction of the differentiated phenotype appear to be mutually exclusive properties in many, if not all, terminally differentiating systems, including myogenic cells.[35] The $L_6$ and $L_8$ rat myoblasts retain the capacity to undergo myogenesis during cultivation at the nonpermissive cell density and nutritive state, while expressing the muscle specific phenotype under the permissive conditions of confluency and nutrient depletion. In the permissive situation,

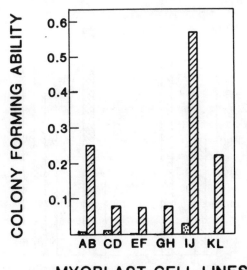

FIGURE 5.   Colony forming abilities of hydroxyurea resistant and sensitive myoblast lines in agar. Cells were added to 60 mm culture plates with growth medium containing agar (0.33% agar on a 0.5% agar base), and incubated at 37°C to allow colonies to form.[36,37] The cell lines are (A) $L_6$WT-1, (B) $L_6$H$^R$-1, (C) $L_6$WT-2, (D) $L_6$H$^R$-2, (E) $L_6$WT-3, (F) $L_6$H$^R$-3, (G) $L_6$WT-4, (H) $L_6$H$^R$-4, (I) $L_6$WT-5, (J) $L_6$H$^R$-5, (K) $L_8$WT-1, (L) $L_8$H$^R$-1.[33]

mononucleated myoblasts fuse to form multinucleated myotubes, and show increases in muscle specific proteins such as creatine phosphokinase. Therefore, both morphological and biochemical differentiation can be monitored and quantitated in these cell lines.[33-35] Six independently isolated hydroxyurea resistant cell lines have been obtained from myogenesis-positive, wild-type clones by single step procedures.[33] Interestingly, every drug resistant line showed absent or reduced capacity for the developmental pathway typical of its wild type clone. These altered differentiated properties were also accompanied by modest but significant elevations in the levels of ribonucleotide reductase activity and modifications in deoxyribonucleotide but not ribonucleotide pools. Drug uptake studies with $^{14}$C-hydroxyurea suggested that resistance was not due to drug permeability modifications.

The change to a more proliferation as opposed to differentiation program by the hydroxyurea resistant myoblast lines suggested that they may also possess altered neoplastic characteristics. In general, a common feature of tumorigenic cell lines is their ability to form colonies in growth medium containing a low percentage of agar.[36,37] As shown in Figure 5, the ability to produce colonies by the drug-resistant myoblast lines in growth medium containing 0.33% agar was significantly enhanced when compared to the parental clones from which they were derived. These results were not influenced by differences in growth rates between cell lines in vitro since the drug-resistant myoblasts exhibited the same or slightly longer doubling times when compared to their wild-type counterparts in normal growth medium. A good correlation is usually found between the ability to form colonies in low percentage agar and tumorigenic abilities in vivo.[36,37] This point was tested by injecting variant and wild type $L_6$ myoblasts subcutaneously into the backs of BALB/c nu/nu mice. Three mice were used for each clone, and the number of tumors and the latency period of each tumor was monitored. A comparison of tumor latency information accumulated for

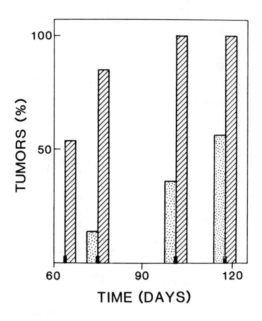

FIGURE 6.    Tumor formation by $L_6WT1$-5 and $L_6H^R1$-5 rat myoblasts in male BALB/c nu/nu mice. Three mice/cell line were injected S.C. in the back with approximately $10^6$ cells. Three mice died prior to developing tumors. Values represent the accumulation of tumor latency results observed with the five resistant (▨) and five parental drug sensitive (▦) $L_6$ myoblast lines.

five of the hydroxyurea-resistant lines and their parental wild type populations is presented in Figure 6. It is clear that as a group these hydroxyurea resistant myoblast lines were more efficient than wild type in forming tumors in BALB/c nu/nu mice. The results obtained with the myoblast lines are reminiscent of previous studies correlating elevations in ribonucleotide reductase with tumorigenic properties of a series of rat hepatoma cell lines.[38,39]

Our working hypothesis is that there is an important link between ribonucleotide reduction, deoxyribonucleotide pools, and the proliferation/differentiation state of normal cells. However, a great deal of caution and more experimentation is required for several reasons. First, it should be mentioned that, although ribonucleotide reductase is the main site of action for hydroxyurea, there is evidence that the drug may affect other important sites as well.[40-42] Therefore, it is possible that some yet undetermined alterations in drug resistant cells may account, at least in part, for the biological changes described above. Also, it is quite likely that mechanisms of hydroxyurea resistance different from those detected in our studies with human fibroblasts and rat myoblasts could have quite different effects upon the biology of the cell than those noted above. Furthermore, whether these observations apply only to hydroxyurea-resistant human diploid fibroblasts and cultured rat myoblasts remains to be determined. Each cell type differs in expression of its genetic content, and these differences should be important in determining the eventual changes that can occur in response to hydroxyurea resistance. This point is evident when considering some recent observations in our laboratory with a hydroxyurea resistant BALB/c 3T3 mouse cell line. This variant cell line exhibited a marked reduction in adipogenic development when compared to its wild-type clone, but unlike the differentiation-defective myoblast lines, the variant 3T3 line was dramatically *less* tumorigenic than the parental line when tested in vivo with BALB/c nu/nu mice. Although more work is required with independently isolated hydroxyurea resistant 3T3 lines before any conclusions can be reached, these studies do suggest that the genetic background of the cell line will play a major role in determining the changes that may be

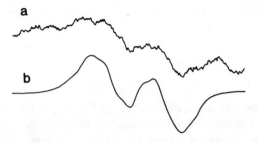

FIGURE 7. Electron paramagnetic resonance at 77K of packed samples of wild type mouse L cells (a) and the hydroxyurea resistant mouse L cell line, LHF (b). The microwave power was 91.5 mW and the modulations were 0.63 and 0.25 mT for wild type and LHF samples, respectively. For the curve shown in (a) the spectrometer amplification was about tenfold greater than in the curve presented in (b).

observed. This point is further supported by studies with hydroxyurea resistant mouse L and CHO cell lines, which lack the rigid growth characteristics exhibited by rat myoblasts and mouse 3T3 cells. In general, both the wild-type and drug-resistant mouse L cell lines and CHO lines were highly tumorigenic. Although some drug resistant mouse L cell lines showed an increase in tumor latency characteristics in preliminary experiments, none of the mouse cell lines examined so far has exhibited an acceleration in tumorigenicity when compared to parental wild type cells, as was observed with the variant myoblast populations. However, several drug resistant CHO cell lines have been isolated which exhibit significantly enhanced tumorigenic properties as judged by elevated tumor growth rates in vivo, suggesting that further cellular and molecular characterization of these cell lines would be worthwhile.

## III. ALTERED EXPRESSION OF RIBONUCLEOTIDE REDUCTASE AND THE ROLE OF GENE AMPLIFICATION IN DRUG RESISTANT CELLS

### A. Protein Elevations

The observation that hydroxyurea-resistant cell lines often contain increased levels of ribonucleotide reductase,[14,27,28,43] suggests that at least one of the protein components of the enzyme (i.e., the one that is rate limiting in concentration) is significantly elevated in drug-resistant cells. Both M1 and M2 components of ribonucleotide reductase are needed for enzyme activity but different mechanisms appear to regulate the levels of these proteins during cell growth.[17,20,21] M2, the target for hydroxyurea is particularly interesting since it varies significantly during the cell cycle, and its short half life suggests that M2 can be limiting for enzyme acitivty.[17] Since this protein contains a tyrosine-free radical necessary for enzyme activity, it is possible to determine the expression of M2 in drug resistant lines by measuring the free radical characteristics of a functional M2 component by EPR. The concentration of free radical is proportional to the amplitude of the EPR signal, and can be used to estimate cellular concentrations of tyrosyl free radical.[17,43-46] These experiments have been performed with hamster, mouse, and rat hydroxyurea resistant and parental wild-type lines. For example, in a recent study, we have observed that out of eight different drug resistant rodent lines, seven had substantial elevations in M2 tyrosine free radical content.[46] Figure 7 shows the results obtained with the hydroxyurea-resistant LHF mouse cell line and its parental wild-type population. Like the SC2 line described earlier, LHF cells are about 35-fold more resistant to hydroxyurea than wild-type cells.[27] The EPR signal was dramatically elevated by about 50-fold in LHF cells, in keeping with the previous drug resistance and enzyme properties reported for this line.[27] Recently, studies have also been carried out with antiserum specific for either the M1 or the M2 component of ribonucleotide reductase.[44,45,47] These studies have confirmed the EPR findings, and have shown that some cell lines exhibiting resistance to very high hydroxyurea concentrations contain elevations in the levels of both enzyme components.

## B. Analysis of M1 and M2 mRNA and DNA

With the recent preparations of cDNAs encoding the two components of ribonucleotide reductase,[44,48] it is now possible to determine the relative amounts of M1 and M2 transcripts in mammalian cells. Recently, studies have been carried out with a variety of mammalian cell lines (hamster, mouse, rat, and human),[44,46,47] and have shown that M1 cDNA hybridizes to a single mRNA species in all wild type and drug-resistant cell lines. Plate 1a* shows results of a Northern blot analysis with RNA isolated from the mouse LHF cell line and its parental wild type population. Very slight or no changes in the M1 transcript was detected when drug resistant and sensitive cells were compared. In contrast to M1, two M2 mRNA bands of different molecular weights were detected in M2 cDNA hybridization studies. They were approximately 3.4 Kb and 1.6 Kb in all species examined except mouse, where the high molecular weight band was about 2.1 Kb and the 1.6 Kb mRNA was present in very low concentrations. Northern blot analysis showed that M2 mRNA was significantly elevated in most hydroxyurea-resistant cell lines. For example, Plate 1b* shows a large increase of approximately 40-fold with M2 mRNA from LHF cells as compared to wild type cells, in keeping with EPR results (Figure 7) and previous enzyme studies.[27]

To compare the relative number of M1 and M2 gene copies in drug resistant and sensitive cell lines, DNA from these lines have been digested with endonucleases, and Southern blots of the digested mixtures were hybridized with $^{32}$P-labeled M1 or M2 cDNA probes.[44-47] In general, amplification of the M2 gene was frequently observed, even in cell lines which were only slightly more resistant to hydroxyurea than parental wild-type cells.[46] An example of M2 gene amplification is presented in Plate 2*, where we show that the LHF cell line contains the same number of M1 genes but about sixfold more M2 genes than the wild-type population. No obvious M1 or M2 gene rearrangements were observed. M1 gene amplification in hydroxyurea-resistant cell lines appear to occur rarely and seem to be associated with only the most highly drug resistant cells.[46,47] Plate 3* shows Southern blot analysis of a series of hamster cell lines selected for increasing drug resistance properties. Note that although each cell line contained an M2 gene amplification (unpublished observations), only the most highly drug-resistant line, 600H, showed an amplification of the M1 gene, which was accompanied by an increase in M1 message. In general, our studies with a variety of mammalian cell lines indicate that a frequent early event in a mechanism leading to hydroxyurea resistance is the amplification of the M2 gene. Further drug resistance may involve M1 gene amplification as well, although elevations in M1 protein in highly drug-resistant mouse cells can occur without increasing the M1 gene copy number.[45] Finally, it should be mentioned that not all hydroxyurea resistant lines examined have exhibited ribonucleotide reductase gene amplification.[46] We have detected two cell lines, one selected for hydroxyurea resistance and one for *N*-carbamoyloxyurea resistance, that do not appear to have an increase in M1 or M2 gene copies. Determining the mechanism(s) underlying resistance in these lines should also prove very interesting.

## IV. SUMMARY

Hydroxyurea, a drug that has found use in clinical situations, is a specific inhibitor of DNA synthesis, and acts by inhibiting the activity of the highly regulated enzyme ribonu-

---

* See Plates 1 — 3 following this page.

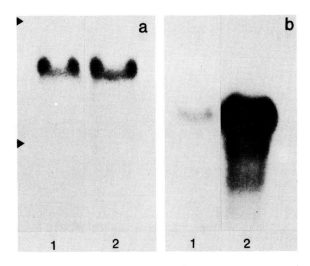

PLATE 1.   Northern blot analysis of (a) M1 and (b) M2 RNA levels in wild-type mouse L cells (lane 1) and the hydroxyurea resistant mouse L cell line, LHF (lane 2). Total cellular RNA was extracted from exponentially growing cells, and experiments were performed with $^{32}$P-labeled Nc01 generated fragments containing the cDNA of clone 65 (M1) or the Pst 1 fragments of clone 10 (M2) essentially as described previously.[43,44] The autoradiograms were exposed for 24 hr at $-70°C$ with intensifying screens. The arrows refer to the positions of 28s and 18s rRNA.

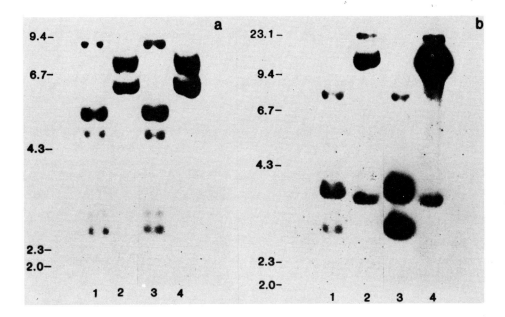

PLATE 2.   Southern blot analysis of (a) M1 and (b) M2 DNA from wild-type mouse L cells (lanes 1 and 2), and from the hydroxyurea-resistant mouse L cell line, LHF (lanes 3 and 4). Genomic DNA was digested to completion with EcoR1 (lanes 1 and 3) or Hind III (lanes 2 and 4), and experiments were performed with the $^{32}$P-labeled M1 or M2 fragments described in Figure 8 essentially as described previously.[43,44] The DNA size markers were Hind III digested lambda DNA (Boehringer Mannheim).

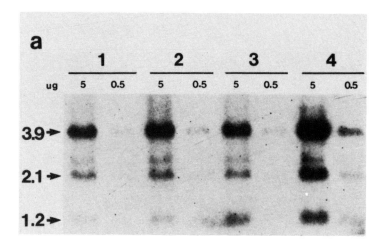

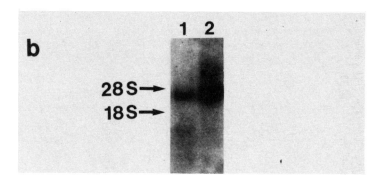

PLATE 3. (a) Southern blot analysis of EcoR1 digested genomic DNA hybridized to [32]P-labeled M1 cDNA.[48] Lane 1, wild-type V79 hamster cells, lane 2, Hyd[R]-4 cells, lane 3, 100H cells, lane 4, 600H cells. Size markers are shown on the left. The resistant lines were derived from a Chinese hamster lung cell line (V79). Chromosomes were purified from a hydroxyurea-resistant V79 clone and used to transform wild-type cells to drug resistance. One transformant was cultivated in the presence of increasing concentrations of hydroxyurea to produce a series of lines with stepwise increases in drug resistance and ribonucleotide reductase activities. The cell lines Hyd[R]-4, 100H, and 600H were selected for growth in 30, 100, and 600 μg/mℓ hydroxyurea, respectively, and the 600H line contained about 80-fold more ribonucleotide reductase activity than wild type cells. (b) Northern blot analysis of M1 RNA from wild type V79 cells (lane 1) and 600H cells (lane 2) performed with [32]P-labeled M1 cDNA.[48] Size markers show the positions of 28s and 18s rRNA.

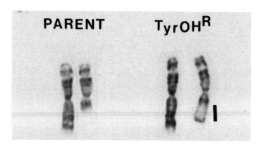

PLATE 4. Chromosomes 2 and Z2 from CHO parental cells and from a Tyrosinol-resistant cell line which contains an HSR on chromosome Z2 (as indicated by the bar).

cleotide reductase. Hydroxyurea, and other drugs whose site of action is at one of the two nonidentical subunits of ribonucleotide reductase (M1 or M2), have been used in cell culture to isolate drug-resistant lines. These lines are useful for studying mammalian drug resistance characteristics, and the regulation of an exceptionally interesting enzyme which plays a central role in DNA synthesis, and therefore, cell proliferation. Hydroxyurea inactivates the M2 subunit by destroying a tyrosine-free radical essential for activity, and cell lines resistant to hydroxyurea exhibit cross resistance to other drugs which have a similar mode of action, such as guanazole and *N*-carbamoyloxyurea. An interesting relationship between ribonucleotide reductase, hydroxyurea, and the commonly used chemotherapeutic agent bleomycin, has been observed. Drug resistant lines containing elevated levels of ribonucleotide reductase have been isolated, which exhibit collateral sensitivity to bleomycin. Furthermore, pretreatment of cells with hydroxyurea-related drugs rapidly converts the reductase to a form hypersensitive to bleomycin. The importance of ribonucleotide reductase in cell proliferation is stressed by observations suggesting that cell cultures altered in this activity can exhibit changes in proliferation-related characteristics, such as in vitro lifespan, cellular differentiation, and tumorigenic properties. Molecular biology studies have indicated that hydroxyurea resistant lines frequently exhibit elevations in the M2 component, M2 mRNA, and M2 gene copy number. The most highly drug-resistant lines may also possess changes in the M1 protein, which may or may not be accompanied by an amplification of the M1 gene. However, not all hydroxyurea resistant lines contain ribonucleotide reductase gene amplification, indicating that other molecular mechanisms are involved in the resistance of some cell lines. Although the molecular studies are relatively recent, it is already clear that the drug resistant lines are capable of providing important new information about the regulation of ribonucleotide reduction, and about cellular mechanisms responsible for resistance to drugs whose target is at a key control point in the synthesis of DNA.

## ACKNOWLEDGMENTS

We thank the M.R.C. of Canada (J.A.W., and W.H.L.), N.C.I. of Canada (J.A.W.), N.S.E.R.C. (J.A.W.) and the American Cancer Society (P.R.S.) for research funds, and the M.R.C. of Canada for a postdoctoral fellowship (G.A.M.). J.A.W. is a recipient of a Terry Fox Cancer Research Scientist Award and W.H.L. is a scholar of the M.R.C. of Canada. Figures 1, 2, and 4 were reprinted from Reference 14 with permission from Pergamon Press, Ltd. J.A.W. and G.A.M. thank L. Thelander for the use of his EPR spectrometer, the cDNA probes for M1 and M2, and for many interesting discussions. The observations on tumorigenicity, including Figures 5 and 6, are from studies in J.A.W.'s laboratory by J. A. Wright, J. S. Morgan, D. C. Creasey, and A. Y. Tagger. W. H. L. acknowledges P. Tonin and E. Wensing for data obtained in his laboratory. J. A. W. is also pleased to acknowledge A. H. Greenberg for advice on tumor experiments, and D. A. Chow, J. C. Jamieson, A. K. M. Chan, A. Y. Tagger, J. Damen, B. Choy, S. E. Egan, and others for their assistance in many ways.

## REFERENCES

1. **Dresler, W. F. C. and Stein, R.** Uber den hydroxylharnstoff, *Justus Liebigs Ann. Chem. Pharmacol.*, 150, 242, 1869.
2. **Stock, C. C., Clarke, D. A., Philips, F. S., Barclay, R. K., and Myron, S. A.**, Sarcoma 180 screening data, *Cancer Res.*, 20, 193, 1960.
3. **Krakoff, I. H., Savel, H., and Murphy, M. L.**, Phase II studies of hydroxyurea (NSC-32065) in adults: clinical evaluation, *Cancer Chemother. Rep.*, 40, 53, 1964.

4. **Engstrom, P. F., MacIntyre, J. M., Mittelman, A., and Klaassen, D. J.,** Chemotherapy of advanced colorectal carcinoma: fluorouracil alone vs. two drug combinations using fluorouracil, hydroxyurea, semustine, dacarbazine, razoxane, and mitomycin, *Am. J. Clin. Oncol.,* 7, 313, 1984.

5. **Bolin, R. W., Robinson, W. A., Sutherland, J., and Hamman, R. F.,** Busulfan versus hydroxyurea in long-term therapy of chronic myelogenous leukemia, *Cancer,* 50, 1683, 1982.

6. **Piver, M. S., Barlow, J. J., Vongtama, V., and Blumenson, L.,** Hydroxyurea: a radiation potentiator in carcinoma of the uterine cervix, *Am. J. Obstet. Gynecol.,* 147, 803, 1983.

7. **Donovan, P. B., Kaplan, M. E., Goldberg, J. D., Tatarsky, I., Najean, Y., Stilberstein, E. B., Knospe, W. H., Laszlo, J., Mack, K., Berk, P. D., and Wasserman, L. R.,** Treatment of polycythemia vera with hydroxyurea, *Am. J. Hematol.,* 17, 329, 1984.

8. **McDonald, C. J.,** The uses of systemic chemotherapeutic agents in psoriasis, *Pharmacol. Ther.,* 14, 1, 1981.

9. **Ashihara, T. and Baserga, R.,** Cell synchronization, in *Methods in Enzymology,* Vol. 58, Jakoby, W. B. and Pastan, I. H., Eds., Academic Press, New York, 1979, 248.

10. **Morgan, J. S., Creasey, D. C., and Wright, J. A.,** Evidence that the antitumor agent hydroxyurea enters mammalian cells by a diffusion mechanism, *Biochem. Biophys. Res. Commun.,* 134, 1254, 1986.

11. **Young, C. W., Schochetman, G., Hodas, S., and Balis, M. E.,** Inhibition of DNA synthesis by hydroxyurea: structure activity relationships, *Cancer Res.,* 27, 535, 1967.

12. **Wright, J. A., Lewis, W. H., and Parfett, C. L. J.,** Somatic cell genetics: a review of drug resistance, lectin resistance and gene transfer in mammalian cells in culture, *Can. J. Genet. Cytol.,* 22, 443, 1980.

13. **Wright, J. A., Hards, R. G., and Dick, J. E.,** Studies of mammalian ribonucleotide reductase activity in intact permeabilized cells: a genetic approach, *Adv. Enzyme Regul.,* 19, 105, 1981.

14. **Wright, J. A.,** Altered forms of mammalian nucleoside diphosphate reductase from mutant cell lines, *Pharmacol. Ther.,* 22, 81, 1983.

15. **Thelander, L. and Reichard, P.,** Reduction of ribonucleotides, *Ann. Rev. Biochem.,* 48, 133, 1979.

16. **Hards, R. G. and Wright, J. A.,** Regulation of ribonucleotide reductase activity in intact mammalian cells, *Arch. Biochem. Biophys.,* 231, 17, 1984.

17. **Eriksson, S., Graslund, A., Skog, S., Thelander, L., and Tribukait, B.,** Cell cycle-dependent regulation of mammalian ribonucleotide reductase. The S-phase-correlated increase in subunit M2 is regulated by *de novo* protein synthesis, *J. Biol. Chem.,* 259, 11695, 1984.

18. **Hopper, S.,** Ribonucleotide reductase of rabbit bone marrow. I. Purification, properties, and separation into two protein fractions, *J. Biol. Chem.,* 247, 3336, 1972.

19. **Thelander, M., Graslund, A., and Thelander, L.,** Subunit M2 of mammalian ribonucleotide reductase. Characterization of a homogeneous protein isolated from M2-overproducing mouse cells, *J. Biol. Chem.,* 260, 2737, 1985.

20. **Eriksson, S. and Martin, D. W., Jr.,** Ribonucleotide reductase in cultured mouse lymphoma cells. Cell cycle-dependent variation in the activity of subunit protein M2, *J. Biol. Chem.,* 256, 9436, 1981.

21. **Cory, J. G. and Fleischer, A. E.,** Noncoordinate changes in the components of ribonucleotide reductase in mammalian cells, *J. Biol. Chem.,* 257, 1263, 1982.

22. **McClarty, G. A., Chan, A. K., Creasey, D. C., and Wright, J. A.,** Ribonucleotide reductase: an intracellular target for the male antifertility agent, gossypol, *Biochem. Biophys. Res. Commun.,* 133, 300, 1985.

23. **Wright, J. A. and Lewis, W. H.,** Evidence of a common site of action for the antitumor drugs, hydroxyurea and guanazole, *J. Cell Physiol.,* 83, 437, 1974.

24. **Lewis, W. H. and Wright, J. A.,** Genetic characterization of hydroxyurea resistance in Chinese hamster ovary cells, *J. Cell Physiol.,* 97, 73, 1978.

25. **Dick, J. E. and Wright, J. A.,** Human diploid fibroblasts with alterations in ribonucleotide reductase activity, deoxyribonucleotide pools and *in vitro* lifespan, *Mech. Aging, Dev.,* 26, 37, 1984.

26. **Hards, R. G. and Wright, J. A.,** N-carbamoyloxyurea-resistant Chinese hamster ovary cells with elevated levels of ribonucleotide reductase activity, *J. Cell Physiol.,* 106, 309, 1981.

27. **McClarty, G. A., Chan, A. K. M., and Wright, J. A.,** Characterization of a mouse cell line selected for hydroxyurea resistance by a stepwise procedure: drug-dependent overproduction of ribonucleotide reductase activity, *Somat. Cell Mol. Genet.,* 12, 121, 1986.

28. **Lewis, W. H. and Wright, J. A.,** Isolation of hydroxyurea-resistant CHO cells with altered levels of ribonucleotide reductase, *Somat. Cell. Genet.,* 5, 83, 1979.

29. **Kjoller Larsen, I., Sjoberg, B.-M., and Thelander, L.,** Characterization of the active site of ribonucleotide reductase of *Escherichia coli,* bacteriophage T4 and mammalian cells by inhibition studies with hydroxyurea analogues, *Eur. J. Biochem.,* 125, 75, 1982.

30. **Ayusawa, D., Iwata, K., and Seno, T.,** Unusual sensitivity to bleomycin and joint resistance to 9-β-D-arabinofuranosyladenine and 1-β-D-arabinofuranosylcytosine of mouse FM3A cell mutants with altered ribonucleotide reductase and thymidylate synthetase, *Cancer Res.,* 43, 814, 1983.

31. **McClarty, G. A., Chan, A. K. M., and Wright, J. A.,** Hydroxyurea-induced conversion of mammalian ribonucleotide reductase to a form hypersensitive to bleomycin, *Cancer Res.,* 46, 4516, 1986.

32. **Blondal, J. A., Dick, J. E., and Wright, J. A.,** Membrane glycoprotein changes during the senescence of normal human diploid fibroblasts in culture, *Mech. Aging Dev.,* 30, 273, 1985.

33. **Creasey, D. C. and Wright, J. A.,** Involvement of ribonucleotide reductase in cellular differentiation, *Biosci. Rep.,* 4, 299, 1984.

34. **Parfett, C. L. J., Jamieson, J. C., and Wright, J. A.,** Changes in cell surface glycoproteins on non-differentiating L$_6$ rat myoblasts selected for resistance to concanavalin A, *Exp. Cell Res.,* 144, 405, 1983.

35. **Nguyen, H. T., Medford, R. M., and Nodal-Ginard, B.,** Reversibility of muscle differentiation in the absence of commitment: analysis of a myogenic cell line temperature-sensitive for commitment, *Cell,* 34, 281, 1983.

36. **MacPherson, I. and Montagnier, L.,** Agar suspension culture for the selective assay of cells transformed by polyoma virus, *Virology,* 23, 291, 1964.

37. **Egan, S. E., McClarty, G. A., Jarolim, L., Wright, J. A., Spiro, I., Hager, G., and Greenberg, A. H.,** Expression of H-*ras* correlates with metastatic potential: evidence for direct regulation of the metastatic phenotype in 10T1/2 and NIH-3T3 cells, *Mol. Cell Biol.,* 7, 830, 1987.

38. **Elford, H. L.,** Functional regulation of mammalian ribonucleotide reductase, *Adv. Enzyme Regul.,* 10, 19, 1972.

39. **Weber, G.,** Biochemical strategy of cancer cells and the design of chemotherapy: G. H. A. Clowes memorial lecture, *Cancer Res.,* 43, 3466, 1983.

40. **Platt, O. S., Orkin, S. H., Dover, D., Beardsley, G. P., Miller, B., and Nathan, D. G.,** Hydroxyurea enhances fetal hemoglobin production in sickle cell anemia, *J. Clin. Invest.,* 74, 652, 1984.

41. **McMillan, T. J., Rao, J., and Hart, I. R.,** Enhancement of experimental metastasis by pretreatment of tumor cells with hydroxyurea, *Int. J. Cancer,* 38, 61, 1986.

42. **Sittman, D. B., Graves, R. A., and Marzluff, W. E.,** Histone mRNA concentrations are regulated at the level of transcription and mRNA degradation, *Proc. Natl. Acad. Sci.,* 80, 1849, 1983.

43. **Lewis, W. H. and Srinivasan, P. R.,** Chromosome-mediated gene transfer of hydroxyurea resistance and amplification of ribonucleotide reductase activity, *Mol. Cell Biol.,* 3, 1053, 1983.

44. **Thelander, L. and Berg, P.,** Isolation and characterization of expressible cDNA clones encoding the M1 and M2 subunits of mouse ribonucleotide reductase, *Mol. Cell Biol.,* 6, 3433, 1986.

45. **McClarty, G. A., Chan, A. K., Engstrom, Y., Wright, J. A., and Thelander, L.,** Elevated expression of M1 and M2 components and drug-induced post-transcriptional modulation of ribonucleotide reductase in a hydroxyurea-resistant mouse cell line, *Biochemistry,* 26, 8004, 1987.

46. **Wright, J. A., Alam, T. G., McClarty, G. A., Tagger, A. Y., and Thelander, L.,** Altered expression of ribonucleotide reductase and the role of M2 gene amplification in hydroxyurea resistant hamster, mouse, rat and human cell lines, *Somat. Cell Mol. Genet.,* 13, 155, 1987.

47. **Cocking, J. M., Tonin, P. N., Stokoe, N. M., Wensing, E. J., Lewis, W. H., and Srinivasan, P. R.,** The gene for the M1 subunit of ribonucleotide reductase is amplified in hydroxyurea-resistant hamster cells, *Somat. Cell Mol. Genet.,* 13, 221, 1987.

48. **Caras, I., Levinson, B., Fabry, M., Williams, S., and Martin, D., Jr.,** Cloned mouse ribonucleotide reductase subunit of M1 cDNA reveals amino acid sequence homology with *Escherichia coli* and herpes virus ribonucleotide reductase, *J. Biol. Chem.,* 260, 7015, 1985.

49. **Muller, W. E. G. and Zahn, R. K.,** Bleomycin, an antibiotic that removes thymine from double-stranded DNA, in *Progress in Nucleic Acid Research and Molecular Biology,* Vol. 20, Cohn, W. E., Ed., Academic Press, New York, 1977, 21.

Chapter 3

APHIDICOLIN

**Chia-Cheng Chang and James E. Trosko**

## TABLE OF CONTENTS

I.      Introduction ................................................................. 30

II.     Effects and Mechanism of Action of Aphidicolin ............................. 30
        A.      Effects on DNA Polymerases ......................................... 30
        B.      Effects on Gene Mutation and Chromosomal Aberrations ............... 31

III.    Isolation and Characterization of Aphidicolin-Resistant Mutants ........... 32
        A.      Aphidicolin-Resistant Mutant with Altered DNA Polymerase ........... 32
        B.      Aphidicolin-Resistant Mutant with Elevated DNA Polymerase
                Level ............................................................. 35
        C.      Aphidicolin-Resistant Mutant with Altered Nucleotide Pools ......... 35
        D.      Aphidicolin-Resistant Mutant with Temperature-Sensitive
                Thymidylate Synthetase ............................................ 35
        E.      Aphidicolin-Resistant Mutant with Unknown Mechanism ............... 36
        F.      Other Mutants Potentially Resistant to Aphidicolin ................ 36

IV.     The Use of Aphidicolin to Solve Some Basic Biological Problems ............ 36
        A.      Functional Roles of DNA Polymerases ............................... 36
        B.      Involvement of DNA Polymerase $\alpha$ in DNA Repair .............. 37

V.      Conclusion ................................................................ 38

Acknowledgments ................................................................. 38

References ...................................................................... 39

# I. INTRODUCTION

Aphidicolin, a tetracyclic diterpenoid (Figure 1) obtained from *Cephalosporium aphidicola* and other fungi, was originally isolated as an antiviral agent.[1,2] It was later found to inhibit the growth of eukaryotic cells,[3-9] of certain animal viruses (SV40,[10] Herpes simplex,[1,4,11] vaccinia,[4,11] and adenoviruses[5,12-14]) and of *Bacillus subtilis* bacteriophage Ø29[15] by inhibiting cellular or viral replicative DNA synthesis without interference with RNA and protein synthesis.[3,6,9,16,17] The target for aphidicolin action in eukaryotes was found to be the DNA polymerase α of animal and plant cells and not the DNA polymerase β or γ.[3,5,8,9,12,17] This specificity makes aphidicolin an extremely useful chemical in elucidating the role of DNA polymerase α and the mechanisms of DNA replication and repair.

Aphidicolin-resistant mutants have been isolated from several rodent cell lines and from some sensitive viruses. Studies of these mutants revealed the existence of diverse mechanisms of resistance and confirmed that the mechanism of action of aphidicolin is mediated directly or indirectly through its effect on DNA polymerase α or viral DNA polymerases. The use of this specific DNA polymerase inhibitor and aphidicolin-resistant mutants in the past has been credited for the progress in our understanding of the basic mechanisms of DNA replication and repair. They will be indispensable for future studies in this area. In this article, we focus our review in three areas: (1) the effect and mechanism of action of aphidicolin; (2) the characterization of aphidicolin-resistant mutants; and (3) the use of aphidicolin to solve some basic biological problems.

# II. EFFECTS AND MECHANISM OF ACTION OF APHIDICOLIN

## A. Effects on DNA Polymerases

Aphidicolin inhibits DNA synthesis of both animal and plant cells.[3,4,18,19] In the presence of the inhibitor, cells that had entered the "S" phase can no longer synthesize the DNA, whereas cells in other phases of the cycle continue the cycle and stop at the $G_1$/S border.[20] However it was observed in Chinese hamster V79 cells that aphidicolin treatment might not stop DNA synthesis immediately but could trigger an extra round of DNA synthesis resulting in endoreduplication and tetraploid cells.[21,22] The inhibition of DNA synthesis and cell proliferation was found to be mediated through inhibition of DNA polymerases by aphidicolin. The DNA polymerases inhibitable by aphidicolin include eukaryotic DNA polymerase α[3,5,8,9,12,17] and yeast DNA polymerase II[23] which, similar to prokaryotic DNA polymerase, has an associated 3' to 5' exonuclease activity.[23] Viral DNA polymerases from Herpes simplex,[1,4,11] vaccinia,[4,11] SV40,[10] and *Bacillus subtilis* bacteriophage Ø29[15] were also inhibited by aphidicolin. Adenovirus DNA replication involves either host γ-polymerase[13] or both α- and γ-polymerase.[5,10,12,14] The viral replication may be weakly inhibited by aphidicolin.[13] Aphidicolin was found to be more effective in inhibiting DNA polymerases from cytosol fraction than those from nuclear and mitochondria fractions.[24] Aphidicolin had no effect on the replication of mitochondrial DNA in HeLa cells.[25] In isolated mitochondria, DNA synthesis was not inhibited by aphidicolin but was completely blocked by dideoxy-cytidine which inhibits DNA polymerase γ but not the α-polymerase.

DNA synthesis in isolated nuclei of sea urchin embryos or of HeLa cells was inhibited by aphidicolin noncompetitively with respect to each of the four dNTPs. This property is different from purified DNA polymerase α which was inhibited by aphidicolin competitively with respect to dCTP and noncompetitively with respect to the other 3 dNTPs.[26,27] In mouse ascites sarcoma cells, the aphidicolin inhibition of DNA synthesis was a mixed type (competitive and noncompetitive) with respect to dCTP, but noncompetitive with the other dNTPs.[28] In a different report, aphidicolin inhibition of purified DNA polymerase α isolated from adenovirus-infected KB cells was also found to be competitive with dCTP.[14] The cytotoxicity

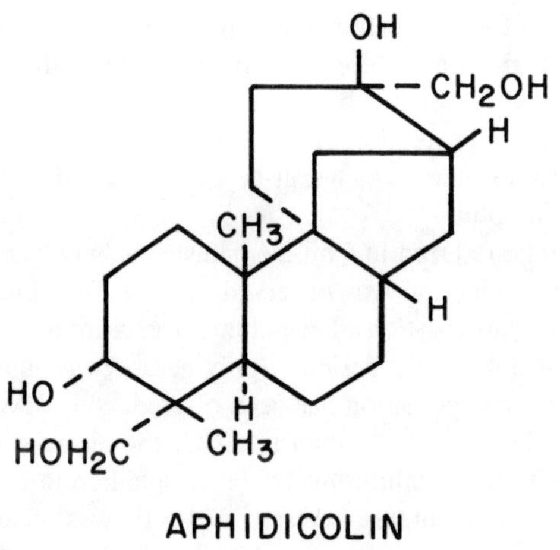

FIGURE 1.   Structure of aphidicolin.

of aphidicolin on mouse FM3A cells can be reversed with the simultaneous addition of all four deoxyribonucleosides to the culture medium.[29] Similarly the inhibition of DNA synthesis by aphidicolin in lysolecithin-permeabilized FM3A cells was reversed by increasing the concentrations of all four dNTPs, but not by increasing the concentrations of three of the four. For purified α-polymerase, it requires 100 times higher concentrations of aphidicolin to inhibit the DNA synthesis and its inhibition was reversed only by dCTP. These results indicate that aphidicolin binds only to a binding site of dCTP, thereby producing a change in the interaction between α-polymerase and the other three dNTPs.[29] DNA synthetic enzymes have been hypothesized to form a multienzyme complex. A supporting evidence for this hypothesis is the observation that aphidicolin can inhibit thymidylate synthetase in S phase of intact cells but not in the soluble extracts.[30]

Aphidicolin and araC were found to exert an inhibitory effect on the DNA chain elongation rate.[31-33] The inhibitory effect was on the synthesis and joining of short DNA fragments but not the union of 10-kb DNA replication intermediates.[34] This is in contrast to a different study which showed that aphidicolin treatment, which inhibited 90 to 95% ³[H]-thymidine incorporation, caused the accumulation of intermediates of nearly the same size as the replicon (2 to 5 × 10⁷ daltons) although the synthesis of short nascent fragments (Okazaki fragments) continued in the presence of aphidicolin.[35] Using aphidicolin and cycloheximide to block DNA synthesis and the size maturation of nascent DNA intermediates, evidence was obtained for the presence of secondary intermediates larger than replicon size (>2 × 10⁷ daltons).[36] It is noted that monoclonal anti-(DNA polymerase α) F(ab) fragments inhibited the discontinuous synthesis of Okazaki DNA, as well as the maturation of Okazaki DNA to larger DNA, thereby implicating DNA polymerase α in both of these processes.[37]

## B. Effects on Gene Mutation and Chromosomal Aberrations

Aphidicolin was not mutagenic in the Ames assay.[38] It did not induce DNA repair synthesis in HeLa cells.[38] The inhibitor can be converted to inactive derivatives by rat liver microsomal oxidases. The metabolites formed were neither mutagenic nor capable of inducing DNA repair synthesis.[38] Frequency of spontaneous or ethyl methane sulfonate induced sister-chromatid exchange was increased by aphidicolin treatment.[39,40] Post-treatment of X-ray irradiated human lymphocytes resulted in an enhanced frequency of chromosomal aberrations.[41,42] A similar synergistic effect of aphidicolin and X-rays was also observed in a Wallaby cell line, Ju56, which also showed enhanced spontaneous chromatid aberrations after aphidicolin treatment.[43] Aphidicolin had a similar effect on inducing sister chromatid exchanges but had a less effect on enhancing chromosomal breakage in cells of Fanconi's anemia compared to normal cells.[44] Deoxycoformycin and aphidicolin act synergistically in causing DNA strand breaks and cell death in unstimulated human lymphocytes.[45] Aphidicolin treatment induced gaps and breaks at common fragile sites in human chromosomes.[46] The fragile site on the x-chromosome, which can be induced by thymidylate stress, however, was not induced by aphidicolin.

Endoreduplication can be induced in Chinese hamster V79 cells by aphidicolin in a dose-dependent manner.[21] The induction was observed only at 37°C but not at 41°C. This was initially explained by the participation of β-polymerase, a more heat-sensitive enzyme, in normal DNA replication during the period α-polymerase was inhibited by aphidicolin.[21] Subsequently, an alternative explanation has been offered. Since cytotoxicity of aphidicolin treatment was greatly reduced at 41°C than at 37°C, the absence of aphidicolin effect at 41°C may be due to the reduced inhibiting effect of aphidicolin on DNA synthesis.[22] The frequency of tetraploid cells in Chinese hamster V79 cells was greatly increased after aphidicolin treatment possibly as a consequence of endoreduplication.[22] Aphidicolin was also capable of inducing gene amplification at the ribonucleotide reductase locus with step-wise increased concentrations of aphidicolin which was also served as the selective agent.[47] Frequencies of methotrexate-resistant mutants were induced by 30 to 50 hr treatment with aphidicolin in a dose-responsive manner.[22] Inhibition of DNA synthesis and over replication of DNA has been hypothesized as features of agents inducing gene amplification.[48] In this regard, aphidicolin is perhaps the best example.

## III. ISOLATION OF APHIDICOLIN-RESISTANT MUTANTS

Aphidicolin-resistant mutants have been isolated from mammalian and Drosophila cells in culture, herpes and vaccinia viruses, and *Bacillus subtilis* bacteriophate Ø29. According to their mechanisms of resistance, they can be classified into three major categories: (1) mutants with an altered DNA polymerase, (2) mutants with an increased DNA polymerase level, and (3) mutants with altered dNTP pools (Table 1).

### A. Aphidicolin-Resistant Mutant with an Altered DNA Polymerase

Chang et al.[49] have reported the isolation of aphidicolin-resistant mutants from Chinese hamster V79 cells following mutagenization with BrdU-black light and UV. Two types of mutants were recovered at a frequency of $4.5 \times 10^{-7}$. Three mutants were found to be resistant to 1-β-D-arabinofuranosylcytosine (araC) and normal in UV sensitivity. One mutant was normal in araC sensitivity but more sensitive to UV radiation. This UV sensitive mutant also exhibits other pleiotropic phenotypes, i.e., slow growth, cytidine sensitive, and elevated frequencies of BrdU-induced chromosome breaks and aphidicolin-induced sister chromatid exchanges. Initial characterization using a nonoptimal assay failed to identify this mutant as a DNA polymerase α mutant.[49] Under correct assay conditions (5 μ*M* instead of 100 μ*M* dCTP), the purified DNA polymerase α from this mutant was found to be resistant to aphidicolin.[50] Furthermore, the apparent Km for dCTP with DNA polymerase α was found to be ten times lower for the mutant enzyme compared to the parental wild-type enzyme. No difference in apparent Km for dATP was found for the mutant enzyme. Therefore, the mechanism of resistance to aphidicolin for the mutant appears to be the high affinity of the mutant DNA polymerase α to dCTP.

This UV-sensitive mutant was also found to be hypermutable for spontaneous[50,51] and UV-induced mutations[49,52] at the ouabain-, 6-thioguanine-, and diphtheria-toxin-resistant loci. These phenotypes of the mutant provide the genetic evidence that DNA polymerase α participates in DNA repair and demonstrate that DNA polymerase α mutant can be a mutator mutant in mammalian cells. The mutant was also sensitive to *N*-methyl-*N*-nitro-*N*-nitroso-

**Table 1**
**MUTANT CELL LINES RESISTANT TO**
**APHIDICOLIN**

| Genetic and biochemical alteration | Cell lines |
| --- | --- |
| Altered DNA polymerase | |
| α-Polymerase | Chinese hamster V79[49,50] |
| | Drosophila[65] |
| Viral polymerase | Herpes simplex[58,61] |
| | Vaccinia virus[59] |
| | Bacillus subtilis bacteriophage Ø29[15] |
| Increased DNA polymerase level | MouseFM 3A[64] |
| | Drosophilia[65] |
| Altered dNTP pools | |
| With altered ribonucleotide reductase | Mouse FM3A[66,67] |
| | Mouse 3T6[68] |
| With increased level of ribonucleotide reductase | CHO[47] |
| | Mouse FM3A[69] |
| With temperature-sensitive thymidylate synthetase | Mouse FM3A[70,71] |
| Mechanism unknown | Chinese hamster V79[49] |
| | Mouse lymphoma L5178Y[73] |

guanidine (MNNG) but normal in sensitivity to X-rays and dimethylsulfate.[53] Treatment with conditioned medium (liquid holding) following UV irradiation increased survival and decreased mutations in wild type cells. The same treatment, however, failed to enhance survival but further increased the already elevated mutability following UV irradiation. This was interpreted as indicating the presence of an error-prone long-patch excision repair in the mutant cells.[53]

Additional characterization provides more information concerning the genotypic structure of the mutant. When the mutant was fused with aphidicolin-sensitive V79 cells, the hybrids showed intermediate sensitivity to aphidicolin between the mutant and the wild type, indicating that aphidicolin resistance of the mutant is a codominant trait. Similar to wild type cells, the hybrid cells were normal in UV and cytidine sensitivity, showing a recessive expression of these characters.[54]

The mutant cells are slow-growing and revertible to fast-growing cells which can be identified as large colonies in the background of small mutant colonies.[49] The revertants regained simultaneously the normal phenotype, not only in their growth rate but also in terms of cytotoxicity to cytidine and mutability to UV. Unlike the wild type cells, the revertants, however, contain the aphidicolin-resistant DNA polymerase α and are intermediate in aphidicolin sensitivity (more resistant than the wild type but more sensitive than the mutant).[54] Based on these results, we postulate that the genotypes for the wild type, the mutant and the revertant as A/A, a/A*, and A/A*, respectively, where A is the wild type allele, A* is the mutant allele, and a is a nonfunctional allele (Table 2).

According to this hypothesis, one normal α-polymerase allele is sufficient for normal growth rate, normal sensitivity to cytidine and UV and normal mutability. Furthermore, by deleting or mutating just one normal allele, the revertants should be readily mutated to slow-growing, aphidicolin-resistant mutants (i.e., A/A* → −/A* or a/A*) by X-rays or other mutagen treatments. Experiments testing this hypothesis, indeed, confirm this prediction.

### Table 2
### PHENOTYPES AND POSTULATED GENOTYPIC CHANGES IN A CHINESE HAMSTER DNA POLYMERASE α MUTANT AND IT'S DERIVATIVES

| | Wild Type | | Mutant | | Revertant | | Aph^r-4-RX | | |
| | | | | | | X-rays | I | II | III |
| | V 79 | → | Aph^r-4 | → | Aph^r-4-R | → | | | |
|---|---|---|---|---|---|---|---|---|---|
| Postulated genotype | A/A | | a/A* | | A/A* | | −/A* or a/A* | A/A* and B→B* | ↑A/A* |
| Phenotype Growth rate | N | | Slow | | N | | Slow | N | N |
| Aph^r α-pol | − | | + | | + | | N.T. | N.T. | N.T. |
| Mutability | N | | M | | N | | N.T. | N.T. | N.T. |
| Sensitivity to | | | | | | | | | |
| Aphidicolin | N | | RR | | R | | RR | RR | RR |
| UV | N | | S | | N | | S | N | N |
| Cytidine | N | | S | | N | | S | N | N |
| Ara-c | N | | N | | N | | N | R | N |

*Note:*  N = normal; S = sensitive; R = resistant; RR = highly resistant; N.T. = not tested; M = mutator; ↑ = increased expression; − = absent; + = present.

Slow-growing, UV-sensitive mutants were readily recovered from the revertant after mutagenization treatment with X-rays (the same treatment yielded no such mutant from wild-type cells). In addition, two other types of mutants highly resistant to aphidicolin were also recovered. One type is characterized by a newly acquired resistance to araC, possibly due to mutations increasing dCTP pools. The other type is similar to normal cells except it is highly resistant to aphidicolin. The molecular defect for this type is not clear. The increase in DNA polymerase α levels is one possibility which may account for this phenotype. The human gene for DNA polymerase α has been located on the X chromosome.[55,56] The postulated two functional genes seem to be contradictory to the hemizygous presence or expression of X-linked genes unless mammalian cells do carry two duplicated DNA polymerase α genes on one X chromosome. The mutant DNA polymerase α gene can be transferred to wild type cells and identified as aphidicolin-resistant cells.[57]

Aphidicolin resistant mutants have been isolated from Drosophila cells in culture. One of the mutant cell lines was reported to contain an aphidicolin-resistant DNA polymerase α.[65] The apparent Ki for the mutant enzyme was about eight times higher than that of the wild-type enzyme, whereas the apparent Km for dCTP was the same for both mutant and wild type enzymes. Therefore, the aphidicolin resistance appears to be due to the reduced affinity of the mutant DNA polymerase to the inhibitor aphidicolin.

Vaccinia and Herpes simplex viruses and *Bacillus subtilis* bacteriophage Ø29 were sensitive to aphidicolin. Mutants resistant to aphidicolin have been isolated from these viruses[58,59] and bacteriophage.[15] A partially purified DNA polymerase from a mutant Herpes simplex type 2 virus exhibited a 7.5-fold lower apparent Km for dCTP and a 3-fold lower apparent Km for dTTP. The apparent Ki for aphidicolin of the mutant polymerase was 6.5-fold higher than that of the wild-type enzyme.[58] For *Bacillus subtilis* bacteriophage Ø29, aphidicolin-resistant mutations have been mapped on gene 2 which encodes Ø29 DNA polymerase.[15] While most aphidicolin-resistant Herpes simplex were sensitive to phosphonoacetic acid (PAA), many PAA-resistant mutants were found to be more sensitive to aphidicolin[60-62] and more resistant to all of four nucleoside analogs.[58] In contrast to the Chinese hamster aphidicolin-resistant DNA polymerase α mutant,[50] the aphidicolin-sensitive Herpes simplex virus type 1 mutant was found to be an antimutator.[63] Hall et al.[63] further showed that purified mutant DNA polymerase from one antimutator exhibits enhanced replication fidelity possibly due to elevated Km values for normal nucleoside triphosphates associated with the mutant enzyme. A hypothesis was proposed that reduced affinity of the polymerase for nucleoside triphosphate accounts for the antimutator phenotype by accentuating differences in base-pair stability, thus facilitating selection of correct nucleotides.[63]

## B. Aphidicolin-Resistant Mutants with an Elevated DNA Polymerase Level

An aphidicolin-resistant mutant isolated from the mouse mammary carcinoma cell line, FM3A, was found to contain an increased activity of DNA polymerase α.[64] The increased activity was observed only when the mutant cells were cultured in the presence of aphidicolin. One aphidicolin-resistant Drosophila mutant was reported to overproduce DNA polymerase α eightfold more than wild-type cells.[65] This mutant was normal in Km and Ki for dNTP and aphidicolin.

## C. Aphidicolin-Resistant Mutants with Altered Nucleotide Pools

This type of mutants has been isolated from various mammalian cell lines. In mutagenized mouse FM3A cells, aphidicolin-resistant mutants were recovered at a frequency of about one per million.[66] All the mutants showed a greatly increased dATP pool and decreased ability to incorporate [³H] deoxycytidine into DNA. They also showed cross resistance to araC and 9-β-D-arabinofuranosyladenine (araA), deoxyadenosine, and excess thymidine.[66,67] In hybrids formed between mutant and wild-type cells, the aphidicolin resistance, as well as this cross-resistance, behaved as codominant traits. Biochemical characterization revealed that the mutants contained an altered ribonucleotide reductase which was desensitized to the allosteric negative effector dATP.[67] Two aphidicolin-resistant mutants isolated from a mouse 3T6 cell line were also found to contain an altered ribonucleotide reductase.[68] One of them overproduces an active M2 subunit and has expanded a dATP pool. The other was found to contain an altered regulatory M1 subunit and have expanded dATP and dCTP pools. Upon exposure to aphidicolin, the dCTP pool rapidly decreased. No effect was found for other dNTP pools.

For Chinese hamster ovary (CHO) cells, serial culture of cells with step-wise increased concentrations of aphidicolin yielded a series of mutants with increasing resistance to aphidicolin.[47] The most resistant mutant isolated (resistant to 5 μg/mℓ aphidicolin) was 44 times more resistant to aphidicolin than the parental cells. No difference was found in sensitivity to aphidicolin or specific activity for the DNA polymerase in mutant cell extracts. The mutants were found to be cross-resistant to araC, deoxythymidine, and deoxyadenosine. The intracellular pools of all four dNTPs in the mutants increased with increasing resistance to aphidicolin. The elevated dNTP pools in the mutant most resistant to aphidicolin appear to be the result of a four- to eightfold increase in the level of ribonucleotide reductase.[47]

Mouse FM3A mutants with cross-resistance to aphidicolin and excess thymidine were isolated by a single step selection for simultaneous resistance to araA and araC with a frequency of about $10^{-5}$ from mutagenized cells.[69] In some of these mutants, the level of ribonucleotide reductase was increased 2 to 5 times than that of the parental cells. These mutants were found to be resistant to hydroxyurea and to contain a ribonucleotide reductase exhibiting normal sensitivity in vitro to the allosteric negative effector dATP. As a consequence, the intracellular pools of dATP and dCTP were expanded in the mutant.[69]

## D. Aphidicolin-Resistant Mutants with Temperature-Sensitive Thymidylate Synthetase

Some aphidicolin-resistant mouse FM3A mutants selected at 33.5°C were unable to grow at 39.5°C.[70] These temperature-sensitive mutants were found to contain a mutant temperature-sensitive thymidylate synthetase. Three of four mutants tested did not show cross-resistance to araC and araA. Aphidicolin-resistance in one of these clones was shown to be a recessive trait in contrast to the aphidicolin-resistant mutants with altered ribonucleotide reductases.[66,67]

Temperature sensitive thymidylate synthetase mutants of mouse FM3A cells can be selected by reduced sensitivity to methotrexate in the presence of 5-methyltetrahydrofolate.[71] This class of mutants shared several common phenotypes with the class of mutants containing an altered ribonucleotide reductase desensitized to deoxyadenosine triphosphate:[66,67] abnormal level of deoxyribonucleoside triphosphate pool, especially those of deoxyadenosine triphosphate; resistance to aphidicolin, 9-β-D-arabinofuranosyladenine, 1-β-D-arabinofuranosylcytosine, and hydroxyurea; sensitivity to bleomycin; and high mutability.[72]

### E. Aphidicolin-Resistant Mutants with Unknown Mechanism

Aphidicolin-resistant mutants with cross-resistance to araC and expanded dCTP pools were isolated from Chinese hamster V79 cells following mutagenization with BrdU-black light and UV irradiation.[49] Two mutant cell lines with high incidence of spontaneous sister chromatid exchanges and chromosome aberrations were obtained from over 400 aphidicolin-resistant mutants isolated from mouse lymphoma L5178Y cells.[73] The biochemical defects of these hamster and mouse lymphoma mutants have not been identified.

### F. Other Mutants Potentially Resistant to Aphidicolin

Mutants with an elevated dCTP pool are potentially aphidicolin-resistant mutants. A common phenotype of these mutants is the resistance to araC. These mutants have been reported in the literature although no information concerning aphidicolin sensitivity is known. The CTP synthetase (CTPS) mutants of Chinese hamster V79 cells[74] and Chinese hamster lung CCL39 cells[75] shared certain common properties. These include (1) joint resistance to araC and excess thymidine, (2) thymidine auxotrophy, (3) cytidine cytotoxicity and its prevention by thymidine, (4) expanded pools of CTP and dCTP, and (5) resistance of CTPS activity to end product feedback inhibition. The thymidine auxotrophy and cytidine cytotoxicity can be explained by the suggestion that the permanently enlarged CTP pool in these cells inhibits UDP reduction.[76] Similar mutants were isolated from CHO cells.[77,78] The nucleotide pools imbalance appear to make these cells mutator mutants.[79,80] In mouse lymphosarcoma S-49 cells, mutator mutants deficient in dCMP deaminase or heterozygous for mutations affecting the M1 subunit of ribonucleotide reductase were reported.[81,82] These mutants have been shown to have elevated dNTP pools and their mutator activity can be modulated by exogenous thymidine.

## IV. THE USE OF APHIDICOLIN TO SOLVE SOME BASIC BIOLOGICAL PROBLEMS

### A. Functional Roles of DNA Polymerases

Mammalian cells have three major DNA polymerases: α-, β-, and γ-polymerase, named in successive order of their discovery.[83] A fourth enzyme, δ-polymerase with 3′ to 5′ exonuclease activity was also described.[84] This enzyme is similar to the α-polymerase in many respects such as sensitivity to aphidicolin and the sulfhydryl blocking agent, N-ethylmaleimide, but can be distinghished from the α-polymerase by two other criteria: highly resistant to inhibition by BuPdGTP (a dGTP analog) and absence of response to neutralizing activity of a monoclonal antibody against the α-polymerase.[84] The roles of the various DNA polymerases have been deduced from other studies without using the aphidicolin. For example, replicative DNA synthesis was found to be strongly inhibited by cytosine arabinoside triphosphate, high KCl, and N-ethylmaleimide, as is DNA polymerase α. DNA repair synthesis was relatively insensitive to these agents, as is the DNA polymerase β activity. These correlations suggested the functional role of α- and β-polymerases in replicative and repair synthesis respectively.[85] A similar conclusion was based on the correlation of peak appearance of replicative and repair activities with the peak α- and β-polymerase activities during the cell cycle.[86] The sole presence of β- or γ-polymerase in neuronal cells and mitochondria respectively were correlated with the presence of DNA repair or replicative activities in these cells and organelles.[87,88] However, the conclusions drawn from these studies need to be validated. The finding of a specific DNA polymerase α inhibitor provided a method to confirm the previous assignments of the functional roles of the three major DNA polymerases. First, since replicative DNA synthesis and cell growth in eukaryotes and SV40 virus[10] replication were stopped only by the DNA polymerase α inhibitor, aphidicolin but not by ddTTP (an inhibitor of both β- and γ-polymerase), the α-polymerase must be responsible for replicative DNA synthesis in eukaryotic cells and SV40.[10] For this type of study, aphidicolin is clearly better than N-ethylmaleimide which inhibit both α- and γ-polymerases. Second, by measuring mutagen induced DNA damage, cytotoxicity and mutations in the presence and absence of aphidicolin, the role of α-polymerase in DNA repair can be determined (see next section). Third, by showing that γ-polymerase is the only DNA polymerase present in the mitochondria, and that mitochondrial DNA synthesis was inhibited by ddTTP but not by aphidicolin, it is clear that mitochondrial DNA synthesis is carried out by γ-polymerase only.[19,25] Fourth, by showing that Adenovirus DNA replication was inhibited by both aphidicolin and ddTTP, it was concluded that Adenovirus DNA replication involves both DNA polymerase α and γ.[10]

## B. Involvement of DNA Polymerase α in DNA Repair

Besides elucidating the functional role of DNA polymerases, the most important contribution made by the use of aphidicolin is the determination whether DNA polymerase α participates in the repair of DNA damage. Both positive and negative evidence has been documented in the literature. But the bulk of evidence seems to implicate the involvement of DNA polymerase α in the DNA repair process. The failure to detect the effect of aphidicolin on bleomycin-, UV-, or X-ray-induced repair synthesis has been reported in mouse sarcoma,[28] HeLa,[89,90] and Ehrlich ascites tumor cells,[91] as well as in protoplasts of Nicotiana.[92] Aphidicolin treatment has even been reported to promote repair of potentially lethal damage in irradiated mouse Ehrlich ascites cells synchronized in the S-phase.[93]

However, positive results indicating that aphidicolin inhibited DNA repair replication are overwhelming.[6,7,32,42,94-118] Most of these studies used human and mammalian cells. The DNA damaging agents used include both physical and chemical mutagens. Various techniques have been used to measure DNA damage and repair, such as mutagen-induced unscheduled DNA synthesis,[6,7,94,106,108,112] rejoining of strand breaks,[95-97,106] dimer removal,[97] density labeling of DNA,[105] and recovery of ribosomal RNA transcription.[99] In human and simian cells, reduced survival after exposure to UV light and post-treatment with aphidicolin has been interpreted as aphidicolin inhibition of DNA repair.[99,107,111] This aphidicolin effect was observed in normal human, and xeroderma pigmentosum (XP) variant cells but not in XP complementation group A cells.[107] It was estimated that α-polymerase may be responsible for 67% of UV repair.[107]

These studies involving aphidicolin have revealed some characteristics of DNA repair. First, the inhibition of DNA repair by aphidicolin may be cell-cycle dependent, e.g., aphidicolin effect, was very efficient in confluent resting cells, but not in rapidly cycling cells.[42,98] This may be due to the difference in dNTP pool between these two types of cells. Second, the aphidicolin effect on the inhibition of UV-induced repair synthesis may be cell-type dependent, e.g., 100 μg/mℓ aphidicolin inhibited 90% of repair synthesis in HeLa cells but 300 μg/mℓ of aphidicolin had no effect on rat liver cells.[112] Third, both α- and β-polymerase are involved in DNA repair. The fraction of repair synthesis mediated by each of the two polymerases is dependent on which DNA damaging agent is administered and on the dose of damaging agent.[110] Low doses of DNA damage induce DNA repair synthesis which is mediated largely by a non-α-polymerase, and with an increasing dose of damage there is increasing participation of α-polymerase in repair synthesis. The maximal level of α-polymerase involvement was estimated to be 80% for UV radiation and N-acetoxy-2-acetylaminofluorene and about 40% for bleomycin.[110] Similarly it was concluded that β-polymerase is primarily responsible for repair synthesis induced by bleomycin or neocarzinostatin (sensitive to ddTTP), whereas α-polymerase plays a major role in repair synthesis induced by UV, dimethyl sulfate, MNNG, and N-nitrosomethyl urea. These alkylating agents and UV induce more DNA damage than the former two mutagens.[101,102,114,115] However, it is the actual type of DNA damage but not the "patch size" that determines which polymerase is used in repair.[103] For UV damage, aphidicolin inhibited the repair induced by UV-B and UV-C (the shorter wavelength) but not that induced by UV-A.[111] In an in vitro base excision DNA repair scheme, a major difference in polymerization function was found for α- and β-polymerase.[113] α-Polymerase does not utilize substrate DNA with gaps smaller than approximately 15. On the other hand, β-polymerase can utilize as primer templates all of the gapped DNA substrate and fills gaps to completion.

A fourth observation related to DNA repair has shown that the α-polymerase may be associated with other enzymes. It was observed that the aphidicolin concentration required to inhibit DNA repair is 20-fold higher than those needed to inhibit replication. This may be explained by the association of different accessory proteins with the α-polymerase involved in repair and replication.[118] Aphidicolin was also reported to block the removal of pyrimidine dimers.[97] The observation is difficult to comprehend, since aphidicolin is known to inhibit the α-polymerase but not the endonuclease and exonuclease which excise pyrimidine dimers. The results, however, can be explained by the formation of a multienzyme complex.

Finally, a human low-density-lipoprotein (LDL) receptor-deficient diploid cell line, GM 1915, was determined to be short patch competent and long patch deficient for DNA excision repair.[119] α-Polymerase in this cell line was not activated by mutagen treatment. The introduction of LDL into the cells resulted in activation of the α-polymerase. The characteristic of this mutant also suggests that α-polymerase involved in repair may be modified by effector molecules. The above observations, especially the cell-cycle and mutagen dependence of aphidicolin effect, might help to explain some of the negative results showing no aphidicolin effect on DNA repair.

## V. CONCLUSION

Aphidicolin, a specific inhibitor of eukaryotic DNA polymerase α and some viral DNA polymerases, has been very useful in elucidating the functional roles of various eukaryotic DNA polymerases. Through the use of this inhibitor, the participation of DNA polymerase α in repair of DNA damage has been firmly established. Studies using this chemical also provided information concerning the mechanism of DNA repair, chromosomal aberrations and gene amplification. Mammalian and viral mutants resistant to aphidicolin have been isolated. They are either due to mutations affecting structure or expression of viral or DNA polymerase α or due to mutations affecting nucleotide pools. Many of these mutants are mutator mutants. These mutants might be very useful in the study of the mechanisms of DNA repair and mutagenesis.

## ACKNOWLEDGMENTS

We thank Darla Conley for her excellent typing assistance in preparing this manuscript. Research upon which this paper was based was supported by a grant from the NCI (CA21104).

# REFERENCES

1. **Bucknall, R. A., Moores, H., Simms, R., and Hesp, B.,** Antiviral effects of aphidicolin, a new antibiotic produced by Cephalosporium aphidicola, *Antimicrob. Agents Chemother.,* 4, 294, 1973.
2. **Brundret, K. M., Dalziel, W., Hesp, B., Javis, J. A. J., and Neidle, S.,** X-ray crystallographic determination of the structure of the antibiotic aphidicolin: a tetracycline diterpenoid containing a new ring system, *J. Chem. Soc. Chem. Commun.,* 18, 1027, 1972.
3. **Ikegami, S., Taguchi, T., Ohashi, M., Oguro, M., Nagano, H., and Mano, Y.,** Aphidicolin prevents mitotic cell division by interfering with the activity of DNA polymerase-α, *Nature,* 275, 458, 1978.
4. **Pedrali-Noy, G. and Spadari, S.,** Effect of aphidicolin on viral and human DNA polymerases, *Biochem. Biophys. Res. Commun.,* 88, 1194, 1979.
5. **Longiaru, M., Ikeda, J., Jarkovsky, Z., Horwitz, S. B., and Horwitz, M. S.,** The effect of aphidicolin on adenovirus DNA synthesis, *Nucleic Acids Res.,* 6, 3369, 1979.
6. **Berger, N. A., Kurohara, K. K., Petzold, S. J., and Sikorski, G. W.,** Aphidicolin inhibits eukaryotic DNA replication and repair — implications for involvement of DNA polymerase α in both processes, *Biochem. Biophys. Res. Commun.,* 89, 218, 1979.
7. **Hanaoka, F., Kato, H., Ikegami, S., Ohashi, M., and Yamada, M.,** Aphidicolin does inhibit repair replication in HeLa cells, *Biochem. Biophys. Res. Commun.,* 87, 575, 1979.
8. **Wist, E. and Prydz, H.,** The effect of aphidicolin on DNA synthesis in isolated HeLa cell nuclei, *Nucleic Acids Res.,* 6, 1583, 1979.
9. **Ichikawa, A., Negishi, M., Tomita, K., and Ikegami, S.,** Aphidicolin: a specific inhibitor of DNA synthesis in synchronous mastocytoma P-815 cells, *Jpn. J. Pharmacol.,* 30, 301, 1980.
10. **Krokan, H., Schaffer, P., and Depamphilis, M. L.,** Involvement of eucaryotic deoxyribonucleic acid polymerase α and γ in the replication of cellular and viral deoxyribonucleic acid, *Biochemistry,* 18, 4431, 1979.
11. **Pedrali-Noy, G. and Spadari, S.,** Mechanism of inhibition of herpes simplex virus and vaccinia virus DNA polymerases by aphidicolin, a highly specific inhibitor of DNA replication in eucaryotes, *J. Virol.,* 36, 457, 1980.
12. **Longiaru, M., Ikeda, J. E., Jarkovsky, Z., Horwitz, S. B., and Horwitz, M. S.,** The effect of aphidicolin on adenovirus DNA synthesis, *Nucleic Acids Res.,* 6, 3369, 1979.
13. **Kwant, M. M. and van der Vliet, P. C.,** Differential effect of aphidicolin on adenovirus DNA synthesis and cellular DNA synthesis, *Nucleic Acids Res.,* 17, 3993, 1980.
14. **Habara, A., Kano, K., Nagano, H., Mano, Y., Ikegami, S., and Yamashita, T.,** Inhibition of DNA synthesis in the adenovirus DNA replication complex by aphidicolin and 2′,3′-dideoxythymidine triphosphate, *Biochem. Biophys. Res. Commun.,* 92, 8, 1980.
15. **Matsumoto, K., Kim, C. I., Urano, S., Ohashi, M., and Hirokawa, H.,** Aphidicolin-resistant mutants of bacteriophage 029: genetic evidence for altered DNA polymerase, *Virology,* 152, 32, 1986.
16. **Huberman, J. A.,** New view of the biochemistry of eucaryotic DNA replication revealed by aphidicolin, an unusual inhibitor of DNA polymerase-α, *Cell,* 23, 647, 1981.
17. **Spadari, S., Focher, F., Sala, F., Ciarrocchi, G., Koch, G., Falaschi, A., and Pedrali-Noy, G.,** Control of cell division by aphidicolin without adverse effects upon resting cells, *Anzneim. Forsch. Drug Res.,* 35, 1108, 1985.
18. **Sala, F., Parisi, B., Burroni, D., Amileni, A. R., Pedrali-Noy, G., and Spadari, S.,** Specific and reversible inhibition by aphidicolin of the α-like DNA polymerase of plant cells, *FEBS Lett.,* 117, 93, 1980.
19. **Geuskens, M., Hardt, N., Pedrali-Noy, G., and Spadari, S.,** An autoradiographic demonstration of nuclear DNA replication by DNA polymerase α and of mitochondrial DNA synthesis by DNA polymerase γ, *Nucleic Acids Res.,* 9, 1599, 1981.
20. **Pedrali-Noy, G., Spadari, S., Miller-Faures, A., Miller, A. O. A., Kruppa, J., and Koch, G.,** Synchronization of HeLa cell cultures by inhibition of DNA polymerase with aphidicolin, *Nucleic Acids Res.,* 8, 377, 1980.
21. **Huang, Y., Chang, C. C., and Trosko, J. E.,** Aphidicolin-induced endoreduplication in Chinese hamster cells, *Cancer Res.,* 43, 1361, 1983.
22. **Mori, T., Chang, C. C., and Trosko, J. E.,** The role of the inhibition of DNA polymerase alpha by aphidicolin in DNA amplification in Chinese hamster V79 cells, in *Accomplishments in Oncology—The Role of DNA Amplification in Carcinogenesis,* Hausen, H. Z. and Schlehofer, J. R., Eds., J. B. Lippincott Co., Philadelphia, 1987, 161.
23. **Plevani, P., Badaracco, G., Ginelli, E., and Sora, S.,** Effect and mechanism of action of aphidicolin on yeast deoxyribonucleic acid polymerases, *Antimicrob. Agents Chemother.,* 18, 50, 1980.
24. **Ohashi, M., Taguchi, T., and Ikegami, S.,** Aphidicolin: a specific inhibitor of DNA polymerases in the cytosol of rat liver, *Biochem. Biophys. Res. Commun.,* 82, 1084, 1978.

25. **Zimmermann, W., Chen, S. M., Bolden, A., and Weissbach, A.,** Mitochondrial DNA replication does not involve DNA polymerase α, *J. Biol. Chem.,* 255, 11847, 1980.

26. **Oguro, M., Suzuki-Hori, C., Nagano, H., Mano, Y., and Ikegami, S.,** The mode of inhibitory action by aphidicolin on eukaryotic DNA polymerase α, *Eur. J. Biochem.,* 97, 603, 1979.

27. **Oguro, M., Shioda, M., Nagano, H., and Mano, Y.,** The mode of action of aphidicolin on DNA synthesis in isolated nuclei, *Biochem. Biophys. Res. Commun.,* 92, 13, 1980.

28. **Seki, S., Oda, T., and Ohashi, M.,** Differential effects of aphidicolin on replicative DNA synthesis and unscheduled DNA synthesis in permeable mouse sarcoma cells, *Biochim. Biophys. Acta,* 610, 413, 1980.

29. **Ayusawa, D., Iwata, K., Ikegami, S., and Seno, T.,** Reversal of aphidicolin-directed inhibition of DNA synthesis in vivo and in vitro by deoxyribonucleosides or their 5′-triphosphates, *Cell Struct. Funct.,* 5, 147, 1980.

30. **Reddy, G. P. V. and Pardee, A. B.,** Inhibitor evidence for allosteric interaction in the replitase multienzyme complex, *Nature,* 304, 86, 1983.

31. **Wist, E.,** Effects of ara C and aphidicolin on DNA chain elongation rate in HeLa $S_3$ cells, *Experimentia,* 36, 405, 1980.

32. **Hill, H. Z. and Hill, G. J.,** Aphidicolin and ara-C inhibit DNA chain elongation more than replicon joining and daughter strand gap repair after UV in B16C14 mouse melanoma cells, *AACR Abstr.,* p. 12, 1982.

33. **Fram, R. J. and Wufe, D. W.,** DNA strand breaks caused by inhibitors of DNA synthesis: 1-β-D-arabinofuranosylcytosine and aphidicolin, *Cancer Res.,* 42, 4050, 1982.

34. **Lonn, U. and Lonn, S.,** Aphidicolin inhibits the synthesis and joining of short DNA fragments but not the union of 10-kilobase DNA replication intermediates, *Proc. Natl. Acad. Sci. U.S.A.,* 80, 3996, 1983.

35. **Yagura, T., Kozu, T., and Seno, T.,** Arrest of chain growth of replicon-sized intermediates by aphidicolin during rat fibroblast cell chromosome replication, *Eur. J. Biochem.,* 123, 15, 1982.

36. **Kozu, T., Yagura, T., and Seno, T.,** Size maturation process of nascent DNA intermediates into chromosomal-sized DNA in Tetrahymena pyriformis macronuclear DNA replication, *Exp. Cell Res.,* 149, 189, 1983.

37. **Miller, M. R., Seighman, C., and Ulrich, R. G.,** Inhibition of DNA replication and DNA polymerase α activity by monoclonal anti-(DNA polymerase α) immunoglobulin G and F(ab) fragments, *Biochemistry,* 24, 7440, 1985.

38. **Pedrali-Noy, G., Mazza, G., Focher, F., and Spadari, S.,** Lack of mutagenicity and metabolic inactivation of aphidicolin by rat liver microsomes, *Biochem. Biophys. Res. Commun.,* 93, 1094, 1980.

39. **Ishh, Y. and Bender, M. A.,** Effect of inhibitors of DNA synthesis on spontaneous and ultraviolet light-induced sister-chromatid exchanges in Chinese hamster cells, *Mutation Res.,* 79, 19, 1980.

40. **Nishi, Y., Hasegawa, M. M., Inui, N., Ikegami, S., and Yamada, M.,** Effect of post-treatment with aphidicolin — a specific inhibitor of DNA polymerase α — on sister chromatid exchanges induced by ethyl methanesulfonate, *Mutation Res.,* 103, 155, 1982.

41. **Degrassi, F., Desalvia, R., Fiore, M., Natarajan, A. T., Palitti, F., and Tanzarella, C.,** Aphidicolin effect on frequency of chromosome aberrations induced by physical and chemical agents, *Atti Assoc. Genet. Ital.,* 27, 145, 1981.

42. **Van Zeeland, A. A., Bussmann, C. J. M., Degrassi, F., Filon, A. R., Van Kesteren-Van Leeuwen, A. C., Palitti, F., and Natarajan, A. T.,** Effects of aphidicolin on repair replication and induced chromosomal aberrations in mammalian cells, *Mutation Res.,* 92, 379, 1982.

43. **Moore, R. C., Randel, C., and Bender, M. A.,** Dose relationships between different effects of aphidicolin in JU56 cells, *Mutation Res.,* 1986.

44. **Porfinio, B., Dallapiccola, B., and Gandini, E.,** The effect of aphidicolin on Fanconi's anemia lymphocyte chromosomes, *Mutation Res.,* 144, 257, 1985.

45. **Brox, L., Hunting, D., and Belch, A.,** Aphidicolin and deoxycoformycin cause DNA breaks and cell death in unstimulated human lymphocytes, *Biochem. Biophys. Res. Commun.,* 120, 959, 1984.

46. **Glover, T. W., Berger, C., Coyle, J., and Echo, B.,** DNA polymerase α inhibition by aphidicolin induces gaps and breaks at common fragile sites in human chromosomes, *Human Genet.,* 67, 136, 1984.

47. **Sabourin, C. L. K., Bates, P. F., Glatzer, L., Chang, C. C., Trosko, J. E., and Boezi, J. A.,** Selection of aphidicolin-resistant CHO cells with altered levels of ribonucleotide reductase, *Somat. Cell Genet.,* 7, 255, 1981.

48. **Schimke, R. T., Sherwood, S. W., Hill, A. B., and Johnston, R. N.,** Over replication and recombination of DNA in higher eukaryotes: potential consequences and biological implications, *Proc. Natl. Acad. Sci. U.S.A.,* 83, 2157, 1986.

49. **Chang, C. C., Boezi, J. A., Warren, S. T., Sabourin, C. L. K., Liu, P. K., Glatzer, L., and Trosko, J. E.,** Isolation and characterization of a UV-sensitive hypermutable aphidicolin-resistant Chinese hamster cell line, *Somat. Cell Genet.,* 7, 235, 1981.

50. **Liu, P. K., Chang, C. C., Trosko, J. E., Dube, D. K., Martin, G. M., and Loeb, L. A.,** Mammalian mutator mutant with an aphidicolin-resistant DNA polymerase α, *Proc. Natl. Acad. Sci. U.S.A.,* 80, 797, 1983.

51. **Liu, P. K., Chang, C. C., and Trosko, J. E.,** Association of mutator activity with UV sensitivity in an aphidicolin-resistant mutant of Chinese hamster V79 cells, *Mutation Res.,* 106, 317, 1982.
52. **Liu, P. K., Trosko, J. E., and Chang, C. C.,** Hypermutability of a UV-sensitive aphidicolin-resistant mutant of Chinese hamster fibroblasts, *Mutation Res.,* 106, 333, 1982.
53. **Liu, P. K., Chang, C. C., and Trosko, J. E.,** Evidence for mutagenic repair in V79 cell mutant with aphidicolin-resistant DNA polymerase-α, *Somat. Cell Mol. Genet.,* 10, 235, 1984.
54. **Chang, C. C., Liu, P. K., Ross, D., Trosko, J. E., and Loeb, L. A.,** Genetic characterization of a UV-sensitive aphidicolin-resistant Chinese hamster DNA polymerase α mutant, submitted for publication.
55. **Wang, T. S. F., Pearson, B., Suomalainen, H. A., Mohandas, T., Shapiro, L. J., Schroder, J., and Korn, D.,** Assignment of the gene for human DNA polymerase α to the x chromosome, *Proc. Natl. Acad. Sci. U.S.A.,* 82, 5270, 1985.
56. **Hanaoka, F., Tandai, M., Miyazawa, H., Hori, T., and Yamada, M.,** Assignment of the human gene for DNA polymerase α to the x chromosome, *Jpn. J. Cancer Res. (Gann),* 76, 441, 1985.
57. **Liu, P. K. and Loeb, L. A.,** Transfection of the DNA polymerase-α gene, Science, 226, 833, 1984.
58. **Nishiyama, Y., Suzuki, S., Yamauchi, M., Maeno, K., and Yoshida, S.,** Characterization of an aphidicolin-resistant mutant of herpes simplex virus type 2 which induces an altered viral DNA polymerase, *Virology,* 135, 87, 1984.
59. **Defilippes, F. M.,** Effect of aphidicolin on vaccinia virus: Isolation of an aphidicolin-resistant mutant, *J. Virol.,* 52, 474, 1984.
60. **Bastow, K. F., Derse, D. D., and Cheng, Y. C.,** Susceptibility of phosphonoformic acid-resistant herpes simplex virus variants to arabinosylnucleosides and aphidicolin, *Antimicrob. Agents Chemother.,* 23, 914, 1983.
61. **Honess, R. W., Purifoy, D. J. M., Young, D., Gopal, R., Cammack, N., and O'Hare, P.,** Single mutations at many sites within the DNA polymerase locus of herpes simplex viruses can confer hypersensitivity to aphidicolin and resistance to phosphonoacetic acid, *J. Gen. Virol.,* 65, 1, 1984.
62. **Coen, D. M., Fleming, H. E., Jr., Leslie, L. K., and Retondo,** Sensitivity of arabinosyladenine-resistant mutants of herpes simplex virus to other anti-viral drugs and mapping of drug hypersensitivity mutations to the DNA polymerase locus, *J. Virology,* 53, 477, 1985.
63. **Hall, J. D., Furman, P. A., St. Clair, M. H., and Knopf, C. W.,** Reduced in vivo mutagenesis by mutant herpes simplex DNA polymerase involves improved nucleotide selection, *Proc. Natl. Acad. Sci. U.S.A.,* 82, 3889, 1985.
64. **Nishimura, M., Yasuda, H., Ikegami, S., Ohashi, M., and Yamada, M. A.,** Aphidicolin resistant mutant of which DNA polymerase α is induced by this drug, *Biochem. Biophys. Res. Commun.,* 91, 939, 1979.
65. **Sugino, A. and Nakayama, K.,** DNA polymerase α mutants from Drosophila melanogaster cell line, *Proc. Natl. Acad. Sci. U.S.A.,* 77, 7049, 1980.
66. **Ayusawa, D., Iwata, K., Kozu, T., Ikegami, S., and Seno, T.,** Increase in dATP pool in aphidicolin-resistant mutants of mouse FM3A cells, *Biochem. Biophys. Res. Commun.,* 91, 946, 1979.
67. **Ayusawa, D., Iwata, K., and Seno, T.,** Alteration of ribonucleotide reductase in aphidicolin-resistant mutants of mouse FM3A cells with associated resistance to arabinosyladenine and arabinosylcytosine, *Somat. Cell Genet.,* 7, 27, 1981.
68. **Nicander, B. and Richard, P.,** Aphidicolin sensitivity of variant 3T6 cells selected for changes in ribonucleotide reductase, *Biochem. Biophys. Res. Commun.,* 103, 148, 1981.
69. **Iwata, K., Ayusawa, D., and Seno, T.,** Increased level of ribonucleotide reductase and associated resistance to 9-β-D-arabinofuranosyladenine and 1-β-D-arabinofuranosylcytosine, *Gann,* 73, 167, 1982.
70. **Ayusawa, D., Iwata, K., and Seno, T.,** Isolation of mouse FM3A cell mutants with thermolabile thymidylate synthetase by resistance to aphidicolin, *Biochem. Biophys. Res. Commun.,* 96, 1654, 1980.
71. **Ayusawa, D., Iwata, K., Seno, T., and Koyama, H.,** Conditional thymidine auxotrophic mutants of mouse FM3A cells due to thermosensitive thymidylate synthetase and their prototrophic revertants, *J. Biol. Chem.,* 256, 12005, 1981.
72. **Ayusawa, D., Iwata, K., and Seno, T.,** Unusual sensitivity to bleomycin and joint resistance to 9-β-D-arabinofuranosyladenine and 1-β-D-arabinofurano-sylcytosine of mouse FM3A cell mutants with altered ribonucleotide reductase and thymidylate synthetase, *Cancer Res.,* 43, 814, 1983.
73. **Tsuji, H., Shiomi, T., Tsuji, S., Tobari, I., Ayusawa, D., Shimizu, K., and Seno, T.,** Aphidicolin-resistant mutants of mouse lymphoma L5178Y cells with high incidence of spontaneous sister chromatid exchanges, *Genetics,* 113, 433, 1986.
74. **Chu, E. H. Y., McLaren, J. D., Li, I. C., and Lamb, B.,** Pleiotropic mutants of Chinese hamster cells with altered cytidine 5'-triphosphate synthetase, *Biochem. Genet.,* 22, 701, 1984.
75. **Robert de Saint Vincent, B., Dechamps, M., and Buttin, G.,** The modulation of the thymidine triphosphate pool of Chinese hamster cells by dCMP deaminase and UDP reductase, *J. Biol. Chem.,* 255, 162, 1980.

76. **Robert de Saint Vincent, B., DeChamps, M., and Buttin, G.,** The modulation of the thymidine triphosphate pool of Chinese hamster cells by dCMP deaminase and UDP reductase, *J. Biol. Chem.,* 255, 162, 1980.

77. **Meuth, M., Trudel, M., and Siminovitch, L.,** Selection of Chinese hamster cells auxotrophic for thymidine by 1-β-D-arabinofuranosyl cytosine, *Somat. Cell Genet.,* 5, 303, 1979.

78. **Trudel, M., Van Genechten, T., and Meuth, M.,** Biochemical characterization of the hamster Thy mutator gene and its revertants, *J. Biol. Chem.,* 259, 2355, 1984.

79. **Meuth, M., Heureux-Huard, N., and Trudel, M.,** Characterization of a mutator gene in Chinese hamster ovary cells, *Proc. Natl. Acad. Sci. U.S.A.,* 76, 6505, 1979.

80. **Meuth, M.,** Sensitivity of a mutator gene in Chinese hamster ovary cells to deoxynucleoside triphosphate pool alterations, *Mol. Cell. Biol.,* 7, 652, 1981.

81. **Weinberg, G. L., Ullman, B., Wright, C. M. and Martin, D. W., Jr.,** The effects of exogenous thymidine on endogenous deoxynucleotides and mutagenesis in mammalian cells, *Somatic Cell Mol. Genet.,* 11, 413, 1985.

82. **Weinberg, G., Ullman, B., and Martin, D. W., Jr.,** Mutator phenotypes in mammalian cell mutants with distinct biochemical defects and abnormal deoxyribonucleoside triphosphate pools, *Proc. Natl. Acad. Sci. U.S.A.,* 78, 2447, 1981.

83. **Weissbach, A.,** The functional roles of mammalian DNA polymerase, *Arch. Biochem. Biophys.,* 198, 386, 1979.

84. **Byrnes, J. J.,** Differential inhibitors of DNA polymerases alpha and delta, *Biochem. Biophys. Res. Commun.,* 132, 628, 1985.

85. **Castellot, J. J., Jr., Miller, M. R., Lehtomaki, D. M., and Pardee, A. B.,** Comparison of DNA replication and repair enzymology using permeabilized baby hamster kidney cells, *J. Biol. Chem.,* 254, 6904, 1979.

86. **Bertrazzoni, V., Stefanini, Pedrali-Noy, G., Guilotto, E., Nuzzo, F., Falashi, A., and Spardari, S.,** Variations of DNA polymerase α and β during prolonged stimulation of human lymphocytes, *Proc. Natl. Acad. Sci. U.S.A.,* 73, 785, 1976.

87. **Hubscher, U., Kuenzle, C. C., and Spadari, S.,** Functional roles of DNA polymerase β and γ, *Proc. Natl. Acad. Sci. U.S.A.,* 76, 2316, 1979.

88. **Waser, J., Hubscher, U., Kuenzle, C. C., and Spadari, S.,** DNA polymerase β from brain neurons is a repair enzyme, *Eur. J. Biochem.,* 97, 361, 1979.

89. **Hardt, N., Pedrali-Noy, G., Focher, F., and Spadari, S.,** Aphidicolin does not inhibit DNA repair synthesis in ultraviolet-irradiated HeLa cells. A radioautographic study, *Biochem. J.,* 199, 453, 1981.

90. **Giulotto, E. and Mondello, C.,** Aphidicolin does not inhibit the repair synthesis of mitotic chromosomes, *Biochem. Biophys. Res. Commun.,* 99, 1287, 1981.

91. **Iliakis, G., Nusse, M., and Bryant, P.,** Effects of aphidicolin on cell proliferation, repair of potentially lethal damage and repair of DNA strand breaks in Ehrlich ascites tumour cells exposed to x-rays, *Int. J. Radiat. Biol.,* 42, 417, 1982.

92. **Sala, F., Magnien, E., Galli, M. G., Dalschaert, X., Pedrali-Noy, G., and Spadari, S.,** DNA repair synthesis in plant protoplasts is aphidicolin-resistant, *FEBS Lett.,* 138, 213, 1982.

93. **Iliakis, G. and Nusse, M.,** Aphidicolin promotes repair of potentially lethal damage in irradiated mammalian cells synchronized in S-phase, *Biochem. Biophys. Res. Commun.,* 104, 1209, 1982.

94. **Ciarrocchi, G., Jose, J. G., and Linn, S.,** Further characterization of a cell-free system for measuring replicative and repair DNA synthesis with cultured human fibroblasts and evidence for the involvement of DNA polymerase α in DNA repair, *Nucleic Acids Res.,* 7, 1205, 1979.

95. **Waters, R., Crocombe, K., and Mirzayans, R.,** The inhibition of DNA repair by aphidicolin or cytosine arabinoside in x-irradiated normal and xeroderma pigmentosum fibroblasts, *Mutation Res.,* 94, 229, 1981.

96. **Waters, R.,** Aphidicolin: an inhibitor of DNA repair in human fibroblasts, *Carcinogenesis,* 2, 795, 1981.

97. **Snyder, R. D. and Regan, J. D.,** Aphidicolin inhibits repair of DNA in UV-irradiated human fibroblasts, *Biochem. Biophys. Res. Commun.,* 99, 1088, 1981.

98. **Snyder, R. D. and Regan, J. D.,** Differential responses of log and stationary phase human fibroblasts to inhibition of DNA repair by aphidicolin, *Biochim. Biophys. Acta,* 697, 229, 1982.

99. **Nocentini, S.,** Effects of aphidicolin on the recovery of ribosomal RNA synthesis and on the repair of potentially lethal damage in UV irradiated simian and human cells, *Biochem. Biophys. Res Commun.,* 109, 603, 1982.

100. **Morita, T., Tsutsui, Y., Nishiyama, Y., Nakamura, H., and Yoshida, S.,** Effects of DNA polymerase inhibitors on replicative and repair DNA synthesis in ultraviolet-irradiated HeLa cells, *Int. J. Radiat. Biol.,* 42, 471, 1982.

101. **Miller, M. R. and Chinault, D. N.,** Evidence that DNA polymerases α and β participate differentially in DNA repair synthesis induced by different agents, *J. Biol. Chem.,* 257, 46, 1982.

102. **Miller, M. R. and Chinault, D. N.,** The roles of DNA polymerases α, β, γ in DNA repair synthesis induced in hamster and human cells by different DNA damaging agents, *J. Biol. Chem.,* 257, 10204, 1982.

103. **Miller, M. and Lui, L.,** Participation of different DNA polymerases in mammalian DNA repair synthesis is not related to "Patch size", *Biochem. Biophys. Res. Commun.,* 108, 1676, 1982.
104. **Mattern, M. R., Paone, R. F., and Day, R. S., III,** Eukaryotic DNA repair is blocked at different steps by inhibitors of DNA topoisomerases and of DNA polymerases α and β, *Biochim. Biophys. Acta,* 697, 6, 1982.
105. **Lonn, U. and Lonn, S.,** Reduced repair of x-ray-induced DNA lesions in cells without functioning DNA polymerase α, *Radiat. Res.,* 102, 71, 1985.
106. **Bohr, V. and Kober, L.,** The effect of aphidicolin on DNA repair in resting and mitogen-stimulated human lymphocytes, *Biochem. Biophys. Res. Commun.,* 108, 797, 1982.
107. **Tyrrell, R. M.,** Specific toxicity of aphidicolin to ultraviolet-irradiated excision proficient human skin fibroblasts, *Carcinogenesis,* 4, 327, 1983.
108. **Seki, S., Hosogi, N., and Oda, T.,** Participation of DNA polymerase α and β in unscheduled DNA synthesis in mammalian cells, *Acta Med. Okayama,* 37, 213, 1983.
109. **Collins, A.,** DNA repair in ultraviolet-irradiated HeLa cells is disrupted by aphidicolin. The inhibition of repair need not imply the absence of repair synthesis, *Biochim. Biophys. Acta,* 741, 341, 1983.
110. **Dresler, S. L. and Lieberman, M. W.,** Identification of DNA polymerases involved in DNA excision repair in diploid human fibroblasts, *J. Biol. Chem.,* 258, 9990, 1983.
111. **Tyrrell, R. M. and Amaudruz, F.,** Alpha polymerase involvement in excision repair of damage induced by solar radiation at defined wavelengths in human fibroblasts, *Photochem. Photobiol.,* 40, 449, 1984.
112. **Seki, S., Hosogi, N., Oda, T.,** Differential sensitivity to aphidicolin of replicative DNA synthesis and ultraviolet-induced unscheduled DNA synthesis in vivo in mammalian cells, *Acta Med. Okayama,* 38, 227, 1984.
113. **Mosbaugh, D. W. and Linn, S.,** Gap-filling DNA synthesis by HeLa DNA polymerase α in an in vitro base excision DNA repair scheme, *J. Biol. Chem.,* 259, 10247, 1984.
114. **Yamada, K., Hanaoka, F., and Yamada, M.,** Effects of aphidicolin and/or 2′,3′-dideoxythymidine on DNA repair induced in HeLa cells by four types of DNA-damaging agents, *J. Biol. Chem.,* 260, 10412, 1985.
115. **Tyrrell, R. M., Keyse, S. M., Amaudruz, F., and Pidoux, M.,** Excision repair in U.V. (254 nm) damaged non-dividing human skin fibroblasts: a major biological role for DNA polymerase α, *Int. J. Radiat. Biol.,* 48, 723, 1985.
116. **Licastro, F., Sarafian, T., Verity, A. M., and Walford, R. L.,** Inhibition of pol-α and -β completely blocks DNA repair induced by UV irradiation in cultured mouse neuronal cells, *Biochem. Biophys. Res. Commun.,* 132, 929, 1985.
117. **Smith, C. A. and Okumoto, D. S.,** Nature of DNA repair synthesis resistant to inhibitions of polymerase α in human cells, *Biochemistry,* 23, 1383, 1984.
118. **Dresler, S. L.,** Comparative enzymology of ultraviolet-induced DNA repair synthesis and semiconservative DNA replication in permeable diploid human fibroblasts, *J. Biol. Chem.,* 259, 13947, 1984.
119. **Joe, C. O., Norman, J. O., Irvin, T. R., and Busbee, D. L.,** DNA polymerase activity in a repair-deficient human cell line, *Biochem. Biophys. Res. Commun.,* 128, 754, 1985.

Chapter 4

## ORNITHINE ANALOGS

**Immo E. Scheffler**

## TABLE OF CONTENTS

I.    The Role of Ornithine Decarboxylase ........................................... 46

II.   Mechanism of Action of the Analogs ........................................... 48
    A.    A Reversible Inhibitor ..................................................... 48
    B.    An Irreversible Inhibitor ................................................. 48

III.  Effects of the Analogs on Cells in Culture ..................................... 48

IV.   Variants of Mammalian Cells Resistant to the Analogs ......................... 49
    A.    The Hepatoma Variant $HMO_A$ ........................................ 49
    B.    Variants with Amplified ODC mRNA .................................... 50
    C.    ODC Overproduction in the Absence of Gene Amplification ............. 53

V.    The Regulation of ODC Activity in Normal and Overproducing Cells ........... 54

VI.   Clinical Uses of the Analogs .................................................... 55
    A.    In Cancer Chemotherapy .............................................. 55
    B.    Against Parasitic Infections .............................................. 55

VII.  Summary ...................................................................... 55

Acknowledgment ................................................................... 56

References ......................................................................... 56

## I. THE ROLE OF ORNITHINE DECARBOXYLASE

All living organisms from prokaryotes to humans require polyamines for cell proliferation, and polyamines may also play a role in differentiation in complex organisms.[1-4] The definition of their precise role in cells is still a subject of much speculation, but it is likely that they have multiple functions as multivalent organic cations in ionic interactions which stabilize the tertiary structure of nucleic acids and proteins. The most common polyamines are putrescine, spermidine, and spermine. The latter two polyamines are derived from the successive addition of propylamine groups to putrescine. Many bacteria and plant cells can derive putrescine by two independent pathways: (1) from the decarboxylation of ornithine, and (2) starting from the decarboxylation of arginine. In contrast, ornithine decarboxylase (ODC) is the exclusive and rate limiting enzyme in the synthesis of putrescine in animal cells and certain other eukaryotic microorganisms.

The essential role of polyamines in cellular proliferation became established only after specific and potent inhibitors of their biosynthesis became available, although genetic experiments aimed at identifying and mutating the corresponding enzymes also contributed to this conclusion.[5-7] With this knowledge it became feasible to consider and test the usefulness of such inhibitors in the control of the multiplication of certain cells such as tumor cells, or pathogens.[8] Inhibitors of ODC were thus expected to deplete mammalian cells completely of their polyamines, while inhibitors of S-adenosylmethionine decarboxylase (SAM decarboxylase) should affect only the synthesis of spermidine and spermine. Alternatively, specific inhibitors of the spermidine and spermine synthases could also be employed. It seems clear now that polyamines are not freely substitutable for each other, and there are some indications that spermine levels may be more critical than putrescine levels. A discussion of experiments delineating the role of individual polyamines is beyond the scope of this article. An expert and comprehensive review of the action of polyamine antimetabolites has been written by Heby and Janne.[9] In the following the emphasis will be on inhibitors of ornithine decarboxylase in mammalian cells. A brief discussion of the properties of this enzyme is therefore in order. It is found in the cytosol of dividing cells representing generally less than 0.001% of the total soluble proteins. In quiescent cells in vivo and in vitro it is often undetectable. In such cells it is inducible by a large variety of treatments including growth factors, certain hormones, tumor promoters, hypotonic shock, etc., depending on the cell type.[1-3] Under such conditions one generally observes a bell-shaped curve of activity, i.e., a sharp rise, a peak, and an equally steep decline. It is now clear that transcriptional activation of the ODC gene plays a role in some systems, for example, in the induction of the enzyme in male mouse kidneys by testosterone.[10,11] However, the rate of translation of the ODC mRNA is also controlled (most likely by endogenous polyamine levels),[12-16] and the unusually high rate of turnover of the enzyme represents another aspect of the control of enzyme levels, which has attracted attention for some time.[2,17] In addition, an inducible, specific protein inhibitor, the ODC antizyme, not only inhibits the activity of ODC by binding tightly and stoichiometrically under physiological conditions,[18,19] but also may contribute to the regulation of its turnover rate.[19]

The mouse enzyme is a homodimer of two identical polypeptides of 51.17 kDa [461 residues].[3,20,21] A required cofactor for its activity is pyridoxal phosphate which forms a Schiff-base with the substrate stabilizing the intermediate carbanion. A likely mechanism for the decarboxylation reaction is outlined in Figure 1.

Efforts in the design of specific inhibitors for this enzyme have focused on analogs of ornithine and putrescine. The extremely high specificty of this enzyme for ornithine (5 carbons) as opposed to lysine (6 carbons) should be noted. Pioneering studies on a variety of ornithine analogs and derivatives were carried out by Bey and co-workers.[22] These workers established that no modifications of the delta amino group of ornithine (e.g.,

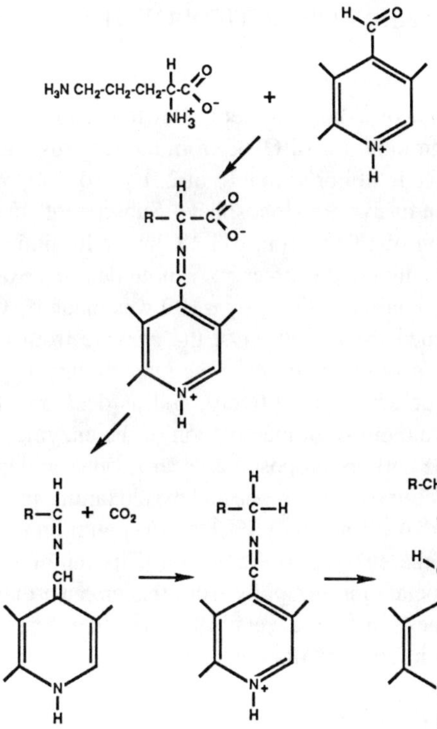

FIGURE 1. Proposed mechanism for the decarboxylation of ornithine by ornithine decarboxylase.

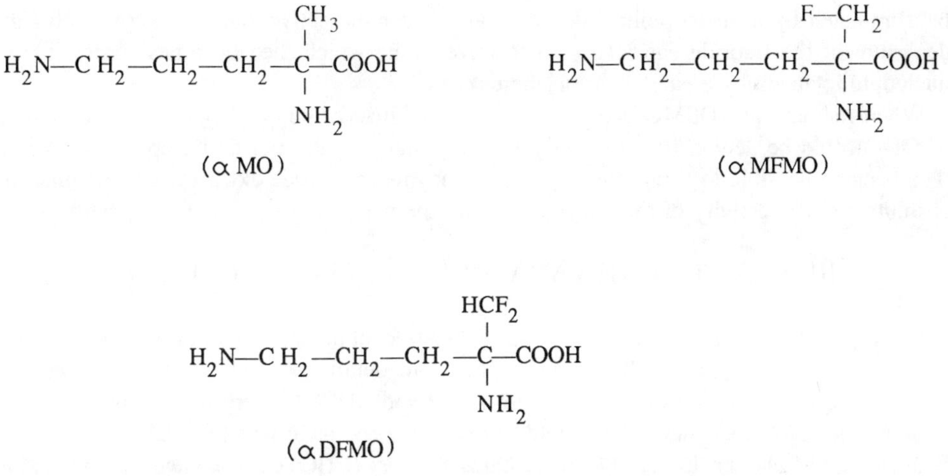

$$H_2N-CH_2-CH_2-CH_2-\underset{\underset{NH_2}{|}}{\overset{\overset{CH_3}{|}}{C}}-COOH$$

( α MO )

$$H_2N-CH_2-CH_2-CH_2-\underset{\underset{NH_2}{|}}{\overset{\overset{F-CH_2}{|}}{C}}-COOH$$

( α MFMO )

$$H_2N-CH_2-CH_2-CH_2-\underset{\underset{NH_2}{|}}{\overset{\overset{HCF_2}{|}}{C}}-COOH$$

( α DFMO )

FIGURE 2. Chemical structures of the analogs of ornithine discussed in the text.

alkylation) were tolerated by the enzyme. Subsequent claims to the contrary by Gilad and colleagues[23] have not been verified elsewhere. By far the most specific and efficient inhibitors of ODC have been compounds with additional substitutions on the alpha carbon of ornithine, such as alpha-methylornithine (αMO), alpha Monofluoromethylornithine (αMFMO), and alpha-difluoromethylornithine (αDFMO) (Figure 2). Very recently, [2R,5R]-6-heptyne-2,5-diamine, and even more potent irreversible inhibitor of ODC has been described.[24]

## II. MECHANISM OF ACTION OF THE ANALOGS

### A. A Reversible Inhibitor

αMO was first synthesized by Abdel-Monem, Newton, and Weeks[25] who also demonstrated its effectiveness as an inhibitor of ODC from the rat prostate gland. Kinetic studies revealed it to be a competitive inhibitor with a $K_i$ of $2.0 \times 10^{-5} M$, which was only slightly affected by the concentration of pyridoxalphosphate. Subsequent studies by the same group failed to detect the formation of $^{14}CO_2$ from α[1-$^{14}$C]methylornithine by crude ODC preparations from a variety of mammalian sources.[26] A more detailed examination of the mechanism of inhibition and inactivation of ODC by αMO was made by O'Leary and Herreid.[27] Although these authors studied the inhibition of the enzyme from Lactobacillus 30a, they noted that their conclusions most likely apply to the mammalian enzymes as well. For short incubation times the analogue acts competitively, and its decarboxylation is undedectable, but upon prolonged exposure there is an inactivation of the enzyme, which can be reversed by pyridoxal phosphate. The authors proposed a decarboxylation-dependent transamination reaction which also yields 5-amino-2-pentanone and pyridoxamine phosphate. Thus the extent of inhibition was found to depend not only on the concentration of the inhibitor, but also on the time of exposure of the enzyme to the analog. The inhibition is reversible because the cofactor appears to dissociate more rapidly from this enzyme than from other pyridoxal phosphate-dependent enzymes. In vivo reversibility may therefore be further complicated by dependence on the concentration of the cofactor.

### B. An Irreversible Inhibitor

The catalytic irreversible inhibition of mammalian ornithine decarboxylase by the substrate analog αDFMO was first described by Metcalf and co-workers.[28] A scheme was postulated in which the analog binds to the active site of the enzyme and becomes decarboxylated. The intermediate carbanion can rearrange to a reactive imine from which the fluoride can be eliminated by a nucleophilic side chain at or near the active site, or alternatively, the departure of the fluoride can lead to a reactive imine which then becomes susceptible to nucleophilic attack by a side chain on the enzyme.

When radioactive αDFMO became available, the inactivation and covalent modification of ODC could be demonstrated directly in crude and partially purified preparations.[20,29] It thus became possible to titrate the amount of enzyme in a crude extract and determine the absolute specific activity of the enzyme without the need for a complete purification.

## III. EFFECT OF THE ANALOGS ON CELLS IN CULTURE

Numerous studies have appeared describing the effect of the ODC inhibitors on mammalian cells in culture, and they will not be reviewed in detail here. The conclusions can be summarized as follows. As expected, both αMO and αDFMO were highly specific ODC inhibitors in vivo, since their effect could be overcome completely by the addition putrescine to the medium. The sensitivity of Chinese hamster ovary (CHO) cells as measured by plating efficiency assays is shown in Figure 3.[30] Relatively high concentrations of αMO were required, consistent with its function as a competitive inhibitor, while an about 100 times lower concentration of the suicide inhibitor was effective. When cells were exposed to a lethal concentration of either inhibitor, their growth rate slowed down gradually over a period of 1 to 2 days, and their viability started to decline after 3 to 5 days. Not surprisingly, an identical behavior was observed when ornithine decarboxylase deficient cells (putrescine auxotrophs) were switched to putrescine deficient medium.[7] An analysis of the polyamine levels in these cells showed that putrescine became undetectable after 24 hr, the spermidine level began to decline towards zero after a 24-hr lag, and intracellular spermine remained

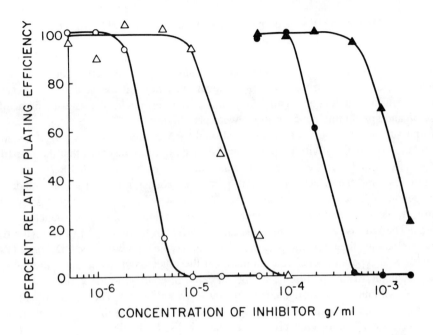

FIGURE 3. Plating efficiency of wild-type and variant cells as a function of inhibitor concentration. Equal aliquots of 100 to 150 cells were plated on 60 mm plates. After 9 to 10 days the plates were stained with crystal violet and colonies with more than 50 cells were counted. Results are plotted as the percent of plating efficiency in control plates with no drug added. Circles: wild-type cells; triangles: variant cells (DF1). Closed symbols: αMO; open symbols: αDFMO.[30]

relatively constant up to the time when cells started to disintegrate. Different cell types may differ slightly with respect to these kinetics, but qualitatively their behaviour is similar. For example, Gerner and Mamont[31] have studied polyamine levels in rat hepatoma (HTC) cells in a comparison of the two potent, irreversible ODC inhibitors αDFMO and [2R,5R]-6-heptyne-2,5-diamine, and found that while putrescine and spermidine levels were depleted within a day, spermine levels remained near control levels. An interesting observation by these authors was that the effect of the diamine could be reversed within 1 day after removal of the drug; in contrast, the recovery from αDFMO took an extra day (see also Section IV. B). In the case of the CHO mutant cells examined by us there was no recognizable accumulation of cells at a particular phase in the cell cycle following polyamine starvation. Similarly, Harada and Morris[32] found that polyamine-limited cells exhibited increases in the length of both the $G_1$ and S phases of the cell cycle. Thus, although ODC has attracted much attention as a marker enzyme for the $G_1$ phase in cells stimulated by growth factors, its activity does not seem to be absolutely obligatory for the traverse of this phase of the cell cycle, as long as the intracellular spermidine/spermine levels are still sufficiently high. Heby and Janne[9] came to a similar conclusion; polyamines enhance the efficiency and fidelity of a variety of steps during the progression of cells through the cell cycle.

## IV. VARIANTS OF MAMMALIAN CELLS RESISTANT TO THE ANALOGS

### 1. The Hepatoma Variant HMO$_A$

The first reported variant of a mammalian cell line partially resistant to an ODC inhibitor was described by Mamont et al.[33] Rat hepatoma cells (HTC) were exposed to 5 m$M$ αMO for 18 days, and survivors were subsequently subcultured for 13 weeks under the same selective pressure. Subcloning yielded several resistant clones of which one, HMO$_A$, has received considerable attention. The phenotype of the variant $HMO_A$ was stable over many generations in the absence of selection. Resistance to the drug could not be ascribed to changes in permeability of the cells. The $K_m$ value for the substrate and the $K_i$ value for the analog were the same for the enzyme from normal and variant cells. The most notable difference in the variant cells was that enzyme levels were not only elevated two- to sevenfold, but they were not modulated significantly during the cell cycle. As a result intracellular putrescine and spermidine concentrations were also higher.

A follow-up of this investigation was published by McCann et al.[13] as part of a study of the regulation of ODC activity by putrescine. A striking discovery was that the half-life of ODC in cells treated with cycloheximide was 22 min in normal cells and 8.2 hr in $HMO_A$ cells. In comparing the effects of different putrescine concentrations it was concluded that low exogenous putrescine concentrations [$10^{-5}M$] mimicked the effect of a protein synthesis inhibitor, while high exogenous concentrations [$10^{-2}M$] led to a rapid induction of the antizyme. The wild type and variant cells did not differ in the induction of antizyme by 10 m$M$ putrescine, and the interactions of the $HMO_A$ antizyme with wild type ODC or of $HMO_A$ ODC with wild type antizyme were similar. On the other hand, some antizyme induction was detectable at $10^{-5}M$ putrescine in normal cells, in contrast to the variant.

The same variant was investigated further by Pritchard et al.[34] The extended half-life of ODC was confirmed, and moreover, it was shown not to be due to a general alteration in the turnover rate of short-lived proteins in these cells. SAM decarboxylase and tyrosine aminotransferase had identical half-lives in normal HTC and $HMO_A$ cells, and the release of radioactive amino acids from prelabeled cells was also unaltered. Elevated ODC activity was correlated with increased ODC protein, as measured by covalent binding of [$^{14}C$] αDFMO. ODC enzymes were purified about 8000-fold from both normal and variant cell types and found to be indistinguishable by several criteria: (1) the conditions for purification with comparable yields were identical; (2) the molecular weights of the subunits were identical; (3) heat inactivation studies revealed no difference; (4) the two proteins were antigenically the same; and (5) titration with rat liver antizyme yielded comparable inactivation curves.

Murakami and Hayashi[19] have recently shown that a good correlation existed between the reciprocal of the half-life of ODC activity in the presence of cycloheximide and the amount of ODC-antizyme complex relative to total ODC, suggesting a role for the antizyme in the control of the degradation of ODC. With these considerations Murakami et al.[35] have re-examined ODC, ODC-antizyme complexes, and free antizyme in HTC and $HMO_A$ cells under various conditions. After a medium change the $HMO_A$ cells had not only more ODC activity, but also seemed to have considerably more ODC-antizyme complex than HTC cells. The increased stability of ODC in $HMO_A$ cells was therefore not explicable in terms of an absence or deficiency of antizyme.

The primary alteration in the $HMO_A$ variant has not been clarified, and Pritchard et al.[34] speculate that a specific deactivation/proteolysis system for ODC is altered in these cells. Antizyme may simply sensitize ODC to this proteolytic system.

## B. Variants with Amplified ODC mRNA

When the analogs αMO and αDFMO became more readily available thanks to the generosity of the Centre de Recherche, Merrell International, in Strasbourg, France, selections for resistant variants were initiated in several laboratories. Choi and Scheffler[30] reported in 1981 the isolation of CHO variants which were resistant to about ten times the lethal concentration of either αMO or αDFMO. (Figure 1). The selection was in a single step following the mutagenesis of the parental cells with 0.4 mg/m$\ell$ ethylmethane sulfonate. This phenotype was codominant in somatic intraspecies hybrid cells, which could be indicative of an altered enzyme, or enzyme overproduction by some mechanism such as gene

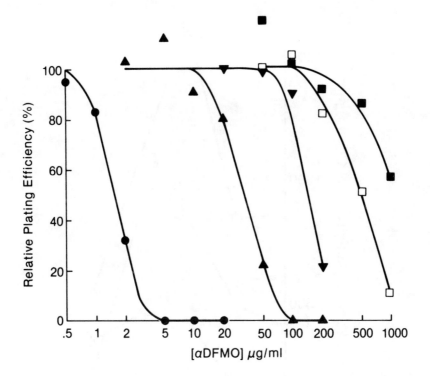

FIGURE 4. Relative plating efficiency in the presence of αDFMO. The experiment is similar to that in Figure 1. The points represent the average of duplicate plates. The closed circles represent the parental CHO cells. The other curves represent the different variants DF1, DF2, DF2.5, and DF3 with increasing levels of resistance.[29]

amplification. It would be interesting to perform a similar test with the $HMO_A$ cells, since a missing function such as the postulated proteolytic activity would likely be expressed as a recessive phenotype.

Starting with this variant, renamed DF1, we selected additional variants, DF2, DF3, with a step-wise increase in the concentration of αDFMO (Figure 4).[29] The variants DF2 and DF3 were resistant to 400 μg/mℓ (2 m$M$) or 1000 μg/mℓ (5 m$M$), respectively, which represents 400 or 1000 times the lethal dose, as measured by determining the plating efficiency.

Like the variant hepatoma cells, these resistant CHO cells had elevated levels of ODC. The more resistant the variant, the higher the inducible ODC activity (Figure 5), although there was no strict proportionality. It is clear that in order to measure the ODC levels in these variants the cells had to be grown in the absence of the inhibitor, but it is less obvious why maximum inducible levels were not obtained until cells had proliferated in the absence of the drug for 5 to 7 days. Even extensive washing of the cells did not reduce this lag period. This observation is reminiscent of that of Gerner and Mamont,[31] and suggests lingering pools of the inhibitor.

We demonstrated that these cells had more ODC protein which was indistinguishable from the normal enzyme by a number of criteria: (1) sensitivity to the inhibitor; (2) $K_m$ with respect to the substrate ornithine; (3) migration in two-dimensional polyacrylamide gels; (4) titration with extracts containing antizyme; (5) determination of the molecular weight of the subunit labeled with [³H] αDFMO, and (6) determination of the absolute specific activity after determining the count of ODC protein by the amount of [³H] αDFMO covalently bound.

In distinct contrast to the hepatoma variants, however, we found that the half-life of the enzyme in these CHO variants was not appreciably different from that of the normal enzyme.

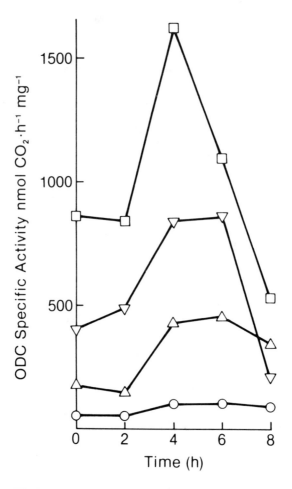

FIGURE 5.    Ornithine decarboxylase activity induced in wild-type ($\bigcirc$) and variant cells (DF1 ($\triangle$), DF2 ($\triangledown$), DF3 ($\square$). The cells were grown in the absence of αDFMO for 7 days, exposed to 2 mg/mℓ αMO for 48 hr, washed, synchronized by serum starvation for 48 hr, and induced by changing to fresh medium with 10% fetal calf serum. The αMO pretreatment changes the absolute amounts but not the relative amounts of inducible ODC.[30]

In fact, we were struck by the perfectly normal kinetics of the induction curves in serum-stimulated cells (Figure 5). The peaks were higher, but occurred at almost the same time in all of these variants.

Another cell line with which selections for resistance to αDFMO were carried out successfully are the S49 mouse lymphoma cells.[36,37] One particular variant, the Z.12 clone, was obtained from nonmutagenized wild-type cells by gradually raising the concentration of αDFMO from 0.02 to 0.4 m$M$ over a period of 13 weeks. The Z.12 line was cloned and subsequently maintained in 0.1 m$M$ αDFMO.

The Z.12 cells had about ten times more ODC activity than the S49 parents. Immuno-precipitations of [$^{35}$S]methionine labeled extracts from wild-type and resistant cells with a specific antiserum[38] were performed. They gave a prominent band in the autoradiograph of one-dimensional SDS polyacrylamide gels with Z.12 extracts; the corresponding band was barely detectable in wild type extracts. Its molecular weight was in agreement with that determined for ODC. The same protein was further identified by two-dimensional gel electrophoresis of total labeled cell extracts. The shift of the spot to a slightly more basic pH when the enzyme was derivatized with the irreversible inhibitor αDFMO served as a confirmation. Thus it could be demonstrated that the increase in activity in the Z.12 variant was due to an increased rate of ODC synthesis relative to the other labeled proteins. Furthermore, its rate of turnover could be determined directly by a pulse-chase experiment and following the weakening of the ODC spot in autoradiograms from the two dimensional gels. A half-life of 45 min was measured. Therefore, the elevated enzyme level was not accounted for by an increased stability of the protein. These data also supported the conclusion that the disappearance of activity was tightly linked to the disappearance of the ODC protein per se, and not the result of some small covalent modification of the protein.

McConlogue and Coffino[37] subsequently extended the step-wise selection to 50 mM αDFMO, which necessitated a reduction in the NaCl concentration in the medium. A clone D4.1 resulted in which the ornithine decarboxylase protein constituted 22% of newly synthesized cytoplasmic protein. This cell line proved to be the ideal starting material for the cloning of an ODC cDNA, since overproduction was due to highly amplified ODC mRNA, as a result of gene amplification.[39]

A similar approach to the cloning of ODC cDNA was taken by Kahana and Nathans.[40,41] αDFMO resistant mouse myeloma cells were selected in 30 mM αDFMO. Differential screening of cDNA libraries from normal and overproducing cells yielded a clone which could be identified as ODC cDNA. When used as a probe it detected an inducible mRNA on Northern blots of RNA from androgen treated mouse kidney or serum stimulated 3T3 cells. An ODC cDNA clone also became available from a differential screening of cDNA libraries from androgen-induced and uninduced mouse kidney.[10] It was made available to us, and we were able to show that ODC overproduction in our CHO DF3 cells was also due to an amplification of an ODC gene (A. Grens, unpublished).

In all of the cases examined so far it has been possible to culture the variant for long periods of time in the absence of any selective pressure without any reversion in their phenotype. This is consistent with a mechanism of gene amplification in a chromosome, not amplification by means of double minute chromosomes. Explicit proof for the existence of a homogeneously staining region as a result of gene amplification is so far available only for the D4.1 clone of McConlogue et al.[37] who found a large HSR on a pair of chromosomes 14 of the mouse. Amplification of the ODC gene can also be achieved by another route not involving the use of inhibitors of ODC. Steglich et al.[42,43] have described ODC-deficient mutants of CHO cells which have a residual amount of activity [2 to 5%]. They required putrescine in the medium. However, in the absence of the polyamine, putrescine-independent clones arose spontaneously at a frequency of 2 to 7 $\times$ 10$^{-5}$ per cell per generation. We interpreted this observed reversion in terms of an amplification of a defective enzyme with partial activity. The spontaneous mechanism raised the level of enzyme activity in these revertants about tenfold. Additional increases could be achieved by further selection in αMO. An analysis with an ODC cDNA probe revealed that higher mRNA levels were responsible for elevated enzyme levels. Evidence for gene amplification was obtained in those cells with the highest levels of activity.[43] Similar observations were published by Pohjanpelto et al.[44]

## C. ODC Overproduction in the Absence of Gene Amplification

In our analysis of reversion of leaky ODC-deficient mutants we noted in some of the cases examined an apparent discrepancy between the mRNA levels and the genomic DNA levels [see Figures 3 and 4 in Steglich et al.[43]] This problem has now been examined in more detail by McConlogue et al.[45] A series of independent variants of S49 cells selected for resistance to 0.1 mM αDFMO were analyzed. All showed increased ODC activity, but the stability (half-life) of the protein was normal in each case. Increased steady state levels of ODC mRNA were also found in all variants. Gene amplification analyzed by Southern analysis, however, could not account for the increased ODC mRNA levels. In fact, the gene copy number was 1-2 in a number of examples chosen, including the original Z.12 clone. Furthermore, in some variants there was no correlation between the mRNA level and the corresponding ODC activity. It was proposed that at least in this class the translatability of ODC mRNA may have been altered. The mechanism giving rise to such phenotypes remains to be established. There are several alternatives. First, the unusually long 5' untranslated leader sequence of mouse ODC mRNA has been proposed to play a role in the translational control of ODC expression by polyamines.[21,41] Changes such as deletions in this part of the message could account for changes in translatability. Second, mutations in the promoter region of the ODC gene may also be involved. Third, the possibility of epigenetic variations should not be discarded. In established, heteroploid cell lines some of the alleles may be silenced by mechanisms that may include DNA methylation, and partial or complete restoration of transcription may occur as a result of changes in methylation patterns. For example, we have described CHO mutants with a complete lack of ODC activity, which could be restored to putrescine independence by treatment with 5 azacytidine.[43]

Genomic Southerns probed with ODC cDNA have revealed that mouse, hamster and human cells contain multiple sequences in the genome which hybridize to the probe. Experiments yet to be completed will have to distinguish between the possibility that this is a multigene family, or that there are a series of pseudogenes in addition to the one active ODC gene.

## V. THE REGULATION OF ODC ACTIVITY IN NORMAL AND OVERPRODUCING CELLS

As expected, when extracts from cells which have been exposed to αDFMO for some time were analyzed for ODC activity, the activity was barely measurable, although large quantities of immunoreactive protein could be detected.[15] The inactive αDFMO-ODC complex appeared to have the same short half life in the presence of a protein synthesis inhibitor. A more puzzling observation was that after removal of the drug and thorough washing of the cells it took up to a week to recover the maximum inducible ODC activity.[29] Such a delayed recovery was also noted by Gerner and Mamont,[31] who contrasted the behavior of αDFMO with that of the other irreversible ODC inhibitor [2R,5R]-6-heptyne-2,5-diamine. A persistent, intracellular pool of the inhibitor has been postulated,[46] and differences in this latency period have been observed between normal and transformed 3T3 cells.[47] The significance of these observations is not yet clear. It was noted earlier that intracellular polyamine levels control the ODC activity by affecting the translation of ODC mRNA and the stability of the protein.[14-16,45] In the presence of sublethal doses of inhibitor one therefore would expect normal levels of polyamines to be maintained by elevated enzyme levels, i.e., the net activity of ODC enzyme would not be above normal. Such reasoning would lead one to expect that upon removal of the inhibitor the enzyme level should fall back to normal levels, but this is not observed. Five to fiftyfold higher enzyme levels can be found in such variants even months after the selective pressure has been removed. It occurred to us[15] and others[14,16] that the limiting factor in such cases was not ODC activity but substrate availability. As predicted, supplementing the medium for such overproducers with $10^{-4}$ *M* ornithine had a dramatic effect on ODC levels and ODC synthesis; they could be completely suppressed. At comparable exogenous concentrations ornithine was much more effective than putrescine, but it was necessary to convert the substrate to putrescine intracellularly. It is still an unresolved question whether putrescine or spermidine or both are the mediators of this control mechanism. Nevertheless, the conclusion seems valid that in such overproducers there is generally no direct proportionality between ODC activity and intracellular putrescine levels. It should also be emphasized that the other enzymes in the pathway of polyamine synthesis, SAM decarboxylase, and spermidine and spermine synthases, are not coordinately overproduced. On the other hand, under conditions of abnormal, distorted polyamine levels their activities may well be affected by mechanisms controlling their synthesis or stability. For example, lack of putrescine has been shown to cause elevation of SAM decarboxylase activity and accumulation of decarboxylated S-adenosyl-L-methionine.[48]

## VI. CLINICAL USES OF THE ANALOGS

### A. In Cancer Chemotherapy

Ornithine decarboxylase activity is generally elevated in rapidly proliferating cell populations, and tumor cells are no exceptions. With its high specificity for ODC, αDFMO therefore became an obvious candidate for applications in cancer chemotherapy, particularly after its antiproliferative effect had been demonstrated successfully in vitro. It is beyond the scope of this article to make a critical appraisal of these studies. Clinical studies revealed that αDFMO was relatively nontoxic to humans and rapidly excreted.[49,50] Repeated oral administrations of significant doses [typically 1.5 g/m² every 6 hr] were therefore required. Upon longer exposure to higher levels side effects included diarrhea, hematologic toxicity (thrombocytopenia) and hearing loss, which was reversible when αDFMO intake was discontinued. By itself αDFMO did not have the desired beneficial effect on human cancer patients. However, preliminary results show promise in the combination of αDFMO with several other cytotoxic agents[49] or leukocyte interferon.[50]

### B. Against Parasitic Infections

Whereas the efficacy of αDFMO in cancer chemotherapy may have been disappointing, these studies provided evidence that humans are relatively tolerant to the analog, and thus paved the way for other very promising applications of αDFMO.

Over 100 patients suffering from a late stage of African trypanosomiasis have been treated with αDFMO by the oral and/or intravenous route, and the results have been most encouraging.[51] Complete cures were achieved in patients which received the drug intravenously. Similar studies with rats infected with *Trypanosoma brucei brucei* have revealed that the success of the treatment may depend on the following series of events; polyamine depletion in the parasite leads to an arrest of cell division without specific cytotoxicity. The long slender bloodstream form is transformed to the short stumpy form. The latter is no longer infectious to the vertebrate host, and also no longer capable of binary fission. At this point an intact immune system of the host can cope with the infection and clear the blood.[52,53]

Another parasitic disease where αDFMO treatment has given encouraging results is *Pneumocystis carinii pneumonia,* the most common lethal infection in AIDS patients in North America.[54] In a clinical trial with patients who had failed to respond to the pentamidine and/or trimethorim/sulfamethoxazole treatment more than 70% could be discharged after several weeks of αDFMO therapy.

## VII. SUMMARY

Highly specific and effective inhibitors of ODC in mammalian cells and other organisms have become available in the last decade. They have been most useful in establishing that polyamines are essential for cell proliferation, and have paved the way for studying the specific role of polyamines in various cellular activities, or their interaction with cellular constituents.

The enzyme-activated suicide inhibitor αDFMO prevents mammalian cell proliferation in tissue culture at around 1 μg/mℓ (50 μ*M*), and it showed some promise in animal tumor models as a potential chemotherapeutic agent. Clinical studies have not lived up to expectations as far as the treatment of cancer patients is concerned, but the drug may yet become a most potent weapon in the fight against certain infectious protozoan parasites such as trypanosomes.

Further examination of the drug in cell culture studies led to the conclusion that variants resistant to elevated drug concentrations arise spontaneously at a significant frequency, perhaps as high as $10^{-4}$ per cell per generation. In all cases examined so far elevated enzyme levels have been associated with this resistance. In the extreme cases of high αDFMO concentrations [$>5$ m$M$] the amplification of an ODC gene was the mechanism responsible for a significant part of this overproduction. On the other hand, lower levels of resistance may result from a variety of genetic or epigenetic changes. Changes in the methylation pattern may alter the rate of transcription of ODC gene(s). A similar result may arise from mutations in the promoter of this gene. Since enzyme levels are subject to translational control by polymines, alterations which affect this mechanism may become responsible for elevated enzyme levels. Finally, the rapid turnover of this enzyme has been a challenging observation for a long time, and in at least one case an increased stability of the enzyme could account for the higher enzyme levels and resistance to the analogs.

## ACKNOWLEDGMENT

The research from our laboratory described in this chapter was supported by a grant from the U.S. Public Health Service (GM 18835). This work would not have been possible without the dedicated and skillful assistance and contributions of ideas from past and present members of my laboratory: J. Choi, C. Steglich, L. Dircks, and A. Grens.

## REFERENCES

1. **Bacharach, V.,** The induction of ornithine decarboxylase in normal and neoplastic cells, in *Polyamines in Biomedical Research,* Gaugas, J. M., Ed., John Wiley and Sons, New York, 1980, 81.
2. **Canellakis, E. S., Madore, D., Kyriakidis, D. A., and Heller, J. S.,** The regulation and function of ornithine decarboxylase and of the polyamines, in *Current Topics in Cellular Regulation,* Horecker, B. L. and Stadtman, E. R., Eds., Academic Press, New York, 1979, 155.
3. **Pegg, A. E. and McCann, P. P.,** Polyamine metabolism and function, *Am. J. Physiol.,* 243, c212, 1982.
4. **Tabor, C. W. and Tabor, H.,** Polyamines, *Ann. Rev. Biochem.,* 53, 749, 1984.
5. **Tabor, H. and Tabor, C. W.,** Polyamine biosynthesis and function in *Escherichia coli,* in *Advances in Polyamine Research,* 4th ed., Bachrach, U., Kaye, A., and Chayen, R., Eds., Raven Press, New York, 1983, 455.
6. **Tabor, C. W., Tabor, H., and Tyagi, A. K.,** Biochemical and genetic studies of polyamines in *Saccharomyces cerevisiae,* in *Advances in Polyamine Research,* 4th ed., Bachrach, U., Kaye, A., and Chayen, R., Eds., Raven Press, New York, 1983, 467.
7. **Steglich, C. and Scheffler, I. E.,** A mutant of Chinese hamster ovary cells with a severe deficiency of ornithine decarboxylase activity and exhibiting auxotrophy for putrescine, *J. Biol. Chem.,* 257, 4603, 1982.
8. **Janne, J., Alhonen-Hongisto, L., Kapyaho, K., and Seppanen, P.,** Experimental approaches to the systemic and topical use of polyamine antimetabolites as antiproliferative agents, in *Advances in Polyamine Research,* 4th ed., Bachrach, U., Kaye, A., and R. Chayen, R., Eds., Raven Press, New York, 1983, 17.
9. **Heby, O. and Janne, J.,** Polyamine antimetabolites: biochemistry, specificity, and biological effects of inhibitors of polyamine synthesis, in *Polyamines in Biology and Medicine,* 8th ed., Morris, D. R. and Marton, L. J., Eds., Marcel Dekker, New York, 1979, 243.
10. **Kontula, K. K., Torkkeli, T. K., Bardin, C. W., and Janne, O. A.,** Androgen induction of ornithine decarboxylase mRNA in mouse kidney as studied by complementary DNA, *Proc. Natl. Acad. Sci. U.S.A.,* 81, 731, 1984.

11. **Janne, O. A., Kontula, K. K., Isomaa, V. V., and Bardin, C. W.,** Ornithine decarboxylase mRNA in mouse kidney: a low abundancy gene product regulated by androgens with rapid kinetics. *Ann. N.Y. Acad. Sci.,* 438, 72, 1984.
12. **Heller, J. S., Chen, K. Y., Kyriakidis, D. A., Fong, W. F., and Canellakis, E. S.,** The modulation of the induction of ornithine decarboxylase by spermine, spermidine and diamines, *J. Cell. Physiol.,* 96, 225, 1978.
13. **McCann, P. P., Tardif, C., Hornsberger, J. M., and Bohlen, P.,** Two distinct mechanisms for ODC regulation in rat hepatoma cells, *J. Cell. Physiol.,* 99, 183, 1979.
14. **Kahana, C. and Nathans, D.,** Translational regulation of mammalian ornithine decarboxylase by polyamines, *J. Biol. Chem.,* 260, 15390, 1985a.
15. **Dircks, L., Grens, A., Slezynger, T., and Scheffler, I. E.,** Posttranscriptional control of ornithine decarboxylase activity, *J. Cell. Physiol.,* 126, 371, 1986.
16. **Holtta, E. and Pohjanpelto, P.,** Control of ornithine decarboxylase in Chinese hamster ovary cells by polyamines. Translational inhibition of synthesis and acceleration of degradation of the enzyme by putrescine, spermidine, and spermine, *J. Biol. Chem.,* in press, 1986.
17. **Russell, D. H. and Snyder, S. H.,** Amine synthesis in regenerating rat liver: extremely rapid turnover of ornithine decarboxylase, *Mol. Pharmacol.,* 5, 253, 1969.
18. **Heller, J. S. and Canellakis, E. S.,** Cellular control of ornithine decarboxylase by its antizyme, *J. Cell. Physiol.,* 107, 20, 1981.
19. **Murakami, Y. and Hayashi, S.,** Role of antizyme in degradation of ornithine dcarboxylase in HTC cells. *Biochem. J.,* 226, 893, 1985.
20. **Pritchard, M. L., Seely, J. E., Poso, H., Jefferson, L. S., and Pegg, A. E.,** Binding of radioactive a-difluoromethyl ornithine to rat liver ornithine decarboxylase, *Biochem. Biophys. Res. Commun.,* 100, 1597, 1981.
21. **Gupta, M. and Coffino, P.,** Mouse ornithine decarboxylase. Complete amino acid sequence deduced from cDNA. *J. Biol. Chem.,* 260, 2941, 1985.
22. **Bey, P., Danzin, C., Van Dorsselaer, V., Mamont, P., Jung, M., and Tardif, C.,** Analogues of ornithine as inhibitors of ornithine decarboxylase. New deductions concerning the topography of the enzyme's active site, *J. Med. Chem.,* 21, 50, 1978.
23. **Gilad, G. M. and Gilad, V. H.,** Visualization of rhodamin-labeled a-difluoromethylornithine in viable neuroblasts: towards in vivo localization of ornithine decarboxylase, in *Advances in Polyamine Research,* 4th ed., Bachrach, U, Kaye, A., and Chayen, R., Eds., Raven Press, New York, 1983, 585
24. **Danzin, C., Casara, P., Claverie, N., Metcalf, B. W., and Jung, M. J.,** (2R,5R)-6-heptyne-2,5-diamine, an extremely potent inhibitor of mammalian ornithine decarboxylase, *Biochem. Biophys. Res. Commun.,* 116, 237, 1983.
25. **Abdel-Monem, M. M., Newton, N. E., and Weeks, C. E.,** Inhibitors of polyamine biosyntheses. I.α-Methyl-( + /-)-ornithine, and inhibitor of ornithine decarboxylase, *J. Med. Chem.,* 17, 447, 1974.
26. **Abdel-Monem, M. M., Newton, N. E., Ho, B. C., and Weeks, C. E.,** Potential inhibitors of polyamine biosynthesis. II. α-Alkyl and benzyl-( + /-)-ornithine, *J. Med. Chem.,* 18, 600, 1975.
27. **O'Leary, R. M. and Herreid, R. M.,** Mechanism of inactivation of ornithine decarboxylase by alpha-methylornithine, *Biochemistry,* 17, 1010, 1978.
28. **Metcalf, B. W., Bey, P., Danzin, C., Jung, M. J., Casara, P., and Vevert, J. P.,** Catalytic irreversible inhibition of mammalian ornithine decarboxylase by substrate and product analogues, *J. Am. Chem. Soc.,* 100, 2551, 1978.
29. **Choi, J. and Scheffler, I. E.,** Chinese hamster ovary cells resistant to alpha-methylornithine are over-producers of ornithine decarboxylase, *J. Biol. Chem.,* 258, 12601, 1983.
30. **Choi, J. and Scheffler, I. E.,** A mutant of Chinese hamster ovary cells resistant to alpha-methyl-and alpha-difluoromethylornithine, *Somat. Cell Genet.,* 7, 219, 1981.
31. **Gerner, E. W. and Mamont, P. S.,** Restoration of the polyamine contents in rat hepatoma tissue-culture cells after inhibition of polyamine synthesis, *Eur. J. Biochem.,* 156, 31, 1986.
32. **Harada, J. J. and Morris, D. R.,** Cell cycle parameters of Chinese hamster ovary cells during exponential, polyamine-limited growth, *Mol. Cell. Biol.,* 1, 594, 1981.
33. **Mamont, P. S., Duchesne, M.-C., Grove, J., and Tardif, C.,** Initial characterization of a HTC cell variant partially resistant to the anti-proliferative effect of ornithine decarboxylase inhibitors, *Exp. Cell Res.,* 115, 387, 1978.
34. **Pritchard, M. L., Pegg, A. E., and Jefferson, L. S.,** Ornithine decarboxylase from hepatoma cells and a variant cell line in which the enzyme is more stable, *J. Biol. Chem.,* 257, 5892, 1982.
35. **Murakami, Y., Fujita, K., Kameji, T., and Hayashi, S.,** Accumulation of ornithine decarboxylase-antizyme complex in HMO-A cells, *Biochem. J.,* 225, 689, 1985.
36. **McConlogue, L. and Coffino, P.,** Ornithine decarboxylase in difluoromethyl ornithine resistant mouse lymphoma cells, *J. Biol. Chem.,* 258, 8384, 1983.

37. **McConlogue, L. and Coffino, P.,** A mouse lymphoma cell mutant whose major protein product is ornithine decarboxylase, *J. Biol. Chem.,* 258, 12083, 1983.
38. **Persson, L.,** Antibodies to ornithine decarboxylase. Immunological crossreactivity, *Acta Chem. Scand.,* 36, 685, 1982.
39. **McConlogue, L., Gupta, M., Wu, L., and Coffino, P.,** Molecular cloning and expression of the mouse ornithine decarboxylase gene, *Proc. Natl. Acad. Sci. U.S.A.,* 81, 540, 1984.
40. **Kahana, C. and Nathans, D.,** Isolation of cloned cDNA encoding mammalian ornithine decarboxylase, *Proc. Natl. Acad. Sci. U.S.A.,* 81, 3645, 1984.
41. **Kahana, C. and Nathans, D.,** Nucleotide sequence of murine ornithine decarboxylase mRNA, *Proc. Natl. Acad. Sci. U.S.A.,* 82, 1673, 1985.
42. **Steglich, C. and Scheffler, I. E.,** An ornithine decarboxylase-deficient mutant of Chinese hamster ovary cells, *J. Biol. Chem.,* 257, 4603, 1982.
43. **Steglich, C., Grens, A., and Scheffler, I. E.,** Chinese hamster cells deficient in ornithine decarboxylase activity: reversion by gene amplification and by azacytidine treatment, *Somat. Cell Mol. Genet.,* 11, 11, 1985.
44. **Pohjanpelto, P., Holtta, E., Janne, O. A., Knuutila, S., and Alitalo, K.,** Amplification of ornithine decarboxylase gene in response to polyamine deprivation in Chinese hamster ovary cells, *J. Biol. Chem.,* 260, 8532, 1985.
45. **McConlogue, L., Dana, S. L., and Coffino, P.,** Multiple mechanisms are responsible for altered expression of ornithine decarboxylase in overproducing variant cells, *Mol. Cell. Biol.,* 6, 2865, 1986.
46. **Alhonen-Hongisto, L., Deen, D. F., and Marton, L. J.,** Time dependence of the potentiation of 1,3-bis(2-chloroethyl)-1-nitrosourea cytotoxicity caused by alpha-difluoromethylornithine-induced polyamine depletion in 9L rat brain tumor cells, *Cancer Res.,* 44, 1819, 1984.
47. **Medrano, E. E., Goldenberg, S. H., and Algranati, I. D.,** Differential effect of alpha-difluoromethylornithine on the proliferation of Balb 3T3 and chemically transformed 3T3 cells, *J. Cell. Physiol.,* 117, 141, 1983.
48. **Mamont, P. S., Danzin, C., Wagner, J., Siat, M., Joder-Ohlenbusch, A.-M., and Claverie, N.,** Accumulation of decarboxylated S-adenosyl-L-methionine in mammalian cells as a consequence of the inhibition of putrescine biosynthesis, *Eur. J. Biochem.,* 123, 499, 1982.
49. **Sunkara, P. S., Prakash, N. J., Mayer, G. D., and Sjoerdsma, A.,** Tumor suppression with a combination of a-difluoromethylornithine and interferon, *Science,* 219, 851, 1983.
50. **Talpaz, M., Plager, C., Quesada, J., Benjamin, R., Kantarijan, H., and Gutterman, J.,** Difluoromethylornithine and leukocyte interferon: a phase I study in cancer patients, *Eur. J. Cancer Clin. Oncol.,* 22, 685, 1986.
51. **Schechter, P. J. and Sjoerdsma, A.,** Difluoromethylornithine in the treatment of African trypanosomiasis, *Parasitol. Today,* 2, 223, 1986.
52. **Giffin, B. F., McCann, P. P., Bitonti, A. J., and Bacchi, C. J.,** Polyamine depletion following exposure to DL-a-difluoromethylornithine both in vivo and in vitro initiates morphologcal alterations and mitochondrial activation in a monomorphic strain of Trypanosoma brucei brucei, *J. Protozool.,* 33, 238, 1986.
53. **Bitonti, A. J., McCann, P. P., and Sjoerdsma, A.,** Necessity of antibody response in the treatment of African trypanosomiasis with difluoromethylornithine, *Biochem. Pharmacol.,* 35, 331, 1986.
54. **McCann, P. P., Clarkson, A. B. Jr., Bey, P., Bacchi, C. J., Sjoerdsma, A., Schechter, P. J., Walzer, P. D., and Barlow, J. L. R.,** Inhibition of polyamine biosynthesis by difluoromethylornithine in African trypanosomes and Pneumocystis carinii as a basis of chemotherapy: biochemical and clinical aspects, *Am. Trop. Med. Hyg.,* in press, 1986.

Chapter 5

# MYCOPHENOLIC ACID

**Buddy Ullman**

## TABLE OF CONTENTS

I.      Introduction .................................................................. 60

II.     Cellular Effects of Mycophenolic Acid ....................................... 60
        A.      Historical Perspective ......................................... 60
        B.      Reversal of Mycophenolic Acid Toxicity by Purines ..................... 61
        C.      Effects of Mycophenolic Acid on Nucleic Acid Synthesis ............... 62
        D.      Effects of Mycophenolic Acid on Purine Nucleotide Synthesis ........... 62
        E.      Effects of Mycophenolic Acid on Nucleotide Pools ..................... 62
        F.      IMP Dehydrogenase ....................................... 63

III.    Mycophenolic Acid-Resistant Mutant Cell Lines .............................. 63
        A.      Chinese Hamster V79 Cells ............................... 64
        B.      Mouse S49 Cells ......................................... 64
        C.      Mouse Neuroblastoma Cells .................................. 65

IV.     Selection for the Bacterial *Ecogpt* Gene Encoding Xanthine-Guanine
        Phosphoribosyltransferase Activity .............................. 65

V.      Conclusions ............................................................... 66

Acknowledgments ................................................................... 67

References ........................................................................ 67

# I. INTRODUCTION

Mammalian cells possess two avenues for the synthesis of purine nucleotides; a *de novo* biosynthetic pathway, which synthesizes purine nucleotides from amino acids and one carbon containing compounds, and a salvage pathway which generates nucleotides from preformed purine nucleosides and nucleobases. The biosynthetic pathway consists of a linear sequence of 11 enzymes which convert ribose-5-phosphate and ATP to inosine 5'-monophosphate (IMP), the first nucleotide synthesized, and four branchpoint enzymes, which convert IMP to adenylate (AMP) and guanylate (GMP). The biosynthetic pathway is diagrammed in Figure 1. The *de novo* pathway is highly regulated. The first two enzymes of purine bio-synthesis, phosphoribosylpyrophosphate (PRPP) synthetase, and PRPP amidotransferase, are subject to feedback inhibition by a variety of nucleotide effectors. The branchpoint enzymes are also highly regulated. GMP and AMP inhibit their own synthesis, and GTP is required for the conversion of IMP to adenylosuccinate (AMPS) and ATP is necessary for xanthosine 5'-monophosphate (XMP) amination to GMP (Figure 1). This reciprocal regulation ensures a balanced supply of purine nucleotides for the cell.

By virtue of the fact that animal cells possess two routes for purine synthesis, the purine pathway in cells in culture is uniquely amenable to both pharmacologic and genetic manipulation. For instance, one can pharmacologically block *de novo* purine synthesis with inhibitors such as methotrexate and amethopterin, and still allow for cell survival and growth by the provision of purines to the culture medium. This is the basis for the widely exploited hypoxanthine-amethopterin-thymidine (HAT) medium initially developed by Littlefield.[1] Moreover, mutant cells can be generated which are genetically deficient in one or more purine salvage enzymes, and the genetically altered cell can still meet its purine requirements via the biosynthetic pathway.

The *de novo* purine nucleotide pathway has proven far less tractable to somatic cell genetic manipulation. Genetic deficiencies in any of the *de novo* enzymes creates an auxotrophy for purines. Nevertheless, Patterson and coworkers have successfully isolated and characterized a series of purine auxotrophs in Chinese hamster ovary (CHO) cells.[2-4] As elegant as Patterson's selections and investigations have proven, however, the auxotrophic hamster cells are not suitable for studies on regulation, since they are dependent on exogenous purines for growth, and their multiple phenotypes and complex selection systems preclude their usefulness as a marker in mutation rate studies.

The isolation of mammalian cells with genetic alterations in purine biosynthetic enzymes which do not convey auxotrophy requires the existence of potent inhibitors which do not bind to catalytic sites. Kaufman has derived a 6-diazo-5-oxo-L-norleucine resistant Chinese hamster V79 cell line which expresses a GMP synthetase activity that is resistant to the selective agent.[5]

Mycophenolic acid (6-[4-hydroxy-6-methoxy-7-methyl-3-oxo-5-phthalanyl]-4-methyl-4-hexenoic acid), an inhibitor of IMP conversion to GMP, offers an approach to the isolation of mutants with genetic alterations in the purine biosynthetic pathway. The structure of mycophenolic acid is depicted in Figure 2. The isolation and characterization of three mycophenolic acid-resistant mammalian cell lines with their unique and interesting phenotypes is the subject of this review.

# II. CELLULAR EFFECTS OF MYCOPHENOLIC ACID

## A. Historical Perspective

Mycophenolic acid was initially isolated from the culture broth of a corn mold, *Penicillium stoloniferum*, by Gozio in 1896.[6] Seventeen years later, Alsberg and Black conferred the name mycophenolic acid to the compound.[7] The structure of mycophenolic acid was pub-

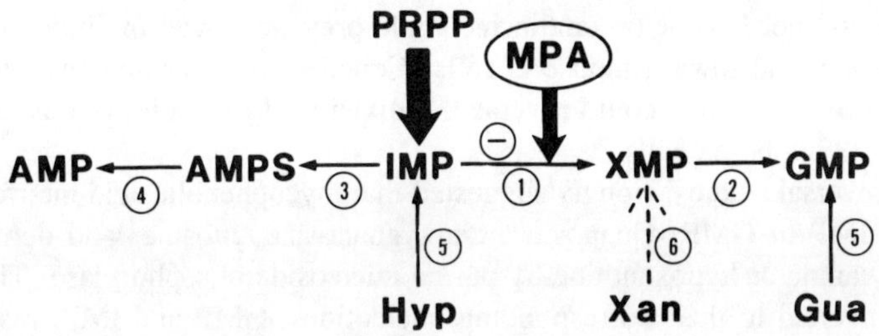

FIGURE 1. Schema of purine nucleotide synthesis and salvage and site of action of mycophenolic acid. The purine biosynthetic pathway is outlined diagramatically and labeled as follows: (1) IMP dehydrogenase, (2) GMP synthetase, (3) adenylosuccinate synthetase, (4) adenylosuccinate lyase, (5) hypoxanthine-guanine phosphoribosyltransferase, (6) xanthine-guanine phosphoribosyl-transferase. PRPP is phosphoribosylpyrophosphate and MPA is mycophenolic acid. The solid lines represent enzyme activities in mammalian cells, whereas the dashed line refers to an enzyme present only in bacteria.

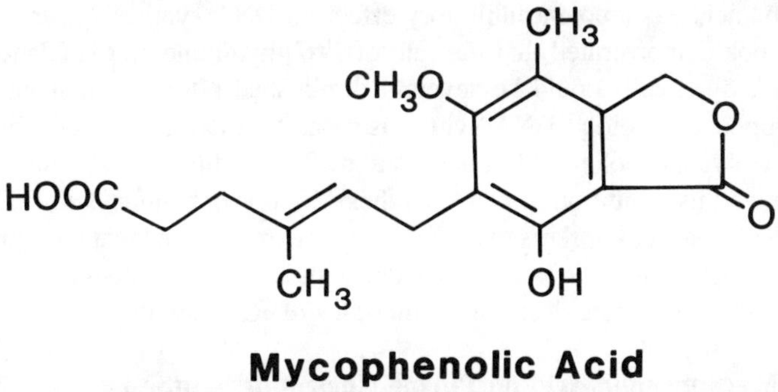

## Mycophenolic Acid

FIGURE 2. Structure of mycophenolic acid.

lished by Birkinshaw et al. in the early 1950s,[8] and Birch and Wright synthesized the compound in 1969.[9] Mycophenolic acid has limited antibacterial and antifungal properties[10,11] but is an effective antiviral agent.[12,13] It is also active against a variety of experimental solid rat and mouse tumors but apparently inactive toward murine leukemias.[12-14] When incubated with cultured mammalian cells, mycophenolic acid is a potent toxin.[15-20] Cohen et al. demonstrated that this toxicity is specific for cells in the S-phase of the cell cycle.[18]

Using [$^{14}$C] mycophenolic acid, Sweeney et al.[15] showed that mycophenolic acid is not incorporated into nucleic acids. The only metabolite of [$^{14}$C]mycophenolic acid detected in humans or animals was mycophenolic acid glucuronide. These workers suggested that the sensitivity of tumors to mycophenolic acid was inversely proportional to their β-glucuronidase activity, since only mycophenolic acid and not mycophenolic acid glucuronide permeated plasma membranes of cells.[15]

## B. Reversal of Mycophenolic Acid Toxicity by Purines

Cline et al. were the first to report that the mycophenolic acid-induced inhibition of viral growth could be reversed by the addition of guanine, guanosine, and GMP to the cell cultures, whereas hypoxanthine, xanthine, and their derivatives had no effect.[21] Franklin and Cook subsequently showed that the mycophenolic acid-induced inhibition of DNA synthesis in mouse L cells could be circumvented by the addition of guanine, but not hypoxanthine, xanthine, or adenine, to the culture medium.[22] Sweeney et al. demonstrated that guanosine, but not inosine or xanthosine could prevent growth inhibition caused by 4.4 μ*M* mycophenolic acid toward mouse L cells. Cohen et al. later demonstrated that either guanosine or deoxyguanosine could reverse the toxicity of mycophenolic acid toward wild type mouse S49 lymphoma cells.[18]

The purine reversal studies strongly suggested that mycophenolic acid interferred with the conversion of IMP to GMP. Guanosine, deoxyguanosine, inosine, and deoxyinosine are converted to guanine or hypoxanthine by purine nucleoside phosphorylase. The two purine bases are reconverted to their corresponding nucleotides, GMP and IMP, respectively, by the enzyme hypoxanthine-guanine phosphoribosyltransferase (Figure 1). Mammalian cells possess a biochemically distinct adenine phosphoribosyltransferase activity, which converts adenine to AMP. Neither xanthine nor xanthosine are metabolized by mammalian cells or tissues, since the purine base is a poor substrate for the mammalian enzyme.[23] *Escherichia coli*, however, possess a phosphoribosylating activity active toward xanthine,[24] xanthine-guanine phosphoribosyltransferase activity (Figure 1). The phosphoribosyltransferases are also depicted in Figure 1.

## C. Effects of Mycophenolic Acid on Nucleic Acid Synthesis

Mycophenolic acid has a potent inhibitory effect on DNA synthesis in mammalian cells. Franklin and Cook demonstrated that the rate of [[14]C]thymidine and [[14]C]adenine incorporation into DNA by L cells could be severely diminished after a 1 hr incubation with 10 μg/mℓ of mycophenolic acid.[22] DNA synthesis came to a halt after a 2-hr incubation with a tenfold lower mycophenolic acid concentration. The addition of guanine to the culture medium prevented this inhibition of DNA synthesis by mycophenolic acid.[22] Careful studies carried out by Sadee and co-workers in the S49 cell system revealed that the growth inhibition produced by mycophenolic acid was associated with a drastic reduction in DNA synthetic capability but only a moderate decrease in the rates of RNA synthesis.[18]

## D. Effects of Mycophenolic Acid on Purine Nucleotide Synthesis

Incubation of Yoshida ascites cells, Landschutz ascites cells, and L cells with mycophenolic acid causes an abrupt disruption of the cellular purine biosynthetic capabilities.[22] Analysis of the acid-soluble and acid-insoluble cell fractions indicated that mycophenolic acid diminished the incorporation of radiolabeled [[14]C]hypoxanthine into guanine residues by 80 to 95% in all cases. The uptake of [[14]C]hypoxanthine into soluble adenylate nucleotides was increased, while that into adenine residues in nucleic acids was either unaffected or slightly diminished.[22] Similar results with wild type and mutant WI-L2 human B lymphoblasts were obtained by Snyder et al. using [[14]C]formate as a precursor.[25] Moreover, these workers demonstrated that mycophenolic acid increased the rate of [[14]C]formate incorporation into hypoxanthine and inosine, 25- and 10-fold, respectively. This suggested that the majority of IMP being produced *de novo* in the presence of mycophenolic acid was dephosphorylated to inosine by intracellular nucleotidases. Under more careful extraction conditions, Ullman later demonstrated that mycophenolic acid caused S49 cells to excrete massive amounts of inosine into the culture medium.[19] Mycophenolic acid elicited a 20 to 30% augmentation in overall rates of purine biosynthesis in the human lymphoblasts[25] and almost a 2-fold increase in the murine cells.[19]

## E. Effects of Mycophenolic Acid on Nucleotide Pools

The reversal of the antiviral and antiproliferative effects of mycophenolic acid by guanine-containing compounds suggested that mycophenolic acid might precipitate a depletion of endogenous guanylate nucleotide pools. In vivo studies by Smith and Henderson with Ehrlich ascites cells[26] and by Nelson et al.[27] with L1210 cells, and in vitro studies by Lowe et al.[16] with the murine L5178Y lymphoma and by Cohen et al.[18] and Ullman[19] with S49 cells, all conclusively demonstrated that mycophenolic acid reduced cellular GTP levels to less than 20% of control levels. GDP and GMP pools were reduced equivalently or to a greater extent when measured.[19,27,28] The excellent correlation between the depletion of the small GMP pool and the inhibition of DNA synthesis in the S49 cell system supports the hypothesis that the limited GMP pool may serve the crucial role in limiting the availability of precursors for DNA synthesis.[28] Consistent with the diminution of guanylate nucleotides, IMP levels were markedly augmented by mycophenolic acid in the L1210 cells in vivo[27] and in the S49 cells in vitro.[19] In all studies, ATP pools were relatively unaffected, while pyrimidine ribonucleoside triphosphate levels were consistently augmented by 80%.[12,16,18,27] The elevation in UTP and CTP pools observed after mycophenolic acid incubation is consistent with a decrease in the inhibition of PRPP synthetase activity as a result of the release from feedback inhibition by guanylate nucleotides. dGTP pools were also diminished considerably, as expected, while TTP concentrations augmented several fold.[16,18] Somewhat surprisingly, Lowe et al. reported a mycophenolic acid-mediated diminution of dCTP in the L5178Y cells,[16] while Cohen et al. reported the opposite effect in S49 cells.[18] The effects on deoxyribonucleoside triphosphate pools are by and large consistent with the known regulatory mechanisms of ribonucleotide reductase, the enzyme that governs deoxyribonucleotide levels in mammalian cells.[29]

### F. IMP Dehydrogenase

The consequences of mycophenolic acid on nucleotide pools, nucleic acid synthesis, and purine synthesis, coupled with the ability of guanine, guanosine, and/or guanylate, but not other purines, to reverse these effects strongly suggested that mycophenolic acid prevented cells from converting IMP to GMP. In numerous in vitro studies on partially purified enzyme preparations, mycophenolic acid was shown to be a potent inhibitor of IMP dehydrogenase (IMP-NAD oxidoreductase, EC 1.2.1.14) activity, the penultimate enzyme in guanylate nucleotide synthesis (Figure 1) The apparent $K_i$ values of mycophenolic acid for the IMP dehydrogenases from Landschutz ascites cells[22] and from Chinese hamster V79 cells[17] were 30-45 n$M$ and 16 n$M$, respectively. The type of inhibition appears to be mixed for the liquid tumor[22] and uncompetitive for the hamster fibroblasts.[17]

IMP dehydrogenase catalyzes the conversion of IMP and $NAD^+$ to XMP and NADH and is the rate limiting step in the conversion of IMP to GMP. The enzyme requires a monovalent cation for maximal activity. Kinetic analyses of the partially purified enzyme from murine Sarcoma 180 cells[30] and human placenta[3] are consistent with an ordered sequential reaction mechanism in which IMP binds prior to NAD, while NADH is the first product released followed by XMP. The apparent $K_m$ values of the murine[30] and human[31] IMP dehydrogenases for IMP were 14 $\mu M$ and 16 $\mu M$, respectively, and 46 $\mu M$ for $NAD^+$. Both end products are inhibitors of the enzyme.

Mycophenolic acid is also a powerful inhibitor of GMP synthetase, the enzyme that converts XMP, the product of the IMP dehydrogenase reaction, to GMP.[15] Mycophenolic acid is a competitive inhibitor of the GMP synthetase enzyme from Landschutz ascites cells with a $K_i$ value of 80 n$M$.[15]

## III. MYCOPHENOLIC ACID-RESISTANT MUTANT CELL LINES

Somatic cell genetic approaches have been exploited to generate a variety of unique mammalian mutants that are resistant to mycophenolic acid. Mycophenolic acid-resistant cells have been isolated from Chinese hamster V79 cells,[17] mouse S49 lymphoma cells,[19] and from mouse neuroblastoma cells.[20] Each of the different classes of mycophenolic acid-resistant cells has a unique phenotype. The derivation and characterization of these mutant cells has made invaluable contributions to understanding the mechanism of action of the drug, the role of IMP dehydrogenase in the regulation of purine synthesis and excretion, and the value of mycophenolic acid resistance as a selective marker. They also constitute the first mutant mammalian cell lines with this type of lesion in an important regulatory nucleic acid biosynthetic enzyme.

## A. Chinese Hamster V79 Cells

Huberman et al. isolated mycophenolic-acid resistant cells from a mutagenized wild type Chinese hamster V79 population in a single step by virtue by their resistance to growth inhibition by 1.0 μg/mℓ drug.[17] The frequency of appearance of these mutants increased with the concentration of the mutagen and with the length of expression time. Six mycophenolic acid-resistant clones were found to be one to two orders of magnitude less sensitive to drug toxicity by clonogenic assays. The resistance to mycophenolic acid was stable in the three cell lines examined 4 weeks later. The degree of resistance correlated with a comparable increment in the specific activity of IMP dehydrogenase activity, which in mutant cells was three- to sixfold higher than the enzyme activity in parental cells. In those cell lines tested, the apparent $K_m$ values for IMP (13 to 22 μM) and NAD$^+$ (29 μM) and the apparent $K_i$ values for mycophenolic acid (12 to 20 nM) were equivalent to the parameters obtained for the wild type IMP dehydrogenase activity. These small increases in IMP dehydrogenase activity without an alteration in kinetic parameters suggested, but did not prove, that IMP dehydrogenase is the target of mycophenolic acid in these cells. Whether a 3- to 6-fold increase in total enzyme activity can explain a 10- to 100-fold increase in cellular growth resistance to mycophenolic acid remains problematic.

The kinetic data indicated that the mutant cells did not possess a structural gene alteration. The phenotypes of the mycophenolic acid-resistant V79 cells are consistent with either an alteration in a regulatory gene function or with a gene amplification event, although the latter is less likely due to phenotypic stability and method of selection. The concept of a mutation in a regulatory gene controlling IMP dehydrogenase levels is intriguing in light of Weber's observations that IMP dehydrogenase activity is enhanced in malignant cells and correlates with cellular growth rate.[32]

## B. Mouse S49 Cells

In order to elucidate the regulatory role of purine biosynthetic enzymes on governing the rate of purine biosynthesis, two phenotypically distinct mutant cell lines with altered IMP dehydrogenase activity were isolated from mutagenized cultures of S49 cells.[19] The first clone, MYCO-1A, was isolated by virtue of its resistance to 1 μM mycophenolic acid. MYCO-1A cells were remutagenized, and a secondary clone MYCO-1A-20 was reselected in 20 μM drug. In comparative growth rate experiments, the MYCO-1A and MYCO-1A-20 cells were 3- and 50-fold less sensitive respectively, to mycophenolic acid toxicity than parental wild-type cells. Interestingly, the MYCO-1A cells, which demonstrated intermediate sensitivity to mycophenolic acid, were much more resistant than either parental or MYCO-1A-20 cells to the toxicity of ribavarin (1-β-D-ribofuranosyl-1,2,3-triazole-3-carboximide or virazole), another known inhibitor of IMP dehydrogenase.[33]

Assays of IMP dehydrogenase activity in cell extracts indicated that the enzyme from both sequentially selected mutant cell lines possessed a $V_{max}$ 10- to 15-fold greater than the wild type enzyme. The apparent $K_m$ values for the two substrates were also altered for the extracted mutant enzymes. $K_m$ values for IMP were 30, 300 to 400, and 300 to 400 μM, for the wild type, MYCO-1A, and MYCO-1A-20 enzyme preparations, respectively. Similarly, apparent $K_m$ values for NAD$^+$ were 45, 12, and 50 μM, respectively, for the enzymes extracted from the wild type, MYCO-1A, and MYCO-1A-20 cells. The mutant enzymes were also much less sensitive to inhibition by mycophenolic acid, although $K_i$ values were not determined. Thus, the phenotypes of the mutant cells constituted genetic proof that the site of mycophenolic acid action, at least in these mouse S49 cells, was IMP dehydrogenase. Moreover, the enzyme, as the intracellular target of ribavarin, was strongly implicated.

Measurements of ribonucleotide levels indicated that the mycophenolic acid-resistant clones possessed slightly elevated levels of both GTP and GMP. Incubation of wild-type cells with 1 $\mu M$ mycophenolic acid caused a depletion of intracellular guanylate nucleotide pools, an increase in the concentration of IMP, an increase in the overall rate of *de novo* purine synthesis by twofold, and a massive excretion of inosine into the culture medium. Similar effects were found for MYCO-1A cells incubated with 5 $\mu M$, but not 1 $\mu M$, mycophenolic acid. However, neither purine overproduction nor nucleotide pool perturbations were observed for MYCO-1A-20 cells incubated with 25 $\mu M$ mycophenolic acid.

These mutations behaved, as expected, in a dominant fashion in intra-species cell-cell hybridization experiments. Tetraploid fusion products between wild type and mutant S49 cells retained their mycophenolic acid-resistant phenotype. The altered kinetic parameters determined for the mutant enzymes implied that the mutants were altered in a structural gene encoding the IMP dehydrogenase activity. These results with mutant mammalian cells genetically altered in IMP dehydrogenase activity provided a powerful genetic demonstration that the physiological consequences of mycophenolic acid on guanylate and other nucleotide pools and on purine synthesis and excretion could be attributed to the drug-mediated inhibition of IMP dehydrogenase activity, and not to effects on other purine biosynthetic enzymes, including GMP synthetase. Furthermore, that mycophenolic acid can induce a purine overproduction and overexcretion in wild type cells but not in mycophenolic acid-resistant mutants suggests that genetic lesions in an allele encoding the IMP dehydrogenase might contribute to the large population of individuals who manifest hyperuricemia and gout.

## C. Mouse Neuroblastoma Cells

In an attempt to generate an amplified phenotype, Hodges et al. have exposed mouse neuroblastoma cells to continuous selection in mycophenolic acid.[25] After 109 passages in growth medium containing progressively 10% incremental increases in mycophenolic acid concentration, the surviving cells were then plated in 200 $\mu M$ mycophenolic acid. Two clones, Myco-0.2A and Myco-0.2B, were shown to be over 5000-fold less sensitive to mycophenolic acid-mediated growth inhibition than parental cells. These cells contained tenfold greater levels of IMP dehydrogenase activity than parental neuroblasts. Similar to the mycophenolic acid-resistant S49 mutants, the apparent $K_m$ values of the enzyme from mutant cells for IMP were also elevated eight- to tenfold over that obtained for wild-type parental cells. However, the $K_i$ values for mycophenolic acid were 5 and 10 $\mu M$ for the IMP dehydrogenase activities from the Myco-0.2A and Myco-0.2B cell lines, respectively, a 1000- and 2000-fold increase over the $K_i$ value obtained for wild-type neuroblastoma cells (6 n$M$). Unlike the previously described hamster and mouse mycophenolic acid resistant-mutants, the specific activities of the IMP dehydrogenase enzymes of Myco-0.2A and Myco-0.2B cells grown 18 days in the absence of selective pressure diminished by 65 to 75%. This unstable phenotype is consistent with a gene amplification-like event. The method of continuous exposure to the drug probably allowed for the selection of mutant cells possessing multiple genetic alterations; one in a structural gene for IMP dehydrogenase conferring biochemical resistance to mycophenolic acid and one resulting in a gene/sequence amplification event. Either molecular event could have preceded the other.

## IV. SELECTION OF THE BACTERIAL *Ecogpt* GENE ENCODING XANTHINE-GUANINE PHOSPHORIBOSYLTRANSFERASE ACTIVITY

The understanding of the mechanism of action of mycophenolic acid has proven to be a considerable asset to modern molecular biology by permitting the selection of the bacterial

*Ecogpt* gene encoding xanthine-guanine phosphoribosyltransferase (XGPRTase) in recipient animal cells. Expression of the *Ecogpt* gene is a stable trait and a dominant-acting genetic marker. The dominance of the expression of *Ecogpt* obviates the requirement for the isolation of specific mutant cell lines, such as thymidine kinase deficiency, for the selection of exogenous DNA sequences. Recombinant DNAs containing *Ecogpt* as a selectable marker have proven extremely efficacious in the cotransformation of nonselectable genes into suitable recipient cells.

Mammalian hypoxanthine-guanine phosphoribosyltransferase (HGPRTase) can catalyze the phosphoribosylation of hypoxanthine and guanine, but not xanthine.[23] This can account for the failure of xanthine to reverse mycophenolic acid toxicity in mammalian cell systems. Mulligan and Berg exploited the toxicity of mycophenolic acid and the substrate specificities of the bacterial XGPRTase and the mammalian HGPRTase activities to develop a strategy for isolating plasmids or vectors encoding the bacterial *Ecogpt* gene.[34] Recipient cells expressing XGPRTase can be selected after transfection or infection with vector-*Ecogpt* DNAs using mycophenolic acid to block endogenous guanylate nucleotide production and exogenous xanthine as a source of XMP, thus circumventing the pharmacologic block. Expression of the XGPRTase activity can then serve as the purine salvage function of cells treated with mycophenolic acid/xanthine. Mammalian cells that fail to express XGPRTase will die under the selective conditions. The mycophenolic acid/xanthine selection is often carried out in the presence of adenine, amethopterin, and thymidine to regulate endogenous production of IMP. The overproduction of IMP *de novo* by mycophenolic acid is prevented by the amethopterin-induced blockade of the purine pathway. Amethopterin, an inhibitor of dihydrofolate reductase, depletes cells of their tetrahydrofolate pools necessary for purine biosynthesis.[35] Thymidine and adenine must be added in order to provide a source of thymidylate and adenylate nucleotides. Optimal concentrations of inhibitors for cytotoxicity, and of purines and pyrimidines for growth restoration, will vary among recipient cell lines.

This selection procedure for the bacterial XGPRTase is often incorrectly referred to as mycophenolic acid resistance. Clearly, cells surviving the mycophenolic acid/xanthine or mycophenolic acid/xanthine/adenine/amethopterin/thymidine selective pressure by virtue of their ability to express the XGPRTase activity are not mycophenolic acid resistant. However, the presence of mutant cells, which are truly mycophenolic acid resistant, should be evaluated in these plasmid transfection or viral infection experiments using *Ecogpt*, because transfection frequencies are $10^{-4}$ to $10^{-5}$, only somewhat higher than the frequency of appearance of a dominant mutation, such as true mycophenolic acid resistance, in many mammalian cells.

## V. CONCLUSIONS

Mutants resistant to mycophenolic acid have been invaluable in defining the mechanism of action of the drug. Three independent studies have demonstrated that the intracellular target of mycophenolic acid is the cellular IMP dehydrogenase, the penultimate enzyme in guanylate nucleotide synthesis. These mutants are the first isolated which express a mutation, other than a deficiency, in a purine biosynthetic enzyme. Characterization of these mutant cells has demonstrated that the effects of mycophenolic acid on nucleotide pools and DNA synthesis can be attributed to a specific effect on IMP dehydrogenase. These somatic cell genetic studies suggest that mycophenolic acid resistance might be a useful selective marker in studies of mutagenesis and carcinogenesis in mammalian cell systems. Furthermore, the genetic characterization of the purine overproduction induced by mycophenolic acid in the murine model suggests that genetic deficiencies in IMP dehydrogenase might contribute to the large population of individuals with overproduction hyperuricemia and gout. Finally, the development of defined selective strategies employing mycophenolic acid and the selectable bacterial *Ecogpt* gene have proven invaluable in selecting for DNA segments containing nonselectable markers in recipient mammalian cells. These foreign DNA fragments can be modified in vitro and reintroduced into appropriate cells by cotransfection with *Ecogpt* and selected exploiting the genetically and biochemically defined cellular toxicity of mycophenolic acid.

## ACKNOWLEDGMENTS

This manuscript was supported by funds provided by the National Institutes of Health grant No. DK38809. The author is a recipient of a Research Career Development Award from the National Institutes of Health.

## REFERENCES

1. **Littlefield, J. W.**, Selection of hybrids from matings of fibroblast *in vitro* and their presumed recombinants, *Science,* 145, 709, 1964.
2. **Patterson, D.**, Biochemical genetics of Chinese hamster cell mutants with deviant purine metabolism: biochemical analysis of eight mutants, *Somat. Cell Genet.,* 1, 91, 1975.
3. **Patterson, D.**, Biochemical genetics of Chinese hamster cell mutants with deviant purine metabolism. III. Isolation and characterization of a mutant unable to convert IMP to AMP, *Somat. Cell Genet.,* 2, 41, 1976.
4. **Patterson, D.**, Biochemical genetics of Chinese hamster cell mutants with deviant purine metabolism. IV. Isolation of a mutant which accumulates adenylosuccinic acid and succinylaminoimidazole carboxamide ribotide, *Somat. Cell Genet.,* 2, 189, 1976.
5. **Kaufman, E. R.**, Isolation and characterization of a mutant Chinese hamster cell line resistant to the glutamine analog 6-diazo-5-oxo-L-norleucine, *Somat. Cell Genet.,* 11, 1, 1985.
6. **Gosio, B.**, Richerche bacteriologiche e chimiche sulle alterazoni del mais. *Riv. Igiene Sanita Publica Ann.,* 7, 825, 1896.
7. **Alsberg, C. L. and Black, O. F.**, Contribution to the study of maize deterioration. *U.S. Department of Agriculture Bureau of Plant Industry,* Bulletin No. 270, 1913.
8. **Birkinshaw, J. H., Raistrick, H., and Ross, D. J.**, Studies in the biochemistry of microorganisms. The molecular constitution of mycophenolic acid, a metabolic product of *Penicillium brevicompactum dierckx.* III. Further observations on the structural formula for mycophenolic acid, *Biochem. J.,* 50, 630, 1952.
9. **Birch, A. J. and Wright, J. J.**, A total synthesis of mycophenolic acid, *Aust. J. Chem.,* 22, 2635, 1969.
10. **Florey, H. W., Gilliver, K., Jennings, M. A., and Sanders, A. G.**, Mycophenolic acid - an antibiotic from *Penicillium brevicompactum dierckx, Lancet,* 1, 46, 1946.
11. **Gilliver, K.**, The inhibitory action of antibiotics on plant pathogenic bacteria and fungi, *Ann. Bot.,* 10, 271, 1946.
12. **Williams, R. H., Boeck, L. D., Cline, J. C., DeLong, D. C., Gerzon, K., Gordee, R. S., Gorman, M., Holmes, R. E., Larsen, S. H., Lively, D. H., Matthews, T. R., Nelson, J. D., Poore, G. A., Stark, W. M., and Sweeney, M. J.**, Fermentation, isolation, and biological properties of mycophenolic acid, *Antimicrob. Agents Chemother.,* 229, 1968.
13. **Williams, R. H., Lively, D. H., DeLong, D. C., Cline, J. C., Sweeney, M. J., Poore, G. A., and Larsen, S. H.**, Mycophenolic acid: antiviral and antitumor properties, *J. Antibiot. Tokyo,* 21, 463, 1968.
14. **Sweeney, M. J., Gerzon, K., Harris, P. N., Holmes, R. E., Poore, G. A., and Williams, R. H.**, Experimental antitumor activity and preclinical toxicology of mycophenolic acid, *Cancer Res.,* 32, 1795, 1972.
15. **Sweeney, M. J., Hoffman, D. H., and Esterman, M. A.**, Metabolism and biochemistry of mycophenolic acid, *Cancer Res.,* 32, 1803, 1972.
16. **Lowe, J. K., Brox, L., and Henderson, J. F.**, Consequences of inhibition of guanine nucleotide synthesis by mycophenolic acid and virazole, *Cancer Res.,* 37, 736, 1977.
17. **Huberman, E., McKeown, C. K., and Friedman, J.**, Mutagen-induced resistance to mycophenolic acid in hamster cells can be associated with increased inosine 5'-phosphate dehydrogenase activity, *Proc. Natl. Acad. Sci. U.S.A.,* 78, 3151, 1981.
18. **Cohen, M. B., Maybaum, J., and Sadee, W.**, Guanine nucleotide depletion and toxicity in mouse T lymphoma (S-49) cells, *J. Biol. Chem.,* 256, 8713, 1981.
19. **Ullman, B.**, Characterization of mutant murine lymphoma cells with altered inosinate dehydrogenase activities, *J. Biol. Chem.,* 258, 523, 1983.

20. **Hodges, S. D., Fung, E., Lin, C. C., and Snyder, F. F.,** Increased inosinate dehydrogenase activity in mycophenolic acid resistant neuroblastoma cells, *Purine and Pyrimidine Metabolism in Man,* Vol. 5, Nyhan, W. L., Thompson, L. F., and Watts, R. W. E., Plenum Press, New York, 271.

21. **Cline, J. C., Nelson, J. D., Gerzon, K., Williams, R. H., and DeLong, D. C.,** *In vitro* antiviral activity of mycophenolic acid and its reversal by guanine-type compounds, *Appl. Microbiol.,* 18, 14, 1969.

22. **Franklin, T. J. and Cook, J. M.,** The inhibition of nucleic acid synthesis by mycophenolic acid, *Biochem. J.,* 113, 515, 1969.

23. **Krenitsky, T. A., Papaioannou, R., and Elion, G. B.,** Human hypoxanthine phosphoribosyltransferase. Purification, properties, and specificity, *J. Biol. Chem.,* 244, 1263, 1969.

24. **Miller, R. L., Ramsay, G. A., Krenitsky, T. A., Elion, G. B.,** Guanine phosphoribosyltransferase from *Escherichia coli,* specificity and properties, *Biochemistry,* 11, 4723, 1972.

25. **Snyder, F. F., Trafzer, R. J., Hershfield, M. S., and Seegmiller, J. E.,** Elucidation of aberrant purine metabolism. Application to hypoxanthine-guanine phosphoribosyltransferase- and adenosine kinase-deficient mutants, and IMP dehydrogenase- and adenosine deaminase-inhibited human lymphoblasts, *Biochim. Biophys. Acta,* 609, 492, 1980.

26. **Smith, C. M. and Henderson, J. M.,** Relative importance of alternative pathways of purine nucleotide biosynthesis in Ehrlich ascites tumor cells *in vivo, Can. J. Biochem.,* 54, 341, 1976.

27. **Nelson, J. A., Rose, L. M., and Bennett, L. L., Jr.,** Effects of 2-amino-1,3,4,-thiadiazole on ribonucleotide pools of leukemia L1210 cells, *Cancer Res.* 36, 1375, 1976.

28. **Nguyen, B. Y. and Sadee, W.,** Compartmentation of guanine nucleotide precursors for DNA synthesis, *Biochem. J.,* 234, 263, 1986.

29. **Thelander, L. and Recihard, P.,** Reduction of ribonucleotides, *Ann. Rev. Biochem.,* 48, 133, 1979.

30. **Anderson, J. H. and Sartorelli, A. C.,** Inosinic acid dehydrogenase of sarcoma 180 cells, *J. Biol. Chem.,* 243, 4762, 1968.

31. **Holmes, E. W., Pehlke, D. M., and Kelley, W. N.,** Human IMP dehydrogenase. Kinetics and regulatory properties, *Biochim. Biophys. Acta,* 364, 209, 1974.

32. **Weber, G.,** Biochemical commitment to replication in cancer cells, *Adv. Enzyme Regul.,* 18, 23, 1980.

33. **Streeter, D. G., Witkawski, J. T., Knare, G. P., Sidwell, R. W., Baver, R. J., Robins, R. K., and Simon, L. N.,** Mechanism of action of 1-beta-D-ribofuranosyl-1,2,4-triazole-3-carboxamide (virazole), a new broad-spectrum antiviral agent, *Proc. Natl. Acad. Sci. U.S.A.,* 70, 1174, 1973.

34. **Mulligan, R. C. and Berg, P.,** Selection for animal cells that express the *Escherichia coli* gene coding for xanthine-guanine phosphoribosyltransferase, *Proc. Natl. Acad. Sci. U.S.A.,* 78, 2072, 1981.

35. **Szybalska, E. H. and Szybalski, W.,** Genetics of human cell lines. IV. DNA-mediated heritable transformation of a biochemical trait, *Proc. Natl. Acad. Sci. U.S.A.,* 48, 2026, 1962.

Chapter 6

# ADENOSINE, DEOXYADENOSINE, AND DEOXYGUANOSINE

**Buddy Ullman**

## TABLE OF CONTENTS

I.      Introduction ................................................................. 70

II.     Inborn Errors of Purine Metabolism ......................................... 70

III.    Nucleoside Metabolism ...................................................... 72
        A.      Adenosine ......................................................... 72
        B.      Deoxyadenosine .................................................... 73
        C.      Deoxyguanosine .................................................... 73

IV.     Nucleoside Toxicity ........................................................ 74
        A.      Adenosine ......................................................... 74
        B.      Deoxyadenosine .................................................... 75
        C.      Deoxyguanosine .................................................... 75

V.      Nucleoside-Resistant Somatic Cell Mutants .................................. 76
        A.      Adenosine ......................................................... 76
                1.      Nucleoside Transport Deficiency ........................... 76
                2.      Adenosine Kinase Deficiency ............................... 78
                3.      Adenosine Deaminase Overproduction ........................ 78
                4.      Augmented Levels of S-Adenosylmethionine .................. 79
                5.      Adenosine Supersensitivity ................................ 79
        B.      Deoxyadenosine .................................................... 80
                1.      Nucleoside Transport Deficiency ........................... 80
                2.      Deoxyadenosine Phosphorylation Deficiency ................. 81
                3.      Cytoplasmic Nucleotidase Augmentation ..................... 82
                4.      Ribonucleotide Reductase Alterations ...................... 82
        C.      Deoxyguanosine Resistant .......................................... 83
                1.      Nucleoside Transport Deficiency ........................... 83
                2.      Deoxycytidine-Mutants Kinase Deficiency ................... 83
                3.      Purine Nucleoside Phosphorylase and Hypoxanthine-
                        guanine Phosphoribosyltransferase Deficiencies ............ 83
                4.      Ribonucleotide Reductase Alterations ...................... 84

VI.     Conclusions ................................................................ 84

Acknowledgments ................................................................... 85

References ........................................................................ 85

# I. INTRODUCTION

There are two avenues by which purine nucleotides are synthesized in mammalian cells and tissues. First, there exists a *de novo* biosynthetic pathway by which purine nucleotides are formed from amino acids and one carbon donors. This biosynthetic pathway begins with ribose 5-phosphate and requires a linear sequence of eleven enzymes to synthesize inosine 5'-monophosphate (IMP), the first purine nucleotide. The synthesis of a single IMP molecule *de novo* is an expensive process, entailing the hydrolysis of six high energy phosphate bonds. Adenylate and guanylate nucleotides are synthesized from IMP by separate routes, each consisting of two enzymes, and each requiring the cleavage of another high energy phosphate bond. Due to the consumption of high energy phosphate bonds, amino acids, and one carbon containing tetrahydrofolate compounds, the purine biosynthetic pathway is highly regulated. Phosphoribosylpyrophosphate (PRPP) synthetase and PRPP glutamine amidotransferase, the first two enzymes of the *de novo* pathway, are inhibited by many of the nucleotide end products of purine synthesis. Moreover, the branchpoint enzymes involved in the conversion of IMP to AMP and GMP are regulated in a fashion to ensure a balanced cellular supply of purine nucleotides. AMP and GMP each inhibit their own synthesis, while GTP is required for AMP synthesis and ATP is obligatory for IMP conversion to GMP. The second mechanism by which purine nucleotides are generated occurs via salvage enzymes in which nucleotides are synthesized from preformed purine nucleobases (bases) and nucleosides. This salvage process is much more energy efficient for the cell and serves to scavenge both dietary purines and dephosphorylated purines arising from the breakdown of nucleotides and nucleic acids that originate from cell lysis.

By virtue of the fact that there exist two pathways for producing purine nucleotides, the purine pathway is uniquely amenable in cells in culture to both pharmacologic and genetic manipulation. For instance, the biosynthetic pathway can be pharmacologically inhibited by a variety of drugs, such as amethopterin (methotrexate) or azaserine, yet cells can survive and proliferate if an exogenous source of purines, such as hypoxanthine, is provided in the culture medium. Conversely, mutants possessing non-lethal genetic deficiencies in one or more of the purine salvage enzymes can be isolated, since the cells can still meet their nucleotide requirements via *de novo* nucleotide synthesis.

The application of somatic cell genetic techniques has provided powerful new tools for analyzing the purine pathway in mammalian cells. No other metabolic pathway in somatic cells in continuous culture can be subjected to the array of genetic and pharmacologic manipulations as the purine pathway. Mutant mammalian cells have been generated and characterized that possess genetic alterations in nucleoside and nucleobase transport functions, in nucleobase phosphoribosyltransferases, in nucleoside kinases, and in other components of the purine salvage system. The isolation and characterization of mutant mammalian cells resistant to the cytotoxicity of three important naturally occurring nucleosides, adenosine, deoxyadenosine, and/or deoxyguanosine, is the subject of this review. The structures of these three nucleosides are shown in Figure 1.

# II. INBORN ERRORS OF PURINE METABOLISM

Adenosine, deoxyadenosine, and deoxyguanosine have been implicated in the cellular toxicities associated with specific inborn errors of metabolism in humans that cause immunological abnormalities, adenosine deaminase (ADA) and purine nucleoside phosphorylase (PNP) deficiencies.[1,2] A deficiency in either enzyme results in an ultimately fatal immune dysfunction. Each is an autosomal recessive disease. ADA catalyzes the effectively irreversible deamination of both adenosine and deoxyadenosine to inosine and deoxyinosine respectively. Children born with ADA deficiency have severe combined immunodeficiency

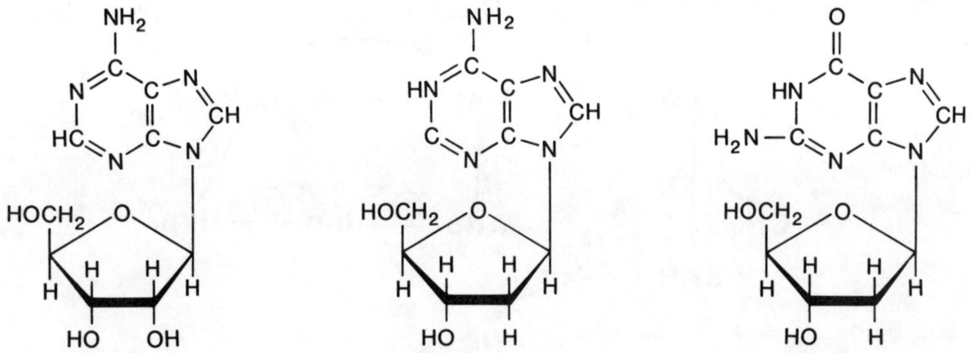

FIGURE 1.    Structures of adenosine, deoxyadenosine, and deoxyguanosine.

disease (SCID) in which both T and B cell number and function are impaired.[1] These children accumulate millimolar concentrations of deoxyATP in their erythrocytes, lymphocytes, and bone marrow cells, and excrete elevated amounts of deoxyadenosine in their urine.[3-6] Transfusions of normal erythrocytes[7] or the intramuscular injection of polyethylene glycol-treated calf intestinal adenosine deaminase[8] into ADA-deficient patients cause the deoxyATP levels to return to normal with a concomitant restoration of transient or partial immunocompetency. Moreover, patients with leukemia or lymphoma that have been treated with deoxycoformycin, a potent inhibitor of ADA activity, also accumulate deoxyATP in their cells and deoxyadenosine in their plasma and urine.[9,10] These data strongly implicate deoxyadenosine as the toxic substrate of ADA, which accumulates abnormally as deoxyATP as a consequence of a genetic or pharmacologic impairment of ADA activity.

A deficiency in PNP, an enzyme that serves as the metabolic sequel to ADA, causes a specific T cell impairment.[2] B cell number and function are normal or at least apparently normal in PNP deficiency. PNP catalyzes the reversible phosphorolysis of inosine, deoxyinosine, guanosine, and deoxyguanosine to the corresponding purine base and either ribose- or deoxyribose-1-phosphate. Children with PNP deficiency have elevated deoxyGTP concentrations in their erythrocytes.[11] Coupled with the observation that deoxyguanosine is the only PNP substrate that is cytotoxic at low concentrations to mouse T cell lymphoblasts genetically deficient in PNP,[12] these data strongly implicate deoxyguanosine as the lymphotoxic substrate of the enzyme, which is consequently converted to deoxyGTP in PNP deficiency.

The precise molecular bases for the selective lymphotoxicities observed in these two inborn errors of purine metabolism have not yet been defined. However, cells derived from the T limb of the immune system are the only nucleated cells capable of accumulating deoxyadenosine and deoxyguanosine intracellularly as the corresponding triphosphate in substantial quantities.[13,14] Moreover, immature thymocytes and T lymphoblasts are uniquely susceptible to deoxyribonucleoside toxicity, including killing by deoxyadenosine and deoxyguanosine.[13-16] It has been suggested that the selective ability of cells of thymic origin to accumulate deoxyribonucleotides is due to the comparatively high deoxyribonucleoside phosphorylating activites and low plasma membrane[18,19] and intracellular[20] deoxyribonucleotide dephosphorylating activities found in these cells. Whether these relatively small comparative differences in enzymatic activities can account for the enormous disparity between the ability of thymic cells and other cells (including B cells) to accumulate deoxyribonucleoside triphosphates remains questionable.

The contrast between B cell function in PNP deficiency and B cell dysfunction in ADA deficiency is even less well understood. Many hypotheses have been advocated. Among

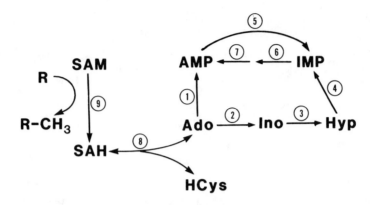

FIGURE 2. Metabolic pathways for adenosine. The pathways for adenosine metabolism are outlined as follows: (1) adenosine kinase; (2) adenosine deaminase; (3) purine nucleoside phosphorylase; (4) hypoxanthine-guanine phosphoribosyltransferase; (5) adenylate deaminase; (6) adenylosuccinate synthetase; (7) adenylosuccinate lyase; (8) S-adenosylhomocysteine hydrolase; and (9) SAM-dependent methylation reactions.

these is that adenosine and/or deoxyadenosine, the substrates of ADA, can interfere with the normal function of S-adenosylhomocysteine (SAH) hydrolase causing accumulation of SAH to levels that inhibit essential S-adenosylmethionine (SAM)-dependent transmethylation reactions in B cells.[21,22] Thus, adenosine, as well as deoxyadenosine might have some role in the B cell impairment in ADA-deficient severe combined immunodeficiency. There is also evidence that adenosine may augment intracellular levels of cyclic AMP,[23,24] a potent antiproliferative agent against certain classes of lymphocytes.[25] Other hypotheses for this functional discrepancy between the lympholytic effects of nucleosides in the two inborn errors of purine interconversion include: (1) sufficient B cell accumulation of deoxyadenosine as deoxyATP, but not of deoxyguanosine as deoxyGTP, to cause B cell death; (2) sensitivity of a T cell subset to deoxyadenosine, but not deoxyguanosine, required for B cell ontogeny or function; or (3) differential developmental sensitivities of T and B cell precursors to deoxyribonucleosides during ontogeny. Although the pathogenic mechanisms by which T and B cell function is obliterated in these inborn errors of purine salvage have not been completely elucidated, the diseases provide a viable clinical correlate to studies using adenosine, deoxyadenosine, and deoxyguanosine in cultured cells. Somatic cell genetics has offered a particularly powerful approach to developing cell culture models for elucidating the pathogenic mechanisms involved in these two inborn errors of purine metabolism.

## III. NUCLEOSIDE METABOLISM

### A. Adenosine

The pathways which convert adenosine to other metabolites are depicted in Figure 2. Adenosine is the preferred substrate for adenosine kinase, an enzyme which converts adenosine to AMP. AMP can subsequently be phosphorylated by adenylate kinase to ADP and then by substrate level or oxidative phosphorylation to the triphosphate level. Alternatively, AMP can also be deaminated by adenylate deaminase (AMP deaminase), an enzyme which plays an important role in balancing adenylate and guanylate nucleotide levels in the cell. Another route of adenosine metabolism is deamination to inosine, a reaction catalyzed by ADA. Inosine is subsequently cleaved to hypoxanthine by PNP and the base reconverted to the nucleotide level via hypoxanthine-guanine phosphoribosyltranferase (HGPRTase) or to uric acid in the liver by xanthine oxidase. Finally, adenosine can also condense with L-

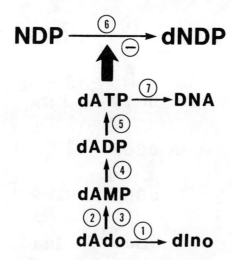

FIGURE 3.   Metabolic pathways for deoxyadenosine. The pathways for deoxyadenosine are depicted as follows: (1) adenosine deaminase; (2) adenosine kinase; (3) deoxycytidine kinase; (4) adenylate kinase; (5) nucleotide kinases; (6) ribonucleotide reductase; (7) DNA polymerase.

homocysteine to form SAH, a reaction catalyzed by SAH hydrolase. SAH is a product of the many essential SAM-dependent transmethylation reactions necessary for the maintenance of cellular homeostasis.

## B. Deoxyadenosine

The metabolic pathways for deoxyadenosine are summarized in Figure 3. Deoxyadenosine can either be phosphorylated directly to deoxyAMP or deaminated by ADA to form deoxyinosine. Two nucleoside kinase enzymes recognize deoxyadenosine as a substrate; adenosine kinase and deoxycytidine kinase. Deoxyadenosine, however, is not a preferred substrate for either kinase.[26] Thus, there is no single deoxyadenosine kinase enzyme, but rather two inefficient deoxyadenosine phosphorylating activities. The relative importance of the two enzymes in deoxyadenosine phosphorylation varies with cell type. In human cells of thymic origin deoxycytidine kinase appears to be the more important enzyme,[27,28] whereas in human B cells adenosine kinase plays a more important functional role in the phosphorylation of deoxyadenosine.[29] It has been hypothesized that the relative distribution and activity of adenosine kinase and deoxycytidine kinase in cells contributes to the lymphotoxicity observed in ADA-deficient immunodeficiency.[20] The base moiety of deoxyadenylates is not subject to further modification by cellular enzymes.

## C. Deoxyguanosine

Deoxyguanosine can be phosphorylated directly to deoxyGMP by deoxycytidine-deoxyguanosine kinase, for which the pyrimidine deoxyribonucleoside is the preferred substrate,[26] or phosphorylyzed to guanine by PNP (Figure 4). It has been proposed that the relatively high level of deoxyguanosine phosphorylating activity in T cells contributes to the T cell deficiency associated with the inherited absence of PNP.[16-18] DeoxyGMP can be converted to the triphosphate level by cellular nucleotide kinases, and deoxyGTP is subsequently incorporated into DNA. Deoxyguanylates are not subject to further modifications on their base moieties.

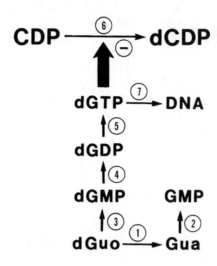

FIGURE 4. Deoxyguanosine metabolism. The routes of deoxyguanosine metabolism are shown as follows: (1) purine nucleoside phosphorylase; (2) hypoxanthine-guanine phosphoribosyltransferase; (3) deoxycytidine kinase; (4) dGMP kinase; (5) nucleoside diphosphate kinase; (6) ribonucleotide reductase; and (7) DNA polymerase.

## IV. NUCLEOSIDE TOXICITY

### A. Adenosine

Adenosine has a multitude of biological and biochemical effects.[30] Adenosine causes cell toxicity, immunosuppression, alters cells morphology, acts as a vasodilator, stimulates hormone secretion, serves as a neurotransmitter and has an assortment of other physiological effects. At a cellular level, adenosine leads to the increased production of cyclic AMP (cAMP), blocks pyrimidine biosynthesis, inhibits PRPP synthesis, and increases intracellular SAH levels.

Adenosine is highly toxic to mammalian cells in culture, especially when ADA function is either genetically or pharmacologically blocked. Two potent inhibitors of adenosine deaminase activity, erythro-9-(2-hydroxy-3-nonyl)-adenine[31] (EHNA) and 2'-deoxycoformycin,[32] have figured prominently in both biochemical and genetic studies on adenosine cytotoxicity. Several mechanisms of adenosine toxicity have been proposed. The first and most likely mechanism for the toxicity of low adenosine concentrations is a depletion of cellular pyrimidine nucleotides.[33-35] Cells exposed to low adenosine concentrations become depleted in UTP and CTP, and the addition of uridine to the culture medium reverses the toxicity of low concentrations of adenosine in several cell types. In addition, S49 cells genetically deficient in either adenylate cyclase or the cAMP-dependent protein kinase are just as sensitive to this pyrimidine directed effect of low adenosine concentrations, indicating that elevation of cAMP content does not mediate adenosine toxicity.[35] Exposure to adenosine also depletes cells of PRPP,[36] a substrate for the penultimate reaction in *de novo* pyrimidine biosynthesis. These data suggest that the excess adenylate nucleotides generated after exposure to exogenous adenosine inhibit the PRPP synthetase activity, diminishing PRPP synthesis to levels inadequate to maintain maximal activity of the orotate phosphoribosyltransferase step of the pyrimidine pathway. The effects of low concentrations of adenosine on growth or on pyrimidine nucleotide levels are not observed in adenosine kinase-deficient cells, indicating that adenosine phosphorylation is required for these effects.[35,36]

A second mechanism for adenosine toxicity was proposed initially by Kredich and Martin.[21] These workers demonstrated in mouse S49 cells that adenosine (+EHNA to inhibit ADA activity) in the presence of L-homocysteine reverses the normal direction of SAH hydrolase activity resulting in the intracellular accumulation of SAH. SAH is a potent inhibitor of SAM-dependent methylation reactions, which are required for proper cell function. This mechanism of adenosine toxicity occurs at concentrations of adenosine considerably higher than those needed to inhibit pyrimidine biosynthesis. Thus, inhibition of pyrimidine synthesis[35] and of transmethylation reactions[21] appear to be the primary and secondary mechanisms of adenosine toxicity in S49 cells. Kredich and Martin further demonstrated that this accumulation of SAH after adenosine/L-homocysteine exposure can occur in cells with an adenosine kinase deficiency or in the presence of uridine in the culture medium.[21] Therefore, SAH accumulation after incubation with adenosine/L-homocysteine is observed in the absence of phosphorylation or deamination. This is often referred to as nucleoside-directed mode of action of adenosine.

## B. Deoxyadenosine

Multiple mechanisms of deoxyadenosine toxicity have also been proposed, all of which require inhibition of the cellular ADA activity. These include inhibition of ribonucleotide reductase,[37-40] inhibition of SAH hydrolase,[22] inhibition of DNA repair processes,[41] and a generalized interference with ATP-dependent reactions by deoxyATP. The primary mechanism by which deoxyadenosine is toxic to dividing mouse T cells is inhibition of ribonucleotide reductase.[38-39] Ribonucleotide reductase in mammalian cells reduces the 2'-hydroxy moiety of all four nucleoside diphosphates, converting them to the corresponding 2'-deoxyribonucleotide diphosphates.[40] Ribonucleotide reductase is the only enzyme in mammalian cells that can synthesize deoxyribonucleotides *de novo*. The enzyme is subject to a variety of complex allosteric regulations among which is that deoxyATP can inhibit the reduction of all four nucleoside diphosphates.[40] DeoxyATP binds to the activity site of ribonucleotide reductase protein M1 and acts as an allosteric inhibitor.[40] In particular, incubation of cells with deoxyadenosine depletes cells of pyrimidine deoxyribonucleotides, and the addition of deoxycytidine to the culture medium can reverse the toxicity of low deoxyadenosine concentrations by supplying a source of cellular deoxyCTP.[37,38] The reversal of deoxyadenosine toxicity by deoxycytidine, however, does not necessarily indicate a replenishment of deoxycytidylate pools. Since deoxycytidine is the preferred substrate for the deoxyadenosine phosphorylating activity of some cells, the pyrimidine deoxyribonucleotide can block deoxyadenosine conversion to deoxyATP.[27,28] However, in murine S49 cells in which adenosine kinase is the major deoxyadenosine phosphorylating activity, deoxycytidine reverses deoxyadenosine-EHNA toxicity without interfering with the expansion of the deoxyATP pool.[38] This ribonucleotide reductase directed mechanism suggest that deoxyadenosine ultimately causes a lethal inhibition of DNA synthesis.

However, Carson et al. demonstrated that deoxyadenosine-EHNA can also kill nondividing peripheral blood lymphocytes.[41] These workers[41,42] and others[43] have proposed that deoxyATP in these resting cells interferes with their ability to repair DNA. Finally, Hershfield has demonstrated that deoxyadenosine is a suicide inactivator of SAH hydrolase,[22] although the apparent $K_i$ value is around 60 $\mu M$, a value much higher than the concentrations of the deoxyribonucleoside circulating in the plasma of ADA-deficient patients.[6] The mechanisms by which deoxyadenosine causes T and B cell dysfunction in ADA deficiency remains controversial.

## C. Deoxyguanosine

The toxicity of deoxyguanosine has been implicated in the T cell lymphotoxicity observed in PNP deficiency.[11,12] Yet, the mechanism by which deoxyguanosine is cytotoxic toward

T cells is different from that by which deoxyguanosine kills other cultured cells. This can be attributed to the unique capacity of T cells to phosphorylate and accumulate deoxyguanosine as deoxyGTP.[14] DeoxyGTP is also a potent allosteric effector of ribonucleotide reductase, although it acts in a different fashion than deoxyATP.[40] DeoxyGTP interacts with the substrate specificity site of ribonucleotide reductase, such that the enzyme recognizes only ADP as a substrate.[40] Consequently, T cells become depleted in pyrimidine deoxyribonucleotides, particularly deoxyCTP, after incubation with deoxyguanosine.[44,45] The addition of deoxycytidine to the culture medium can provide a source of deoxyCTP and reverses deoxyguanosine toxicity in T cells. This reversal of deoxyguanosine toxicity by deoxycytidine, however, does not rigorously prove that ribonucleotide reductase inhibition is the mechanism of deoxyguanosine toxicity, since deoxycytidine also blocks deoxyguanosine phosphorylation by competition for the deoxycytidine-deoxyguanosine kinase.[44,45]

There is a secondary mechanism by which deoxyguanosine is lethal to T lymphoblasts,[44,45] which is also the only mechanism of deoxyguanosine toxicity toward other cultured cells, including B cells and mature T cells.[14,44-46] This involves the metabolism of deoxyguanosine to guanylate ribonucleotides, a process requiring the sequential activities of PNP and HGPRTase[46] (see Figure 4). In effect this is really a guanine-mediated toxicity. This mode of deoxyguanosine cytolysis, therefore, is not observed in PNP-deficient patients. Upon exposure to deoxyguanosine, cells other than immature T cells or T lymphoblasts have greatly elevated GTP pools.[14,46] The addition of adenine or hypoxanthine to the culture medium prevents this toxicity of deoxyguanosine or guanine, either by circumventing a block in the early steps of the purine pathway or by depleting cellular PRPP pools necessary for HGPRTase activity.[44,45]

## IV. NUCLEOSIDE-RESISTANT SOMATIC CELL MUTANTS

### A. Adenosine

There are a variety of biochemically defined and undefined mutations which cause cells to become resistant to adenosine or to adenosine analogs, such as tubercidin (7-deazaadenosine) or cordycepin (3'-deoxyadenosine). Among these are mutants defective in adenosine transport, in adenosine phosphorylation, or in a cellular function which confers a phenotype that circumvents adenosine toxicity. In addition, there are other mutants which have developed a collateral supersensitivity toward adenosine. Mutant somatic cells which are resistant or supersensitive to adenosine are described below.

### 1. Nucleoside Transport Deficiency

Kinetic evidence has suggested that all purine and pyrimidine nucleosides are substrates for the nucleoside transporter of mammalian cells.[47,48] Several classes of nucleoside transport systems have been identified on the basis of their sensitivity to specific powerful inhibitors of nucleoside transport.[49,50] In addition, sodium-dependent nucleoside permeases have been recently identified in kidney and intestinal epithelia.[51,52] In 1979, Cohen et al. isolated from a mutagenized culture of wildtype murine S49 lymphoma cells, a clone, AE$_1$, by virtue of its resistance to the cytoxicity of 0.2 mM adenosine and 10 μM EHNA.[53] In comparative growth rate experiments, the AE$_1$ clone was approximately 200-fold less sensitive to the cytotoxic effects of adenosine. The AE$_1$ cell line was also cross-resistant to a spectrum of cytotoxic nucleosides including 6-thioguanosine, 5-fluorouridine, 5-fluorodeoxyuridine, guanosine, arabinosylcytosine, deoxyadenosine (+ 10 μM EHNA), deoxyguanosine, 6-mercaptoguanosine, 6-azauridine, and 5-bromodeoxyuridine.[53] Interestingly, the AE$_1$ cells were normally sensitive to growth inhibition by either thymidine[54] or arabinosyladenine.[55] The molecular basis for the resistance of the AE$_1$ cells to all these nucleosides is a genetic deficiency in their ability to take up purine and pyrimidine ribonucleosides and deoxyribonucleosides from the culture medium. In long term incorporation studies for intervals up to 1 hr, $AE_1$ cells incorporated adenosine, inosine, and uridine, at a rate less than 2% of that of wild type cells. The levels of five of the rate limiting enzymes in purine and pyrimidine nucleoside metabolism were equivalent in wild type parental and $AE_1$ cells. Furthermore, kinetic analyses of radiolabeled nucleoside incorporation into wild-type cells revealed that inosine, uridine, and adenosine could interefere with the uptake of each other. The subsequent application of rapid sampling kinetic assays to nucleoside transport measurements in mutant cells have now adequately demonstrated that the phenotype of the $AE_1$ cell line can be attributed to a genetic defect in its ability to translocate nucleosides across the plasma membrane.[55,56]

Subsequent to the characterization of the $AE_1$ clone, approximately 15 other independent nucleoside transport-deficient cells have been generated from wild-type S49 cells. The nucleoside transport-deficient cells are all resistant to adenosine, deoxyadenosine, deoxyguanosine, and a multitude of other normally cytotoxic nucleosides to which the $AE_1$ cell line was also resistant. The mutations in all nucleoside transport-deficient cell lines have been analyzed by intraspecies complementation. Examination of the phenotypes of the tetraploid fusion progeny between wild type and nucleoside transport-deficient diploid parents isolated subsequent to polyethylene-glycol fusion indicated that the deficiencies in nucleoside transport in all cell lines behaved in a recessive fashion[53] (unpublished data). This recessive behavior of nucleoside transport deficiency is consistent with a structural gene mutation. Tetraploid cell lines generated between two independently isolated nucleoside transport-deficient parents indicated that all the nucleoside transport-deficient cell lines belonged to a single complementation group. Thus, the genetic lesion in the 15 independently isolated nucleoside transport-deficient mutants occurs in the same genetic locus. Whether this genetic locus is a structural gene for the nucleoside transporter, a gene regulating nucleoside transport, or some genetic function that regulates membrane composition or architecture, remains to be resolved.

Cass et al. established that the nucleoside transport-deficient $AE_1$ cells failed to bind [$^3$H]nitrobenzylthioinosine (NBMPR),[55] a powerful inhibitor of nucleoside transport in many mammalian cells.[57,58] The treatment of S49 cells with NBMPR simulates a genetic deficiency in nucleoside transport in that NBMPR treatment prevents nucleoside toxicity and radiolabeled nucleoside entry into the cells.[54,56] [$^3$H] NBMPR has also been exploited to identify the nucleoside transporter in a variety of cells and tissues by photoaffinity labeling.[56,59-62] The nucleoside transport-deficient S49 cells have been especially useful for this purpose, because they fail to bind NBMPR.[55] Incubation of [$^3$H] NBMPR with plasma membranes prepared from wild-type S49 cells photolabels a broad band on SDS polyacrylamide gels with a molecular weight of 45 to 66 kDa.[56,62] This broad band probably reflects the heterogeneous glycosylation of the wild-type S49 nucleoside transporter. That the photolabeled band is the nucleoside transporter of wild-type S49 cells can be demonstrated genetically by the lack of a similarly photolabeled protein in membranes prepared from $AE_1$ cells.[56,62]

The derivation of mutant mammalian cells genetically deficient in nucleoside transport function have unequivocally established that the transport of all nucleosides requires a common genetic component. Moreover, the somatic cell genetic analysis of nucleoside transport in genetically altered cells has provided a plethora of invaluable information concerning the multiplicity, substrate specificity, binding site determinants, and mechanisms by which nucleosides are translocated across the plasma membrane of mammalian cells. Finally, the generation of adenosine-resistant cells deficient in transport establishes unequivocally, at least in mouse S49 cells, that adenosine must enter cells in order to exert its cytotoxic effects. This is an important observation since mammalian cells possess cell surface receptors for adenosine and other purines.[63]

## 2. Adenosine Kinase Deficiency

A major class of mutant cells that have been derived by virtue of their growth resistance to adenosine or adenosine analogs is deficient in adenosine kinase activity. This enzyme catalyzes the direct phosphorylation of adenosine to AMP (Figure 2). These mutants indicate, therefore, that adenosine phosphorylation can initiate adenosine toxicity in mammalian cells. The isolation and characterization of adenosine kinase-deficient cell lines is the subject of another article in this volume.

## 3. Adenosine Deaminase Overproduction

ADA serves a detoxification function in cells by converting both adenosine and deoxyadenosine to inosine and deoxyinosine, respectively. Neither nucleoside is particularly toxic toward mammalian cells in culture in the presence of functional ADA activity, while both nucleosides are extremely toxic if an ADA inhibitor, such as EHNA or deoxycoformycin, is supplied in the culture medium. Thus, adenosine kinase serves to initiate adenosine toxicity, while ADA is the chief detoxification mechanism.

Kellums and co-workers have exploited this detoxification of adenosine by ADA to isolate mutant cell lines which contain enormous quantities of ADA protein.[64-66] Since ADA activity is not required for cell growth, a selection protocol was devised which requires ADA expression for survival. This was accomplished by modifying a selection system that had been devised previously by Chan et al. for isolating adenosine kinase-positive revertants of adenosine kinase-deficient cells.[67] This modified selection system was termed 11AAU and selects for the simultaneous expression of adenosine kinase and ADA activity. The 11AAU selection medium contained 50 $\mu M$ alanosine, an inhibitor of the penultimate enzyme in AMP biosynthesis, 1.1 m$M$ adenosine, which provided a source of cellular adenylate nucleotides via adenosine kinase phosphorylation, and 1 m$M$ uridine to alleviate the adenosine-induced block in the pyrimidine biosynthetic pathway. The selection system is predicated on the fact that ADA activity is obligatory to detoxify this concentration of adenosine by converting it to inosine. Yeung et al. exploited this 11AAU selection system in conjunction with stepwise increasing doses of deoxycoformycin, the ADA inhibitor, to isolate mouse fibroblast Cl-1D cells which contained a 6000-fold increased amount of ADA protein.[64] Remarkably, ADA accounted for over 50% of the total soluble protein in the mutant cells. The ADA protein from these 11AAU/deoxycoformycin-resistant cells was indistinguishable from the wild-type ADA by isoelectric focusing, by electrophoretic mobility on starch gels, and by deoxycoformycin binding studies. In a later publication by the same group, Ingolia et al. reported that continued selective pressure resulted in the selection of cells in which ADA accounted for 75% of the total soluble protein, an 11,000-fold increase over the amounts of ADA protein in wild type Cl-1D cells.[66] This is the highest level of protein amplification ever observed after genetic selection in animal cells. The huge quantities of enzyme produced facilitated subsequent protein purification and the generation of specific antibodies.[66]

Preliminary genetic analysis revealed the presence of numerous double minute chromosomes in the ADA overproducing cells, cytogenetic structures indicative of the presence of amplified DNA sequences.[64] Incubation of these 11AAU-deoxycoformycin-resistant cells in the absence of selective pressure for 12 cell divisions resulted in a 90% decrease in ADA activity and the simultaneous loss of the double minutes. Later, Yeung et al. subsequently demonstrated that messenger RNA encoding ADA was greatly elevated in one Cl-1D derived cell line which overproduced ADA 3,200-fold.[65] A cDNA library was constructed from the poly(A$^+$) RNA from these ADA overproducing cells, and cDNA clones isolated using $^{32}$P-labeled cDNA probe synthesized from amplified mRNA that had been prehybridized to an excess of DNA from wild-type cells. cDNA clones encoding ADA hybridized with three poly(A$^+$) RNA species of 1.5, 1.7, and 5.2 kb in length.[65] All three poly(A$^+$) RNA species were overproduced in the mutant cells. Dot blot analyses indicated that the gene for ADA was amplified in the ADA overproducing cells approximately 2600-fold, a figure that correlated quite closely with the 3200-fold increase in ADA protein. These mutants should prove to be extremely useful in studying the regulation of expression and the structure of the ADA gene.

### 4. Augmented Levels of S-Adenosylmethionine

Kredich and Martin initially proposed that unmetabolized adenosine could also kill cells by condensing with L-homocysteine to form SAH, a reaction catalyzed by SAH hydrolase.[21] In addition, a variety of adenosine analogs with anticancer and antiviral activity, such as 3-deazaadenosine, 3-deazaaristeromycin, and S-isobutylthioadenosine, also do not appear to require the cellular metabolic apparatus in order to exert their cytotoxic effects.[68-70] In order to probe the nucleoside-related toxicity of adenosine and these related analogs, Kajander et al. isolated adenosine-resistant cells from an adenosine kinase-deficient derivative of a murine T lymphoma line, R1.1.[71,72] The adenosine kinase-deficient genetic background was essential for this selection, since adenosine toxicity at the nucleoside level occurs at higher concentrations of adenosine than those which inhibit pyrimidine biosynthesis.[21] The pyrimidine-directed toxicity requires adenosine phosphorylation and does not occur in adenosine kinase-deficient cells. Adenosine resistant cells were isolated by culturing cells in increasing adenosine concentrations from 50 $\mu M$ to 1.0 m$M$ in the presence of 5 $\mu M$ deoxycoformycin and single cell cloning under nonselective conditions. One clone, AKR4, was analyzed further.[71] The AKR4 clone contained a six- to sevenfold greater level of SAM than the parental cell line and the SAM to SAH ratio in the mutant cells was also elevated six- to sevenfold over that in parental cells. The mutant cells were cross resistant to a variety of agents postulated to cause accretion of SAH, formation of SAH analogs, impairment of SAM synthesis, or interference with SAM-dependent transmethylations. The biochemical basis for the phenotype of the AKR4 cells was an elevation of the cellular methionine adenosyltransferase activity over that in parental cells. The enzyme from mutant cells was also slightly less sensitive to heat inactivation and to inhibition by dimethyl sulfoxide than the enzyme from parental cells. The characterization of these interesting and unique somatic cells provided a powerful genetic demonstration that unmetabolized adenosine and many adenosine analogs could interfere with methylation reactions involving SAM and thereby inhibit cell proliferation. This, in turn, authenticated the hypothesis that adenosine reversal of the flux through SAH hydrolase could have lethal effects to somatic cells.

### 5. Adenosine Supersensitivity

The plethora of adenosine-resistant mutants have somewhat overshadowed the interesting phenotypes associated with mutant mammalian cells which had developed collateral supersensitivity to adenosine. These include the AMP deaminase-deficient S49 cells isolated by Buchwald et al.[73] and the biochemically undefined baby hamster kidney cells selected by Juranka and Chan.[74] The AMP deaminase-deficient mutant was selected by continuous selection of wild-type S49 cells in increasing concentrations of arabinosyl 2,6-diaminopurine.[73] A clone, 100-10, was subsequently isolated by plating in 0.1 m$M$ of the selective agent. The 100-10 cell line, compared to the wild-type S49 cell line, was much more sensitive to growth inhibition by both adenosine-EHNA and adenine but surprisingly less sensitive to thymidine, deoxyadenosine-EHNA, arabinosyl 2,6-diaminopurine, arabinosylguanine, and arabinosyladenine. The complex growth phenotype of the 100-10 cells could be attributed to two separate mutations. The 100-10 cells express an AMP deaminase activity with altered kinetic properties, including a lower $V_{max}$, a higher $K_m$ for AMP, increased sensitivity to inhibition by inorganic phosphate, and a tenfold higher $K_i$ for GTP. The genetically altered AMP deaminase activity could account for the supersensitivity of 100-10 cells to both adenosine-EHNA and adenine. In cells deficient in AMP deaminase activity, adenylate nucleotides accumulate subsequent to exposure to either adenine or adenosine-EHNA and feedback on the early steps of the purine pathway, starving cells for guanylate. In wild-type parental cells, however, AMP is deaminated efficiently to IMP, which is the precursor nucleotide for the guanylate nucleotide branchpoint pathway. Thus, AMP deaminase serves to detoxify adenylate by providing a source of guanylate nucleotides. The addition of hypoxanthine or guanine to the culture medium of the 100-10 cells provided a source of guanylate nucleotides and ameliorated the supersensitivity to adenosine-EHNA and adenine. In addition, the 100-10 cells possess a ribonucleotide reducatse activity with decreased sensitivity to feedback inhibition by deoxyATP.[73] The latter mutation accounted for the resistance of the 100-10 cell line to deoxyribonucleosides and arabinosides. The independence of the AMP deaminase and ribonucleotide reductase mutations was demonstrated by the isolation of an adenosine-resistant clone from 100-10 cells, which had reverted its AMP deaminase, but not its ribonucleotide reductase, phenotype.

The second class of mutant cells that had developed a collateral supersensitivity to adenosine were selected by Chan and Juranka on the basis of their resistance to arabinosyladenine.[74] These arabinosyladenine-resistant mutants, as exemplified by the spontaneously derived ara-S10d cell line, were cross resistant to deoxyadenosine, but were approximately two orders of the magnitude more sensitive than the parental baby hamster kidney cells to adenosine-EHNA cytotoxicity. ADA and deoxyadenosine and adenosine phosphorylating activities were equivalent in wild-type and ara-S10d cells, and thus could not account for the unique phenotype of the mutant cells. That the arabinosyladenine/deoxyadenosine resistance and the adenosine supersensitivity could be attributed to a single mutation was demonstrated definitively genetically by isolating an adenosine-resistant revertant from the ara-S10d cell line. The adenosine-resistant revertant was normally sensitive to arabinosyladenine. Thus, the adenosine supersensitivity and the arabinosyladenine/deoxyadenosine resistance could be ascribed to a lesion in a single genetic locus. When ara-S10d cells were exposed to adenosine, they displayed a substantial elevation of SAH, SAM, and methylthioadenosine, a byproduct of polyamine metabolism.[75] Wild-type cells under similar conditions elevated their SAH levels 50% higher than mutant cells without a concurrent elevation of SAM or methylthioadenosine.

These workers attributed the bizarre phenotype of the ara-S10d cells to a mutation that caused increased expression of SAH hydrolase activity.[75] However, the SAH hydrolase enzyme levels were not measured. This presumably increased SAH hydrolase activity could, nevertheless theoretically, account for the growth phenotype of the mutant cells, since both arabinosyladenine and deoxyadenosine are potent suicide inhibitors of the hydrolase, and adenosine is a substrate for the enzyme. Therefore, adenosine would be more rapidly converted to SAH by mutant cells, while higher concentrations of both arabinosyladenine and deoxyadenosine would be required for abrogation of hydrolase activity. Subsequent investigations revealed that the methylation of DNA and transfer RNA was more sensitive to derangements by exogenous adenosine in mutant cells than in wild-type parental cells.[75] Levels of 5-methylcytosine, 5-methyluracil, 7-methylguanine and, $N^2$-dimethylguanine in tRNAs and 5-methylcytosine in DNA were considerably lower in ara-S10d cells exposed 24 hr to adenosine as compared to wild-type cells incubated in parallel. The particular methylation enzymes that are adversely affected by abnormal SAM metabolism in the mutant cells have not been identified.

## B. Deoxyadenosine

### 1. Nucleoside Transport Deficiency

Deoxyadenosine has also been taken advantage of as a selective agent for the derivation of nucleoside transport-deficient clones in the mouse S49 cell line. The phenotypes of these nucleoside transport-deficient cells are essentially identical to those previously described above. That nucleoside transport-deficient cells are resistant to deoxyadenosine-EHNA toxicity indicates that deoxyadenosine must permeate the plasma membrane in order to exert its cytotoxic effects.

## 2. Deoxyadenosine Phosphorylation Deficiency

Kinetic studies have revealed that both adenosine kinase and deoxycytidine kinase are capable of recognizing deoxyadenosine as a substrate, although the deoxyribonucleoside is not a particularly effective substrate for either enzyme. The relative contribution that each enzyme makes to deoxyadenosine phosphorylation in vivo varies among different cell lines.[27-29,38] Moreover, the preferred enzyme in vitro is not necessarily the same as the preferred enzyme in vivo. In mouse S49 cells, the majority of deoxyadenosine phosphorylation both in vitro and in vivo is catalyzed by adenosine kinase.[38] Adenosine kinase-deficient S49 cells are approximately sixfold less sensitive to deoxyadenosine-mediated growth inhibition and accumulate deoxyATP from deoxyadenosine inefficiently.[38] The introduction of a secondary mutation in deoxycytidine kinase activity to the adenosine kinase-deficient cells confers virtually complete resistance to deoxyadenosine and obliterates the residual accumulation of deoxyATP from deoxyadenosine. Deoxycytidine kinase deficiency has no effect on deoxyadenosine toxicity and immeasurable effects on the extent of deoxyATP accumulation, if adenosine kinase is intact. Thus, adenosine kinase plays a primary role and deoxycytidine kinase a secondary role in deoxyadenosine phosphorylation by S49 cells.

Genetic studies using the human WI-L2 B lymphoblast cell line have indicated that adenosine kinase is the major deoxyadenosine phosphorylating activity in vivo, while deoxycytidine kinase appears to be more active toward deoxyadenosine in vitro.[29] Cell extracts prepared from deoxycytidine kinase-deficient WI-L2 mutants possess less than 10% of the deoxyadenosine phosphorylating activity of wild-type cell extracts.[29] However, growth sensitivity experiments indicated that the deoxycytidine kinase-deficient cells were just as sensitive as the wild type cells to deoxyadenosine toxicity and just as capable of accumulating deoxyATP from exogenous deoxyadenosine. A second WI-L2 mutant cell line deficient in adenosine kinase contained wild-type amounts of deoxyadenosine phosphorylating activity when measured in extracts. However, this adenosine kinase-deficient cell line was twofold less sensitive than the wild-type cell line to deoxyadenosine and accumulated far less intracellular deoxyATP from exogenous deoxyadenosine. A double mutant lacking both adenosine kinase and deoxycytidine kinase activity was the least sensitive of all the WI-L2 cell lines to deoxyadenosine toxicity and accumulated no deoxyATP. Thus, it appears that the major deoxyadenosine phosphorylating activity in cell extracts is associated with deoxycytidine kinase, although the physiologically important enzyme for deoxyadenosine phosphorylation in intact WI-L2 cells is adenosine kinase.

Kinetic studies by Carson have implicated deoxycytidine kinase as the primary determinant in deoxyadenosine phosphorylation by human T cells.[13] Since these data suggested that deoxyadenosine phosphorylation by human T cells occurs via a different enzyme than that used by mouse T cells or human B cells, somatic cell genetic approaches were applied by several groups, some in a collaborative effort, to define the relative importance of the two deoxyadenosine phosphorylating activities to deoxyadenosine phosphorylation in a human T cell line, CEM.[27,28] These studies of deoxyadenosine phosphorylation in human T cells are particularly relevant clinically, since it is the human T cell which is adversely affected in both inborn errors of purine metabolism associated with immunodeficiency. Both Verhaef et al.[27] and Hershfield et al.[28] isolated deoxycytidine kinase-deficient CEM cells that had lost 75 to 90% of their deoxyadenosine phosphorylating capacities in vitro. These deoxycytidine kinase-deficient cells were approximately threefold less sensitive to deoxyadenosine toxicity than parental cells. The introduction of a secondary mutation in adenosine kinase into the deoxycytidine kinase-deficient parents obliterated the remaining in vitro deoxyadenosine phosphorylating catalytic activity. These double mutants genetically deficient in both kinase activities were approximately 250-fold more resistant to the cytotoxic effects of deoxyadenosine than wild-type cells. These independent genetic analyses of deoxyadenosine phosphorylating activities in the human T cell line were particularly important in that they determined the relative roles of the two important deoxyribonucleoside phosphorylating activities in initiating the toxicity of deoxyadenosine toward growing T cells. Moreover, these deoxycytidine kinase-deficient mutants have been subsequently exploited in defining the in vivo determinants responsible for the metabolic activation of a variety of deoxyadenosine analogs with anticancer activity.

### 3. Cytoplasmic Nucleotidase Augmentation

The mutants generated from the somatic cell genetic investigations of deoxyadenosine phosphorylating activities described above were isolated by virtue of their resistance to cytotoxic analogs of adenosine and deoxycytidine. Carson and co-workers used a more direct approach to analyze deoxyadenosine phosphorylation by isolating mutants resistant to the selective pressure of deoxyadenosine.[76] Mutagenized CEM T lymphoblasts were grown in medium supplemented with gradually increasing concentrations of deoxyadenosine and single cell cloned on plates containing 10 $\mu M$ deoxyadenosine. One clone was found to be cross resistant to deoxyguanosine and arabinosylcytosine but had not lost any of its deoxycytidine kinase activity.[76] These deoxyadenosine-resistant cells formed minimal amounts of deoxyATP and deoxyGTP after exposure to the corresponding deoxyribonucleoside and excreted substantial quantities of deoxycytidine into the culture medium. The phenotype of the deoxyadenosine-resistant mutant cells could be attributed to a three- to fourfold elevation in an ATP-activated cytosolic nucleotidase activity.[76] The elevated cytoplasmic nucleotidase could account for the growth phenotype, the inability to accumulate nucleoside triphosphates, and the elevated deoxycytidine excretion. In a certain sense, the elevated soluble nucleotidase activity essentially conferred a B cell like phenotype on the mutant T cells, i.e., high levels of intracellular deoxyribonucleotide dephosphorylating activities. These genetic studies demonstrated the role of intracellular deoxyribonucleotidase activities in regulating cellular growth sensitivity toward deoxyribonucleosides.

### 4. Ribonucleotide Reductase Alterations

Mutants genetically deficient in nucleoside transport or deoxyadenosine phosphorylating activities implicated deoxyATP as the toxic metabolite of deoxyadenosine. The ultimate cellular target for deoxyATP toxicity, however, has been a subject of some controversy. In order to determine the molecular mechanism of deoxyadenosine toxicity in S49 cells, Ullman et al. isolated a mutant cell line which possessed a ribonucleotide reductase activity that was refractory to complete inhibition by deoxyATP.[39] This cell line, dGuo-200-1, was fivefold less sensitive to the growth inhibitory and cytotoxic effects of deoxyadenosine in the presence of EHNA.[39] This growth resistance could be accounted for by the fact that the ribonucleotide reductase activity in the dGuo-200-1 cells, in contrast to its parent, is not normally sensitive to feedback inhibition by deoxyATP, although the specific activities of the enzyme were equivalent in parental and mutant cells. Purification of the enzyme from mutant cells proved that dGuo-200-1 cells possessed two different ribonucleotide reductase protein M1 subunits that could be separated by deoxyATP-agarose chromatography.[77] One protein M1 was as sensitive as wild-type ribonucleotide reductase to deoxyATP inhibition, while the other was completely refractory to any inhibition by deoxyATP, whatsoever.[77] Thus, dGuo-200-1 cells are heterozygous for their expression of ribonucleotide reductase activity, possessing one allele coding for a wild-type enzyme and one allele encoding a ribonucleotide reductase activity that is completely insensitive to inhibition by deoxyATP. This study demonstrated genetically that the activity site of ribonucleotide reductase is located on the protein M1 subunit.[77]

The intracellular levels of all four deoxyribonucleoside triphosphates in exponentially growing dGuo-200-1 cells are two- to fivefold greater than those in parental cells.[39] The markedly deranged nucleotide pools confer a mutator pheontype on dGuo-200-1 cells.[78] The rate of spontaneous mutation of dGuo-200-1 cells to two independent markers, dexamethasone and 6-thioguanine resistance, was 100-fold greater than wild-type cells. Indeed, this mutant cell line displays the highest rate of spontaneous mutation of any diploid mammalian cell line yet described.

Another cell line possessing a mutation in ribonucleotide reductase was isolated by Kubota et al. from a human histiocytic lymphoma cell line (DHL-9).[79] The mutant lymphoma clone was isolated for increased resistance to deoxyadenosine and exhibited a phenotype somewhat similar to the dGuo-200-1 cell line described above. The mutant DHL-9 cell line was cross resistant to a spectrum of deoxyribonucleosides, possessed elevated deoxyribonucleoside triphosphate pools, and excreted large amounts of deoxyadenosine and thymidine into the culture medium.[79] That the mutant DHL-9 cells failed to accumulate deoxyATP efficiently from exogenous deoxyadenosine could be attributed to the end product inhibition on the cellular deoxyadenosine phosphorylating activities as a consequence of the elevated cellular deoxyribonucleoside triphosphate pools. The specific activity of the ribonucleotide reductase activity of the mutant cells, when assayed with either ADP or CDP as a substrate, was 2.5-fold elevated over that in wild type cells. The sensitivity of the mutant enzyme to allosteric effectors was not reported. Thus, it appears that the biochemical aberration in ribonucleotide reductase in the mutant DHL-9 cells was different from that in the dGuo-200-1 cells. The elevated ribonucleotide reductase activity could account for the elevated deoxyribonucleoside triphosphate pools, which in turn, could explain the reduced ability of the mutant cells to form deoxyATP, the excessive deoxyribonucleoside excretion, and the abnormal growth phenotype.

## C. Deoxyguanosine Resistant Mutants

### 1. Nucleoside Transport Deficiency

The nucleoside transport-deficient mutants described earlier are also cross resistant to deoxyguanosine. Additional mutants have been isolated by their resistance to deoxyguanosine directly, which are also nucleoside transport-deficient.[12] Their phenotypes are similar to other nucleoside transport-deficient cells. The ability to generate nucleoside transport-deficient cells resistant to deoxyguanosine indicated that the deoxyguanosine toxicity observed both in cultured cells and in PNP deficiency occurs subsequent to cell entry.

### 2. Deoxycytidine Kinase Deficiency

Deoxyguanosine is a substrate for deoxycytidine kinase. Consequently, deoxycytidine kinase-deficient human and mouse T cells are resistant to deoxyguanosine and fail to accumulate deoxyguanosine as deoxyGTP.[27,45] This mechanism of resistance toward deoxyguanosine, however, is observed exclusively in cultured T cell lines in which the primary mechanism of deoxyguanosine toxicity is dependent upon deoxyguanosine accumulation into deoxyGTP.

### 3. Purine Nucleoside Phosphorylase and Hypoxanthine-Guanine Phosphoribosyltransferase Deficiencies

The primary mechanism of deoxyguanosine toxicity in cultured cell lines of nonthymic origin requires the conversion of deoxyguanosine to guanylate nucleotides. This requires the sequential cleavage of deoxyguanosine to guanine by PNP, followed by the PRPP-dependent phosphoribosylation of guanine, a step catalyzed by HGPRTase. Thus, B cell lymphoblasts derived from PNP-deficient patients and either naturally occurring or mutationally induced HGPRTase-deficient B lymphoblasts are completely resistant to deoxyguanosine toxicity.[80]

This mechanism of deoxyguanosine toxicity is also observed in T cells, although at higher concentrations than required for deoxyGTP mediated toxicity.[44,45] S49 cells genetically deficient in deoxycytidine kinase are only several-fold more resistant to deoxyguanosine. If a secondary mutation in HGPRTase is inserted into these deoxycytidine kinase-deficient cells, they become much more resistant to deoxyguanosine toxicity. These genetic studies were useful in differentiating mechanisms of toxicity of deoxyguanosine toward human T and B cells and could explain the specific T cell lymphotoxicity observed in PNP deficiency.

### 4. Ribonucleotide Reductase Alterations

To analyze PNP deficiency in a genetic cell culture model, Ullman et al. isolated a PNP-deficient S49 T cell line, NSU1.[12] In order to delineate the biochemical processes necessary for the sensitivity of the PNP-deficient cell line to deoxyguanosine, a series of secondary mutants resistant to deoxyguanosine were inserted into NSU1 cells. One class of mutants cells was defective in deoxyguanosine transport. A second lacked the deoxycytidine-deoxyguanosine kinase activity. A third type of mutant, dGuo-L, however, could transport and phosphorylate deoxyguanosine and accumulate deoxyGTP normally.[12] However, unlike its parental cell line, this mutant cell line did not become depleted of deoxyCTP or TTP upon exposure to exogenous deoxyguanosine. This observation could be accounted for by the fact that the ribonucleotide reductase activity of the dGuo-L cells was not normally sensitive to feedback inhibition by deoxyGTP, or for that matter TTP.[12] The ribonucleotide reductase from dGuo-L cells possesses two ribonucleotide reductase protein M1 components separable by affinity chromatography, one similar to the wild-type protein M1, while the second had a mutation in the substrate specificity site of the enzyme, which conferred complete insensitivity to the allosteric deoxyGTP and TTP.[81] Thus the dGuo-L cells, like the dGuo 200-1 cells, were also heterozygous for ribonucleotide reductase expression, possessing a wild-type allele and an allele encoding an enzyme with a genetically altered substrate specificity site. That ribonucleotide reductase was the ultimate target for deoxyguanosine toxicity in this cell culture model led these workers to hypothesize that ribonucleotide reductase was the pathogenic target for deoxyguanosine toxicity in T cells from PNP-deficient children. A proposed mechanism to account for the specific T cell lymphotoxicity is that deoxyguanosine is selectively accumulated by T cells to deoxyGTP. DeoxyGTP interacts with the substrate specificity site, located on the protein M1 subunit of ribonucleotide reductase, preventing the enzyme from recognizing CDP and consequently depleting the cellular deoxyCTP pools below those adequate for the maintenance of DNA synthetic or repair functions.

## VI. CONCLUSIONS

These investigations on mutant mammalian cell lines resistant to adenosine, deoxyadenosine, and/or deoxyguanosine have allowed somatic cell geneticists to dissect the *in situ* factors involved in the toxicity of the three naturally occurring nucleosides, adenosine, deoxyadenosine, and deoxyguanosine. These studies have also provided invaluable information on the biochemical properties of the determinants involved in the cellular metabolism of these nucleosides and have made significant contributions to the elucidation of the pathogenic targets involved in two inborn errors of deoxyribonucleoside metabolism associated with immunological dysfunction. For instance, the phenotypes of the nucleoside transport-deficient S49 cells conclusively demonstrate that permeation of the plasma membrane is required for the effects of these three nucleosides on cultured cells. This is significant in light of the observation that cells possess purinergic receptors and other nucleoside binding components on their cell surface. Moreover, these cells altered in their nucleoside transport function have proven invaluable in characterizing the multiplicity, substrate specificity, binding site determinants, and mechanisms by which nucleosides are translocated across the mammalian plasma membrane. Second, mutants genetically deficient in one or several kinases have been useful in assigning substrate specificities to phosphorylating enzymes, for evaluating the contributions of phosphorylating capacities to nucleoside toxicity in various cell types, and for studying the cellular metabolism of anticancer drugs. These studies have indicated that: (1) the toxicity of low adenosine concentrations requires adenosine phosphorylation, while higher adenosine concentrations cause a nucleoside-directed toxicity; (2) deoxyadenosine is phosphorylated primarily by deoxycytidine kinase in human T cells but by adenosine kinase in intact human B cells and mouse T cells; and (3) deoxyguanosine is phosphorylated by deoxycytidine kinase, which initiates cellular toxicity in T cells but not in other cell types. Third, the primary mechanisms of deoxyadenosine and deoxyguanosine toxicities in dividing T cells have been established genetically by the isolation and characterization of mutant cell lines containing ribonucleotide reductase activities that are refractory to complete inhibition by deoxyATP and deoxyGTP, respectively. These mutants have also proven of great advantage in understanding the regulation of this critical enzyme of nucleic acid synthesis. Moreover, the lymphospecificities of the two inborn errors of metabolism can be understood in terms of their unique sensitivities and unique mechanisms of resistance to deoxyadenosine and deoxyguanosine. Finally, mutations in other cellular functions influencing nucleoside metabolism, such as SAM synthetase, SAH hydrolase, nucleotidase, and ADA have all provided important confirmatory information concerning the toxic mechanisms and the metabolic pathways of these three important endogenous nucleosides.

## ACKNOWLEDGMENTS

This article was supported by funds provided by the National Institutes of Health grant No. DK38809. The author is a recipient of a Research Career Development Award from the National Institutes of Health.

## REFERENCES

1. **Giblett, E. R., Anderson, J. E., Cohen, F., Pollara, B., and Meuwissen, H. J.,** Adenosine-deaminase deficiency in two patients with severely impaired immunity, *Lancet,* 2, 1067, 1972.
2. **Giblett, E. R., Ammann, A. J., Wara, D. W., Sandman, R., and Diamond, L. K.,** Nucleoside phosphorylase deficiency in a child with severely defective T-cell immunity and normal B cell immunity, *Lancet,* 1, 1010, 1975.
3. **Cohen, A., Hirschhorn, R., Horowitz, S. D., Rubinstein, A., Polmar, S. H., Hong, R., and Martin, D. W., Jr.,** Deoxyadenosine triphosphate as a potentially toxic metabolite in adenosine deaminase deficiency, *Proc. Natl. Acad. Sci. U.S.A.,* 75, 426, 1978.
4. **Coleman, M. S., Donofrio, J., Hutton, J. J., Hahn, L., Daoud, A., Lampkin, B., and Dyminski, J.,** Identification and quantitation of adenine deoxynucleotides in erythrocytes of a patient with adenosine deaminase deficiency and severe combined immunodeficiency, *J. Biol. Chem.,* 253, 1619, 1978.
5. **Donofrio, J., Coleman, M. S., Hutton, J. J., Daoud, A., Lampkin, B., and Dyminski, J.,** *J. Clin. Invest.,* 62, 884, 1978.
6. **Hirschhorn, R., Roegner, V., Rubinstein, A., and Papagergious, P.,** *J. Clin. Invest.,* 65, 768, 1980.
7. **Polmar, S. H., Stern, R. C., Schwartz, A. L., Wetzler, E. M., Chase, P. A., and Hirschhorn, R.,** Enzyme replacement therapy for adenosine deaminase deficiency and severe combined immuno-deficiency, *New Engl. J. Med.,* 295, 1337, 1976.
8. **Hershfield, M. S., Buckley, R. H., Greenberg, M. L., Melton, A. L., Hatem, C., Kurtzberg, J., Markert, M. L., and Abuchowski, A.,** Treatment of adenosine deaminase deficiency with polyethylene glycol-modified adenosine deaminase (PEG-ADA), *New Engl. J. Med.,* in press.

9. **Grever, M. R., Siaw, M. F. E., Jacob, W. F., Neidhart, J. A., Wiser, J. S., Coleman, M. S., Hutton, J. J., and Balcerzak, S. P.,** The biochemical and clinical consequences of 2'-deoxycoformycin in refractory lymphoproliferative malignancy, *Blood,* 57, 406, 1981.

10. **Koller, C. A. and Mitchell, B. S.,** Alterations in erythrocyte adenine nucleotide pools resulting from 2'-deoxycoformycin therapy, *Cancer Res.,* 43, 1409, 1983.

11. **Cohen, A., Gudas, L. J., Ammann, A. J., Staal, G. E. J., and Martin, D. W., Jr.,** Deoxyguanosine triphosphate as a possible toxic metabolite in purine nucleoside phosphorylase deficiency, *J. Clin. Invest.,* 61, 1405, 1978.

12. **Ullman, B., Gudas, L. J., Clift, S. M., and Martin, D. W., Jr.,** Isolation and characterization of purine-nucleoside phosphorylase-deficient T-lymphoma cells and secondary mutants with altered ribonucleotide reductase: Genetic model for immunodeficiency disease, *Proc. Natl. Acad. Sci. U.S.A.,* 76, 1074, 1979.

13. **Carson, D. A., Kaye, J., and Seegmiller, J. E.,** Differential sensitivity of human leukemic T cell lines and B cell lines to growth inhibition by deoxyadenosine, *J. Immunol.,* 121, 1726, 1978.

14. **Ullman, B. and Martin, D. W., Jr.,** Specific cytotoxicity of arabinosyl-guanine toward cultured T lymphoblasts, *J. Clin. Invest.,* 74, 951, 1984.

15. **Mitchell, B. S., Meijas, E., Daddona, P. E., and Kelley, W. N.,** Purinogenic immunodeficiency disease: selective toxicity of deoxyribonucleosides for T cells, *Proc. Natl. Acad. Sci. U.S.A.,* 75, 5011, 1978.

16. **Gelfand, E. W., Lee, J. J., and Dosch, H.-M.,** Selective toxicity of purine deoxynucleosides for human lymphocytes growth and function, *Proc. Natl. Acad. Sci. U.S.A.,* 76, 1998, 1979.

17. **Carson, D. A., Kaye, J., and Seegmiller, J. E.,** Lymphospecific toxicity in adenosine deaminase deficiency and purine neucleoside phosphorylase deficiency: possible role of nucleoside kinase(s), *Proc. Natl. Acad. Sci. U.S.A.,* 74, 5677, 1977.

18. **Carson, D., Kaye, J., Matsumoto, S., Seegmiller, J. E., and Thompson, L.,** Biochemical basis for the enhanced susceptibility of human malignant T cell lines to deoxyribonucleosides, *Proc. Natl. Acad. Sci. U.S.A.,* 76, 2430, 1978.

19. **Wortmann, R. L., Mitchell, B. S., Edwards, N. L., and Fox, I. H.,** Basis for differential deoxyadenosine toxicity to T- and B-lymphoblasts: a role for 5'-nucleotidase, *Proc. Natl. Acad. Sci. U.S.A.,* 76, 2434, 1978.

20. **Carson, D. A., Kaye, J., and Wasson, D. B.,** The potential importance of soluble deoxynucleotidase activity in mediating deoxyadenosine toxicity in human lymphoblasts, *J. Immunol.,* 126, 348, 1981.

21. **Kredich, N. M. and Martin, D. W., Jr.,** Role of S-adenosylhomocysteine in adenosine-mediated toxicity in cultured mouse T lymphoma cells, *Cell,* 12, 931, 1977.

22. **Hershfield, M. S.,** Apparent suicide inactivation of human lymphoblast S-adenosylhomocysteine hydrolase by 2'-deoxyadenosine and adenine arabinoside, *J. Biol. Chem.,* 254, 11, 1979.

23. **Wolberg, G., Zimmerman, T. P., Hiemstra, K., Winston, M., and Chu, L.-C.,** Adenosine inhibition of lymphocyte-mediated cytolysis: possible role of cyclic adenosine monophosphate, *Science,* 187, 957, 1975.

24. **Zenzer, T. V.,** Formation of adenosine 3',5'-monophosphate from adenosine in mouse thymocytes, *Biochim. Biophys. Acta,* 404, 202, 1975.

25. **Bourne, H. R., Lichtenstein, L. M., Melmon, K. L., Henney, C. S., Weinstein, Y., and Shearer, G. M.,** Modulation of inflammation and immunity by cyclic AMP, *Science,* 184, 19, 1974.

26. **Anderson, E. P.,** Nucleoside and nucleotide kinases, *Enzymes,* 9, 49, 1973.

27. **Verhoef, V., Sarup, J., and Fridland, A.,** Identification of the mechanism of activation of 9-beta-D-arabinofuranosyladenine in human lymphoid cells using mutants deficient in nucleoside kinases, *Cancer Res.,* 41, 4478, 1981.

28. **Hershfield, M. S., Fetter, J. E., Small, W. C., Bagnara, A. S., Williams, S. R., Ullman, B., Martin, D. W., Jr., Wasson, D. B., and Carson, D. A.,** Effects of mutational loss of adenosine kinase and deoxycytidine kinase on deoxyATP accumulation and deoxyadenosine toxicity in cultured CEM human T-lymphoblastoid cells, *J. Biol. Chem.,* 257, 6380, 1982.

29. **Ullman, B., Levinson, B. B., Hershfield, M. S., and Martin, D. W., Jr.,** A biochemical genetic study of the role of specific nucleoside kinases in deoxyadenosine phosphorylation by cultured human cells, *J. Biol. Chem.,* 256, 848, 1981.

30. **Fox, I. H. and Kelley, W. N.,** The role of adenosine and 2'-deoxyadenosine in mammalian cells, *Annu. Rev. Biochem.,* 47, 655, 1978.

31. **Schaeffer, J. J. and Schwender, C. F.,** Enzyme inhibitor. 26 bridging hydrophobic and hydrophilic regions on adenosine deaminase with some 9-(2-hydroxy-3-alkyl) adenines, *J. Med. Chem.,* 17, 6, 1974.

32. **Agarwal, R. P., Spector, T., and Parks, R. E.,** Tight-binding inhibitors. IV. Inhibition of adenosine deaminase by various inhibitors, *Biochem. Pharmacol.,* 26, 259, 1979.

33. **Green, H. and Chan, T. S.,** Pyrimidine starvation induced by adenosine in fibroblasts and lymphoid cells: role of adenosine deaminase, *Science,* 182, 836, 1973.

34. **Ishii, K. and Green, H.,** Lethality of adenosine for cultured mammalian cells by interference with pyrimidine biosynthesis, *J. Cell Sci.,* 13, 429, 1973.

35. **Ullman, B., Cohen, A., and Martin, D. W., Jr.,** Characterization of a cell culture model for the study of adenosine deaminase- and purine nucleoside phosphorylase-deficient immunologic disease, *Cell*, 9, 205, 1976.

36. **Gudas, L. J., Cohen, A., Ullman, B., and Martin, D. W., Jr.,** Analysis of adenosine mediated pyrimidine starvation using cultured wild type and mutant mouse T-lymphoma cells, *Somat. Cell Genet.*, 4, 201, 1978.

37. **Morris, N. R., Reichard, P., and Fischer, G. A.,** Studies concerning the inhibition of cellular reproduction by deoxyribonucleosides. II. Inhibition of the synthesis of deoxycytidine by thymidine, deoxyadenosine, and deoxyguanosine, *Biochim. Biophys. Acta*, 68, 93, 1963.

38. **Ullman, B., Gudas, L. J., Cohen, A., and Martin, D. W., Jr.,** Deoxyadenosine metabolism and cytotoxicity in cultured mouse T lymphoma cells: a model for immunodeficiency disease, *Cell*, 14, 365, 1978.

39. **Ullman, B., Clift, S. M., Gudas, L. J., Levinson, B. B., Wormsted, M. A., and Martin, D. W., Jr.,** Alterations in deoxyribonucleotide metabolism in cultured cells with ribonucleotide reductase activities refractory to feedback inhibition by 2'-deoxyadenosine triphosphate, *J. Biol. Chem.*, 255, 8308, 1980.

40. **Thelander, L. and Reichard, P.,** Reduction of ribonucleotides, *Annu. Rev. Biochem.*, 48, 133, 1979.

41. **Carson, D. A., Wasson, D. B., Lakow, E., and Kamatani, N.,** Possible metabolic basis for the different immunodeficient states associated with genetic deficiencies of adenosine deaminase and purine nucleoside phosphorylase, *Proc. Natl. Acad. Sci. U.S.A.*, 79, 3848, 1982.

42. **Seto, S., Carrera, C. J., Kubota, M., Wasson, D. B., and Carson, D. A.,** Mechanism of deoxyadenosine and 2-chlorodeoxyadenosine toxicity to nondividing human lymphocytes, *J. Clin. Invest.*, 75, 377, 1985.

43. **Brox, L., Ng, A., Pollock, E., and Belch, A.,** DNA strand breaks induced in human T-lymphocytes by the combination of deoxyadenosine and deoxycoformycin, *Cancer Res.*, 44, 934, 1984.

44. **Chan, T.-S.,** Deoxyguanosine toxicity on lymphoid cells as a cause for immunosuppression in purine nucleoside phosphorylase deficiency, *Cell*, 14, 523, 1978.

45. **Gudas, L. J., Ullman, B., Cohen, A., and Martin, D. W., Jr.,** Deoxyguanosine toxicity in a mouse T lymphoma: relationship to purine nucleoside phosphorylase-associated immune dysfunction, *Cell*, 14, 531, 1978.

46. **Sidi, Y. and Mitchell, B. S.,** 2-Deoxyguanosine toxicity for B and mature T lymphoid cell lines is mediated by guanine ribonucleotide accumulation, *J. Clin. Invest.*, 74, 1640, 1984.

47. **Oliver, J. M. and Paterson, A. R. P.,** Nucleoside transport, I. A mediated process in human erythrocytes, *Can. J. Biochem.*, 49, 262, 1971.

48. **Taube, R. A. and Berlin, R. D.,** Membrane transport of nucleosides in rabbit polymorphonuclear leukocytes, *Biochim. Biophys. Acta*, 255, 6, 1972.

49. **Belt, J. A.,** Heterogeneity of nucleoside transport in mammalian cells. Two types of activity in L1210 and other cultured neoplastic cells, *Mol. Pharmacol.*, 24, 479, 1983.

50. **Plagemann, P. G. W. and Wohlhueter, R. M.,** Nucleoside transport in cultured mammalian cells. Multiple forms with different sensitivity to inhibition by nitrobenzylthioinosine or hypoxanthine, *Biochim. Biophys. Acta*, 773, 39, 1984.

51. **Le Hir, M. and Dubach, U. C.,** Sodium gradient-energized concentrative transport of adenosine in renal brush border vesicles, *Pflugers Arch. Eur. J. Physiol.*, 401, 58, 1984.

52. **Schwenk, M., Hegazy, E., and Lopez del Pino, V.,** Uridine uptake by isolated intestinal epithelial cells of guinea pig, *Biochim. Biophys. Acta*, 805, 370, 1984.

53. **Cohen, A., Ullman, B., and Martin, D. W., Jr.,** Characterization of a mutant mouse lymphoma cell with deficient transport of purine and pyrimidine nucleosides, *J. Biol. Chem.*, 254, 112, 1979.

54. **Aronow, B. and Ullman, B.,** Thymidine incorporation in nucleoside transport-deficient lymphoma cells, *J. Biol. Chem.*, 260, 16274, 1985.

55. **Cass, C. E., Kolassa, N., Uehara, Y., Dahlig-Harley, E., Harley, E. R., and Paterson, A. R. P.,** Absence of binding sites of the transport inhibitor nitrobenzylthioinosine on nucleoside transport-deficient mouse lymphoma cells, *Biochim. Biophys. Acta*, 649, 769, 1981.

56. **Aronow, B., Allen, K., Patrick, J., and Ullman, B.,** Altered nucleoside transporters in mammalian cells selected for resistance to the physiological effects of inhibitors of nucleoside transport, *J. Biol. Chem.*, 260, 6226, 1985.

57. **Paterson, A. R. P. and Oliver, J. M.,** Nucleoside transport. II. Inhibition by p-nitrobenzylthioguanosine and related compounds, *Can. J. Biochem.*, 49, 271, 1971.

58. **Aronow, B. and Ullman, B.,** Genetic analysis of the 6-thiobenzylpurine binding site of the nucleoside transporter in mouse lymphoblasts, *Proc. Soc. Exp. Biol. Med.*, 179, 463, 1985.

59. **Young, J. D., Jarvis, S. M., Robins, M. J., and Paterson, A. R. P.,** Photoaffinity labeling of the human erythrocyte nucleoside transporter by $N^6$-(p-azidobenzyl)adenosine and nitrobenzylthioinosine, *J. Biol. Chem.*, 258, 2202, 1983.

60. **Kwan, K. F. and Jarvis, S. M.,** Photoaffinity labeling of adenosine transporter in cardiac membranes with nitrobenzylthioinosine, *Am. J. Physiol.*, 246, 710, 1984.

61. **Wu, J.-S. R., and Young, J. D.,** Photoaffinity labeling of nucleoside transport proteins in plasma membranes isolated from rat and guinea pig liver, *Biochem. J.,* 20, 499, 1984.

62. **Young, J. D., Jarvis, S. M., Belt, J. A., Gati, W. P., and Paterson, A. R. P.,** Identification of the nucleoside transporter in cultured mouse lymphoma cells, *J. Biol. Chem.,* 259, 8363, 1984.

63. **Bruns, R. F., Daly, J. W., and Snyder, S. H.,** Adenosine receptors in brain membranes: binding of $N^6$-cyclohexyl[$^3$H]adenosine and 1,3-diethyl-8-[$^3$H]phenylxanthine, *Proc. Natl. Acad. Sci. U.S.A.,* 77, 5547, 1980.

64. **Yeung, C.-Y., Ingolia, D. E., Bobonis, C., Dunbar, B. S., Riser, M. E., Siciliano, M. J., and Kellems, R. E.,** Selective overproduction of adenosine deaminase in cultured mouse cells, *J. Biol. Chem.,* 258, 8338, 1983.

65. **Yeung, C.-Y., Frayne, E. G., Al-Ubaidi, M. R., Hook, A. G., Ingolia, D. E., Wright, D. A., and Kellems, R. E.,** Amplification and molecular cloning of murine adenosine deaminase gene sequences, *J. Biol. Chem.,* 258, 15179, 1983.

66. **Ingolia, D. E., Yeung, C.-Y., Orengo, I. F., Harrison, M. L., Frayne, E. G., Rudolph, F. B., and Kellems, R. E.,** Purification and characterization of adenosine deaminase from a genetically enriched mouse cell line, *J. Biol. Chem.,* 260, 13261, 1985.

67. **Chan, T., Creagan, R. P., and Reardon, M. P.,** Adenosine kinase as a new selective marker in somatic cell genetics: isolation of adenosine kinase-deficient mouse cell lines and human-mouse hybrid cell lines containing adenosine kinase, *Somat. Cell Genet.,* 4, 1, 1978.

68. **Bader, J. P., Brown, N. R., Chiang, P. K., and Cantoni, G. L.,** 3-Deazaadenosine, an inhibitor of adenosylhomocysteine hydrolase, inhibits reproduction of Rous sarcoma virus and transformation of chick embryo cells, *Virology,* 89, 494, 1978.

69. **DeClercq, E. and Cools, M.,** Antiviral potency of adenosine analogues: correlation with inhibition of S-adenosylhomocysteine hydrolase, *Biochem. Biophys. Res. Commun.,* 129, 306, 1985.

70. **Montgomery, J. A., Clayton, S. J., Thomas, H. J., Shannon, W. M., Arnett, G., Bodner, A. J., Kion, I.-K., Cantoni, G. L., and Chiang, P. K.,** Carbocyclic analogue of 3-deazaadenosine: a novel antiviral agent using S-adenosylhomocysteine hydrolase as a pharmacological target, *J. Med. Chem.,* 25, 626, 1982.

71. **Kajander, E. O., Kubota, M., Carrera, C. J., Montgomery, J. A., and Carson, D. A.,** Resistance to multiple adenine nucleoside and methionine analogues in mutant murine lymphoma cells with enlarged S-adenosylmethionine pools, *Cancer Res.,* 46, 2866, 1986.

72. **Kajander, E. O., Kubota, M., Willis, E. H., and Carson, D. A.,** S-Adenosylmethionine metabolism as a target for adenosine toxicity, in *Purine and Pyrimidine Metabolism in Man,* Vol. 5, Nyhan, W. L., Thompson, L. F., and Watts, R. W. E., Eds., Plenum Press, New York, 1986, 221.

73. **Buchwald, M., Ullman, B., and Martin, D. W., Jr.,** Biochemical and genetic analysis of AMP deaminase deficiency in cultured mammalian cells, *J. Biol. Chem.,* 256, 10346, 1981.

74. **Chan, V. L. and Juranka, P.,** Isolation and preliminary characterization of 9-beta-D-arabinofuranosyladenine-resistant mutants of baby hamster cell, *Somat. Cell Genet.,* 7, 147, 1981.

75. **Skinner, M. A., Ho, H. J., and Chan, V. L.,** Inhibition of methylation of DNA and tRNA by adenosine in an adenosine-sensitive mutant of the baby hamster kidney cell line, *Arch. Biochem. Biophys.,* 246, 725, 1986.

76. **Carson, D. A., Carrera, C. J., Kubota, M., Wasson, D. B., and Iizasa, T.,** Genetic analysis of deoxyadenosine toxicity in dividing human lymphoblasts, *Purine and Pyrimidine Metabolism in Man,* Vol. 5, Nyhan, W. L., Thompson, L. F., and Watts, R. W. E., Eds., Plenum Press, New York, 1986, 207.

77. **Eriksson, S., Gudas, L. J., Ullman, B., Clift, S. M., and Martin, D. W., Jr.,** DeoxyATP-resistant ribonucleotide reductase of mutant mouse lymphoma cells. Evidence for heterozygosity for the protein M1 subunits, *J. Biol. Chem.,* 256, 10184, 1981.

78. **Weinberg, G. L., Ullman, B., and Martin, D. W., Jr.,** Mutator phenotypes in mammalian cell mutant with distinct biochemical defects and abnormal deoxyribonucleoside triphosphate pools, *Proc. Natl. Acad. Sci. U.S.A.,* 78, 2447, 1981.

79. **Kubota, M., Carrera, C. J., Wasson, D. B., and Carson, D. A.,** Deoxynucleoside overproduction in deoxyadenosine-resistant adenosine deaminase-deficient human histiocytic lymphoma cells, *Biochim. Biophys. Acta,* 804, 37, 1984.

80. **Ochs, U. H., Chen, S.-H., Ochs, H. D., Osborne, W. R. A., and Scott, C. R.,** Deoxyribonucleoside toxicity on adenosine deaminase and purine nucleoside phosphorylase positive and negative cultured lymphoblastoid cells, *Inborn Errors of Specific Immunity,* Pollara, B., Pickering, R. J., Meuwissen, H. J., and Porter, I. H., Eds., Academic Press, New York, 1979, 191.

81. **Ullman, B., Gudas, L. J., Caras, I. W., Eriksson, S., Weinberg, G. L., Wormsted, M. A., and Martin, D. W., Jr.,** Demonstration of normal and mutant protein M1 subunits of deoxyGTP-resistant ribonucleotide reductase from mutant mouse lymphoma cells, *J. Biol. Chem.,* 256, 10189, 1981.

Chapter 7

## PURINE NUCLEOSIDE ANALOGS

**R. S. Gupta**

### TABLE OF CONTENTS

I.      Introduction.................................................................... 90

II.     Biochemical Effects of Different Nucleoside Analogs ......................... 90
        A.      Toyocamycin, Tubercidin, Sangivamycin, and the Tricyclic
                Nucleoside, Pentaazaacenaphthylene ................................... 90
        B.      6-Methylmercaptopurine Riboside (6-MeMPR).......................... 92
        C.      Formycin A, Formycin B, and other C-Nucleoside Analogs ............. 92

III.    Cellular Resistance to Purine Nucleoside Analogs ............................ 94
        A.      Characteristics of Different Types of Mutants Affected in
                Adenosine Kinase ...................................................... 94
        B.      Immunological Studies with the Mutants .............................. 100
        C.      Cross Resistance Studies with the Mutants toward other Purine
                and Pyrimidine Derivatives............................................ 101
        D.      Selection and Characteristics of Second-Step Mutants Resistant
                to Toyocamycin ....................................................... 101
        E.      Revertant Selection................................................... 104

IV.     Usefulness of the AK⁻ Mutant Selection System in Quantitative
        Mutagenesis Studies ........................................................ 104

V.      Summary and Prospects...................................................... 105

References...................................................................... 106

# I. INTRODUCTION

Nucleoside analogs constitute an important group of antimetabolites, many of which possess very useful biochemical and medicinal properties.[1-5] This chapter examines the mechanism of cellular resistance to a number of nucleoside analogs, all of which have in common the property that their initial phosphorylation is carried out via the enzyme adenosine kinase (AK). This group of compounds include the pyrrolopyrimidine nucleosides toyoca-mycin, tubercidin, and sangivamycin; the pyrazolopyrimidine nucleosides formycin A, for-mycin B, and a large number of other C- and N-nucleoside derivatives including 6-methyl mercaptopurine riboside (MeMPR), pyrazofurin, 8-azaadenosine, 2-fluoroadenosine, the tricyclic nucleoside, 3-amino-1,5-dihydro-5-methyl-1-β-D-ribofuranosyl-1,4,5,6,8-pentaa-zaacenaphthylene (TCN), bredinine, 9-deazaadenosine, 6-methyl aminopurine riboside (MeAPR), etc. All of these analogs require initial phosphorylation before their biological/ cellular activities are manifested. The enzyme AK which is involved in their phosphorylation, is the major purine nucleoside phosphorylating enzyme of mammalian cells and it carries out the following reaction:[6-9]

$$\begin{array}{c}\text{Adenosine} \\ \text{or} \\ \text{Adenosine} \\ \text{analogs (AA)} \end{array} + \text{ATP} \xrightarrow{\overset{\text{adenosine}}{\text{kinase}}} + \text{AMP (or AA-5}'\text{-monophosphate)} + \text{ADP}$$

Following phosphorylation the phosphorylated derivatives of the above mentioned nu-cleoside analogs affect/participate in diverse cellular reactions and a brief account of the biological effects of some of these analogs is given below.

# II. BIOCHEMICAL EFFECTS OF DIFFERENT NUCLEOSIDE ANALOGS

## A. Toyocamycin, Tubercidin, Sangivamycin, and Tricyclic Nucleoside Pentaazaace-naphthylene

The nucleoside analogs toyocamycin, tubercidin, and sangivamycin (referred to as pyr-rolopyrimidine nucleosides), are 7-deazaderivatives of adenosine (see Figure 1 for chemical structures).[2,4,10,11] These antibiotics were originally isolated form *Streptomyces* cultures and their chemical structures have been elucidated by degradative as well as synthetic methods.[11] These compounds exhibit a broad spectrum of biological activities including antibacterial, antifungal, antiparasitic, antineoplastic, and antiviral.[1,4,5] Because of their close structural relationship to adenosine, these analogs are excellent substrates for AK, but are not subject to phosphorolysis or deamination.[4,8,11-13] After phosphorylation, the phosphorylated derivatives can substitute for AMP, ADP, and ATP, in a wide variety of cellular re-actions.[4,10-12] The metabolism and the mechanism of action of these compounds have been reviewed by Acs and Reich,[10] Suhadolnik,[4,11] and Ritch and Glazer.[12]

Studies with toyocamycin show that its phosphorylated derivatives are rapidly incorporated into RNA which cause selective inhibition of mature rRNA formation.[10-12,14,15] The incor-poration of drug does not have much effect on the processing of 45S RNA to the 38S RNA, but formation of mature 28S and 18S RNA is markedly inhibited.[4,10-12,15] The drug has been reported to interfere with methylation of adenosine residues which could account for the aberrant processing of rRNA.[4]

Tubercidin nucleotides have been shown to be incorporated into both RNA and DNA of mammalian cells.[4,10-12,16] Treatment with the drug leads to pleiotropic effects on cells in-

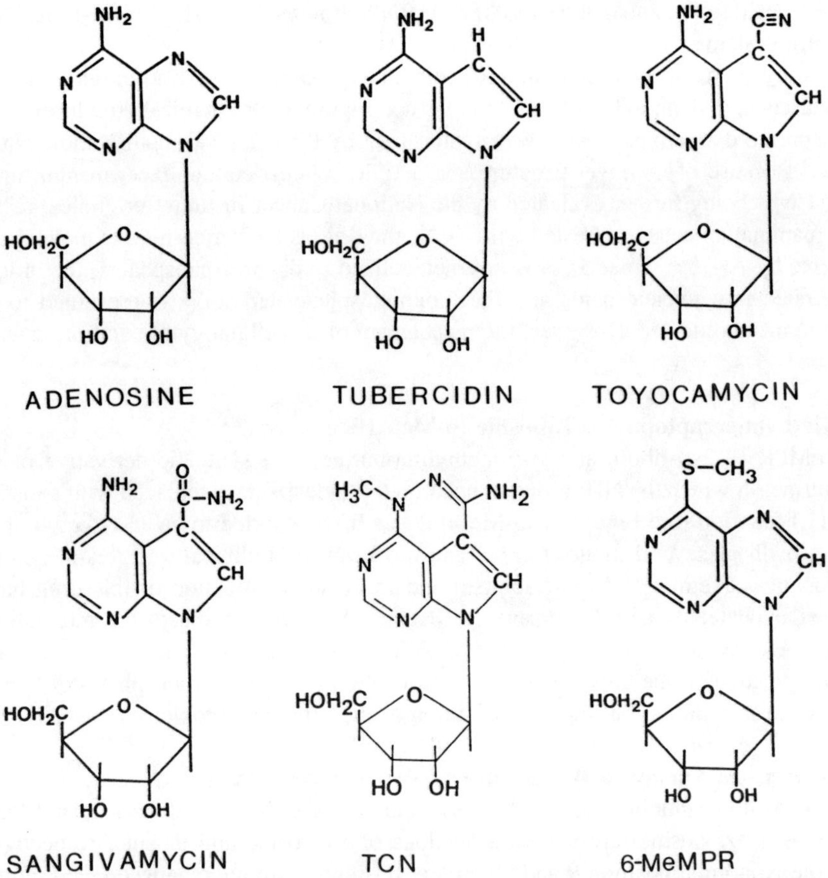

FIGURE 1. Chemical structures of adenosine, and the N-nucleoside analogs tubercidin, toyocamycin, sangivamycin, tricyclic nucleotide (TCN), and 6-methylmercaptopurine riboside (6-MeMPR).

cluding inhibition of protein and nucleic acid biosynthesis, inhibition of rRNA processing,[17] inhibition of methylation of nuclear RNA and tRNA,[18] inhibition of polyamine biosynthesis, inhibition of mitochondrial respiration as well as visible nuclear damage (see Reference 4 and references cited therein). Numerous other effects of tubercidin have been observed in studies where it substitutes for adenosine in either nicotineamide adenine dinucleotide, cyclic AMP, S-adenosylmethionine, or S-adenosyl-homocystein.[4] Studies on the time course of inhibition of macromolecular synthesis by pyrrolopyrimidine nucleosides indicate that in comparison to toyocamycin, which initially caused greater inhibition of RNA synthesis, tubercidin had a more pronounced effect on DNA and protein synthesis.[19,20] Since cytotoxic effects of tubercidin correlate with both inhibition of protein synthesis as well as processing of rRNA,[17] it is unclear which of these effects is primarily responsible for the drug's cytotoxicity.

Sangivamycin, which shows strong antileukemic activity and is currently undergoing clinical trials,[5,21] is incorporated into both RNA and DNA of mammalian cells. Treatment with the drug has been reported to cause inhibition of *de novo* purine synthesis, inhibition of RNA synthesis, and interference with amino acids activation.[4,10-12] In L1210 cells, transcription of several species of messenger RNA (mRNA) is reported to be inhibited by the drug.[22] Recently, it has been reported that sangivamycin is selectively incorporated into polyadenylated RNA, and that the modified mRNA shows a diminished translational capacity in in vitro systems.[23]

The 'tricyclic nucleoside' 3-amino-1,5,-dihydro-5-methyl-1-β-D-ribofuranosyl-1,4,5,6,8-pentaazaacenapthylene (TCN, NSC-154020; see Figure 1 for chemical structure), is also a 7-deazapurine derivatives, which was synthesized by the chemical modification of toyocamycin.[24] Because of its novel structure and activity against certain experimental tumors in vivo, TCN is being further evaluated by the National Cancer Institute for clinical activity.[25] When mammalian cells are treated with TCN, the drug is converted into its monophosphate derivative by AK.[26-28] Since TCN is not metabolized to di- or triphosphates, the drug is not incorporated into nucleic acids and the monophosphate derivative is presumed to be the cytotoxic metabolite.[26-28] However, the mechanism of its cellular cytotoxicity remains to be elucidated.

## B. 6-Methylmercaptopurine Riboside (6-MeMPR)

6-MeMPR (9-β-D-ribofuranosyl-6-methylthiopurine) is a synthetic derivative of 6-mercaptopurine, in which the $NH_2$ group at position 6 of adenosine is replaced with a methylthio ($-SCH_3$) function (see Figure 1). 6-MeMPR has been reported to be an effective inhibitor of the growth of several mouse tumors and has been used clinically in treatment of acute granulocytic leukemia.[29] The metabolism and mechanism of action of this drug has been reviewed by Paterson and Tidd[30] and Le Page.[31] After conversion to the monophosphate form via AK, the drug has been shown to inhibit phosphoribosylamino-transferase, thereby blocking *de novo* purine biosynthesis.[30,31] Intracellularly di- and triphosphates of 6-MeMPR have also been reported but their contribution to the drug's cytotoxicity is unclear.[30,31]

## C. Formycin A, Formycin B, and other C-Nucleoside Analogs

The pyrazolopyrimidine nucleosides formycin A (8-aza-9-deazaadenosine) and formycin B (8-aza-9-deazainosine) are structural analogs of adenosine and inosine, respectively, in which the N-atom at position 9 and C-atom at position 8 are interchanged (see Figure 2 for chemical structures). Unlike adenosine, inosine and most other nucleosides (referred to as N-nucleosides) which possess a N-C glycosyl bond, both formycin A and formycin B contain a C-C glycosyl bond and such compounds are generally referred to as C- nucleosides.[32,33] As a result of this structural difference, these nucleosides are hydrolytically (i.e., hydrolysis of the base from the sugar) stable, and they could also exist in an equilibrium of *syn-anti* forms, which differs from adenosine that exists predominantly in the *anti*-conformation only.[4,32,33] The chemistry, biochemistry, and cellular metabolism of C-nucleosides has been reviewed by Suhadolnik,[4] Daves and Cheng,[32] and Hacksell and Daves.[33]

Formycin A has been shown to be phosphorylated enzymatically to the 5'-mono-, di-, and triphosphates and deaminated to formycin B in mammalian cells.[34] Due to its close structural similarity to adenosine, formycin A derivatives are incorporated in place of adenine nucleotides in a wide variety of cellular reactions including incorporation into DNA, various types of RNA, cAMP, $NAD^+$, etc.[4,32,33] Although the exact mechanism of formycin A cytotoxicity remains to be elucidated, the drug's incorporation into DNA has been reported to correlate closely with its lethal effects on mammalian cells.[35]

Earlier studies on formycin B (7-hydroxy-3-β-D-ribofuranosyl-pyrazolo [4,3-d] pyrimidine), which is an inosine analog, indicated that unlike other nucleoside analogs, formycin B was not phosphorylated in mammalian cells.[34] The drug is a potent inhibitor of aldehyde oxidase and purine nucleoside phosphorylase,[36] although these effects do not appear to be related to the drug's cytotoxicity.[4,32] Since formycin B shows potent growth inhibitory activity against *Leishmania donovani*, a protozoan that causes visceral disease in humans, there has been much interest in its metabolism in *Leishmania* and mammalian species. Recently several groups of investigators have shown that formycin B is phosphorylated to its 5'-monophos-

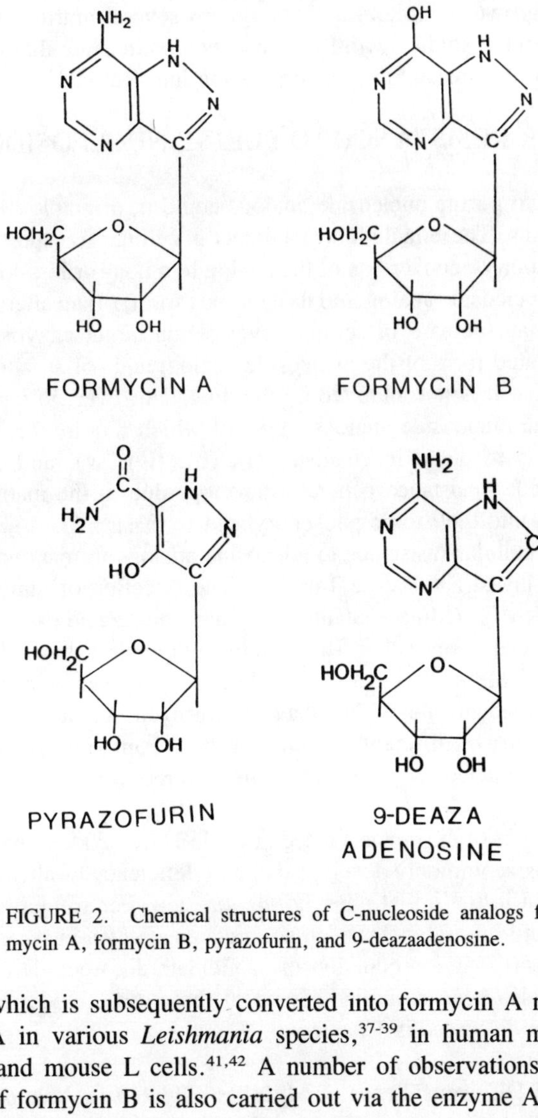

FIGURE 2. Chemical structures of C-nucleoside analogs formycin A, formycin B, pyrazofurin, and 9-deazaadenosine.

phate derivative which is subsequently converted into formycin A nucleotides and incorporated into RNA in various *Leishmania* species,[37-39] in human macrophages,[40] and in Chinese hamster and mouse L cells.[41,42] A number of observations indicate that cellular phosphorylation of formycin B is also carried out via the enzyme AK. These include: (1) increased resistance and reduced phosphorylation of formycin B in AK⁻ mutants of CHO cells,[42] (2) reduced cellular toxicity of formycin B in presence of adenosine which is a more efficient substrate of AK; (3) structural alteration in AK in formycin B-resistant mutants of CHO cells;[43,44] and (4) inhibition of phosphorylation of formycin B by 5-iodotubercidin which is a specific inhibitor of AK.[42] Although it is established that formycin B is phosphorylated, the exact mechanism by which its cytotoxic effects are produced remain unclear at present.

Pyrazofurin (PF) (3,β-D-ribofuranosyl,4-hydroxypyrazole-5-carboxamide) is another C-nucleoside, isolated from cultures of *Streptomyces candidus*, which exhibits a broad spectrum of antiviral as well as antitumor activity.[46] Although PF is not a purine nucleoside analog (see Figure 2 for chemical structure), its phosphorylation is also carried out by AK.[46-48] The 5'-monophosphate of pyrazofurin is a potent and specific inihbitor (Ki = 5 × 10⁻⁹ M) of the pyrimidine biosynthetic pathway enzyme orotidine decarboxylase.[46,48] As a result of this inhibition, cellular toxicity of pyrazofurin is due to pyrimidine nucleotide starvation of cells and can be overcome by addition of either uridine, cytidine, or thymidine.[46] Lim and Klein[49] have recently synthesized another C-nucleoside (viz. 9-deazaadenosine, Figure 2) which shows highly potent growth inhibitory activity against several murine and human leukemia cell lines in vitro. Limited studies with 9-deazaadenosine indicate that its cytotoxicity may result from inhibition of translation via incorporation into RNA.[50,51]

## III. CELLULAR RESISTANCE TO PURINE NUCLEOSIDE ANALOGS

Cellular resistance to purine nucleoside analogs could in principle develop by a number of different mechanisms. These include: (1) a defect in cellular transport of the nucleosides, (2) increased inactivation or conversion of the analog to a non- or less-toxic form; (3) a lack of conversion of the nucleoside analog into its cytotoxic form; (4) an alteration in intracellular nucleotide pools; (5) an increase in cellular level of the target enzyme/function which is inhibited by the activated form of the nucleoside analog; and (6) an alteration in the target enzyme/function so that it is not inhibited by the drug. However, in terms of development of resistance to purine nucleoside analogs, most of which require phosphorylation before they become cytotoxic to cells, mechanisms (i), (ii), (iv), (v), and (vi) have not been commonly encountered. Resistance generally develops due to the inability of the cells to convert these analogs into their toxic phosphorylated forms.[2,52-56]

The mechanism of cellular resistance to adenosine analogs in mammalian cells has been studied by numerous investigators (see Table 1). The selection of mutants resistant to the adenosine analog 6-MeMPR (Mmp$^r$ mutants) in human epidermoid carcinoma cells was first reported by Bennett et al.[6] Since then such studies employing many different purine nucleoside analogs viz. 6-MeMPR, kinetin riboside (KR), toyocamycin, tubercidin, pyrazofurin, bredinin, 2-fluoroadenosine, TCN, ribavirin, formycin A, and formycin B, have been carried out with a number of different cell lines derived from various species. A survey of mutants resistant to the nucleoside analogs that are covered in this review is given in Table 1.

From the characteristics of the mutants listed in Table 1, it is evident that cellular resistance to most of these analogs commonly develops due to a deficiency or alteration in the enzyme AK, which is involved in the initial phosphorylation step. For some of these nucleosides, viz. adenosine, pyrazofurin, arabinosyl adenine, mutants affected in other cellular functions, viz, nucleoside transport,[78] overproduction of orotidylate decarboxylase[79-80] adenosine deaminase,[81] etc. have also been described. Some of these other modes of resistance to the nucleoside analogs are discussed in Chapters 6, 9, and 12.

### A. Characteristics of Different Types of Mutants Affected in Adenosine Kinase

The properties of the mutants resistant to purine nucleoside analogs, which are affected in AK, has been most thoroughly investigated in CHO cells.[19,20-44,62,69,70,72,82-84] Based upon their genetic and biochemical characteristics, three different types of mutants affected in AK have been isolated in CHO cells.[44,82,83] Representative results for two mutants of each of these three groups are presented in Table 2 and Figure 3.

The most common of these mutants (which we refer to as class A) could be selected using any of a number of adenosine analogs including 6-MeMPR, toyocamycin, tubercidin, pyrazofurin, TCN, etc. in different cell types. The characteristics of this class of mutants are

1.   These mutants exhibit high degree of cross resistance to various N-adenosine analogs (e.g., toyocamycin, tubercidin, 6-MeMPR, 8-azaadenosine), as well as C-adenosine analogs (e.g., formycin A, 9-deazaadenosine etc.) which are phosphorylated via AK (Table 2).[44,82,83]

2.   In comparison to the parental cells, the mutant cells show greatly reduced phosphorylation of both N- as well as C-adenosine analogs such as tubercidin and formycin A (Figure 3). However, they are able to phosphorylate adenosine at about 10 to 15%

## Table 1
## SELECTION OF MUTANTS RESISTANT TO PURINE NUCLEOSIDE/ ADENOSINE ANALOGS IN MAMMALIAN CELLS

| Selective drug | Cell line and species | Mutant frequency | Biochemical defect | Ref. |
|---|---|---|---|---|
| 6-MeMPR | Human epidermoid carcinoma | Serial passage | AK deficiency | 6 |
| 6-MeMPR | Ehrlich ascites carcinoma | Serial passage | AK deficiency | 57—59 |
| Kinetin riboside | Mouse sarcoma 180 | Serial passage | AK deficiency | 60 |
| 6-MeMPR | Mouse 3T6 | Serial passage | AK deficiency | 61 |
| | CHO cells | $10^{-3} - 10^{-4}$ | AK deficiency | 19, 62 |
| | Chinese hamster V79 cells | $6.0 \times 10^{-6}$ | AK deficiency | 63, 64 |
| | Human cervical, HeLa cells | $1.0 \times 10^{-6a}$ | AK deficiency | 65 |
| Toyocamycin | Chinese hamster GMA32 cells | Not determined | AK deficiency | 66 |
| | CHO | $0.1 - 2 \times 10^{-3}$ | AK deficiency | |
| | CHW | $2.0 \times 10^{-4}$ | AK deficiency | 19, 62, 64 |
| | V79 | $2 - 10 \times 10^{-6}$ | AK deficiency | |
| | M3-1 | $<1 \times 10^{-7}$ | AK deficiency | |
| | Mouse CAK cells | $5 - 10 \times 10^{-7}$ | AK deficiency | 67 |
| | Mouse terato-carcinoma | $7 \times 10^{-6a}$ | AK deficiency | 68 |
| | Human, HeLa cells | $1 \times 10^{-6a}$ | AK deficiency | 65 |
| Tubercidin | CHO cells | $10^{-3} - 10^{-4}$ | AK deficiency | 19, 62, 69, 70 |
| | HeLa cells | $1.0 \times 10^{-6a}$ | AK deficiency | 65 |
| | V79 cells | $1.0 \times 10^{-6a}$ | AK deficiency | 64 |
| Pyrazofurin | Mouse L5178Y cells | Not reported | AK deficiency | 48 |
| | Morris rat Hepatoma 3924A cells | Not reported | AK deficiency | 71 |
| | CHO cells | $10^{-3} - 10^{-4}$ | AK deficiency | 62 |
| Adenosine | CHO cells | $2.0 \times 10^{-3}$ $2.0 \times 10^{-4}$ | AK deficiency | 72 |
| Bredinin | Mouse mammary carcinoma FM3A cells | $<1.0 \times 10^{-7}$ $5.8 \times 10^{-5a}$ | AK deficiency | 73 |
| 2-Fluoroadenosine | Mouse 3T6 cells | Serial passage | AK deficiency | 74 |
| TCN | Novikoff rat hepatoma cells | Not reported | AK deficiency | 26 |
| Formycin A/ formycin B | CHO cells | $<1 \times 10^{-6}$ $1.0 \times 10^{-5a}$ | AK deficiency | 43 |
| Formycin B | CHO cells | $1 - 5 \times 10^{-6a}$ | Biochemically altered AK | 44 |
| Arabinosyl adenine | Syrian hamster BHK 21 cells; Mouse L1210 cells | $4 - 8 \times 10^{-5}$ | AK deficiency[b] | 75, 76 |
| Ribavirin | CHO cells | Not reported | AK deficiency | 77 |

[a]   Frequency in mutagen-treated cells.
[b]   Mutants affected in other functions are also obtained.

## Table 2
### CROSS RESISTANCE PATTERNS OF REPRESENTATIVE CLASS A (TOY$^r$), CLASS B (FOM$^R$) AND CLASS C (FOM$^r$)AK$^-$ MUTANTS TOWARD SELECTED NUCLEOSIDE ANALOGS

| Nucleoside Analogs | D$_{10}$ value for[a] the WT cells (ng/m$\ell$) | Relative resistance of the mutant cell lines | | | | | |
|---|---|---|---|---|---|---|---|
| | | Toy$^r$4 (A) | Toy$^r$5 (A) | Fom$^R$2 (B) | Fom$^R$4 (B) | Fom$^r$10 (C) | Fom$^r$12 (C) |
| N-Nucleosides | | | | | | | |
| Toyocamycin | 0.4 | 500 | 400 | 1 | 2 | 3 | 5 |
| Tubercidin | 2.0 | 1000 | 1000 | 2 | 3 | 2 | 3 |
| 8-Azaadenosine | 3.0 | >1000 | >1000 | 1 | 1 | N.D.[d] | N.D.[d] |
| 6-MeAPR | 200 | > 500 | > 500 | 2 | 2 | 50 | 70 |
| 6-MeMPR | 250 | > 400 | > 400 | 3 | 3 | 15 | 30 |
| C-Nucleosides | | | | | | | |
| Formycin A | 1.0 | > 500 | > 500 | 70 | 150 | 15 | 20 |
| Formycin-B | 2500 | 2 | 2 | 3 | 8 | 5 | 7 |
| Bbb-73[c] | 2000 | 50 | 50 | > 50 | > 50 | 10 | 55 |
| Bbb-85[c] | 20 | 1250 | >1000 | 100 | 350 | 25 | 70 |
| Pyrazofurin | 15 | 1000 | 1000 | 20 | 45 | 5 | 10 |
| 9-Deazaadenosine | 0.5 | > 200 | > 200 | 30 | 80 | 5 | 15 |
| Tiazofurin | 200 | 1 | 1 | 1 | 1 | 1 | 1 |

[a]   The D$_{10}$ values represent the concentration of the analog which reduces plating efficiency of the cells to 10% of that observed in the absence of any drug.

[b]   Assuming the D$_{10}$ value of an analog for the parental wild-type WT cells as 1, the relative degrees of resistance of the mutant cell lines were determined from the ratios of the D$_{10}$ values of the mutant cell lines compared to the WT cell.

[c]   Bbb-73 — (N$^7$-benzylformycin A) and Bbb-85 — (N$^7$-($\Delta^2$-isopentenyl)formycin A).[89]

[d]   N.D. — not determined.

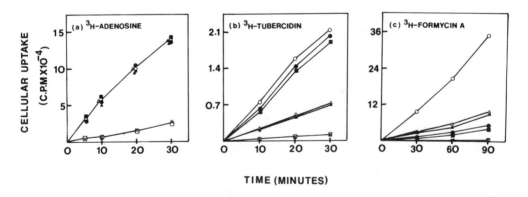

TIME (MINUTES)

FIGURE 3.   Cellular uptake of [$^3$H]-adenosine, [$^3$H]-tubercidin, and [$^3$H]-formycin A by representative Class A (Toy$^r$4 and Toy$^r$5), Class B (Fom$^R$2 and Fom$^R$4), and Class C (Fom$^r$10 and Fom$^r$12) AK mutants.[82,103] (a) [$^3$H]-adenosine; (b) [$^3$H]-tubercidin; (c) [$^3$H]-formycin A. Symbols: (○), WT; (●), Fom$^R$2; (■), Fom$^R$4; (X), Toy$^r$4; (□), Toy$^r$5; (△), Fom$^r$10; (▲), Fom$^r$12.

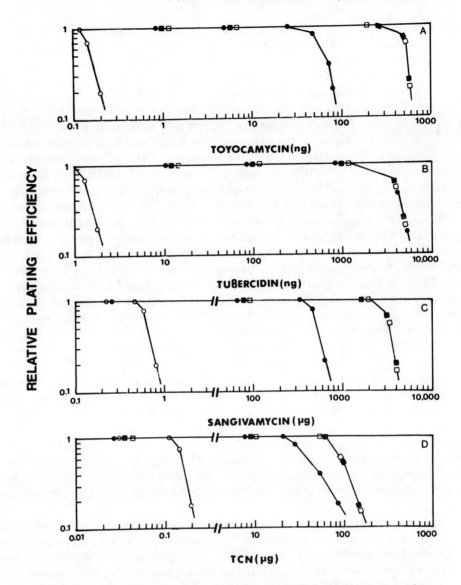

FIGURE 4.   Dose response curves of the parental sensitive cells and the first- and second-step toyocamycin resistant mutants in presence of increasing concentrations (per milliliter of growth medium) of various 7-deazapurine nucleoside analogs.[20] (A), Toyocamycin; (B), tubercidin; (C) sangivamycin; (D), TCN. Symbols: (O), Toy[s] cell line; (●), Toy[r]-16; (□), Toy[rII]-1; (ss), Toy[rII]-2.

of the rate observed in the parental, wild-type (WT) cells.[70,82,83] Plagemann and Wholhueter[70] have shown that this phosphorylation occurs via conversion of adenosine into adenine, which is then metabolized via the enzyme adenine phosphoribosyltransferase (APRT).

3.   Cell extracts of these mutants contain no significant amount (<1% of WT level) of AK activity (Table 1 and Figure 4).[62-70]
4.   The drug resistant phenotype of these mutants behaves recessively in somatic cell hybrids formed with sensitive cells.[19,43,69] In other words, the cell hybrids formed between resistant and sensitive cells contain about 50% of AK activity and are sensitive to the cytotoxic effect of the nucleoside analogs.[19,43,69]

The various properties of the class A mutants are consistent with a genetic lesion that leads to complete loss of the enzymic activity (viz., mutation, deletion, chromosomal loss, or failure of expression of the gene). Based on their reported characteristics, nearly all of the mutants affected in AK (Table 1), except for those selected for formycin A and formycin B, (other exceptions are discussed below) appear to be of this kind. The frequency of class A mutants differs greatly among various cell lines. In CHO cells, the class A mutants are obtained at an unusually high spontaneous frequency of between $1 \times 10^{-3}$ and $1 \times 10^{-4}$.[19,62,69,70,72,73] This high spontaneous mutant frequency is not due to a particular selective drug, as similar high frequency in CHO cells is observed using either toyocamycin, tubercidin, pyrazofurin, or 6-MeMPR as selective agents.[19,62,69,70] Luria-Delbruck fluctuation analysis of the Toy[r] and Tub[r] mutants in CHO cells has established that this type of mutational event occurs spontaneously at a very high rate ($10^{-4}$ to $10^{-5}$ mutations/cell/generation).[19,69] In contrast to CHO cells, in other mammalian cell lines including those derived from Chinese hamster (viz. V79, M3-1), mouse (CAK), and human (HeLa), the frequency of similar mutants is at least 100- to 10,000-fold lower.[19,63-65,67,68] The genetic basis for the large variation in the frequency of this class of mutants in different cell lines is not yet completely clear. However, since the genetic locus for AK has been mapped to an autosome (chromosome 1 in Chinese hamster, chromosome 14 in mouse and chromosome 10 in humans)[67,74,85] variations in the number of functional gene copies for this locus in different cell lines could contribute to the observed differences in mutant frequencies.[86-88] The high spontaneous frequency of AK[−] mutants in CHO cells is also consistent with the presence of a mutational hot spot within the gene (see section C2).[85]

The second type of mutants (class B) resistant to purine nucleoside analogs which are affected in AK have been obtained in CHO cells after selection in presence of formycin A/ formycin B.[43] (Although selection was carried out in presence of formycin A, under the condition employed, i.e., in absence of any adenosine deaminase inhibitor, the drug was gradually converted to formycin B.) In contrast to the unusually high mutant frequency of class A mutants in CHO cells, the class B mutants are obtained at a frequency of $1 \times 10^{-5}$ in mutagen-treated cells, which is comparable to other genetic loci in these cells.[43,48] These mutants (which are also referred to as Fom[R] mutants) exhibit the following characteristics.

1.    The class B (Fom[R]) mutants exhibit increased resistance to various C-nucleosides (viz., formycin A, formycin B, pyrazofurin, 9-deazaadenosine, N[7]-benzylformycin A, and N[7]-($\Delta^2$-isopentenyl)formycin A)[89] which are phosphorylated via AK, but they show no significant cross-resistance to different N-adenosine analogs (viz., toyocamycin, tubercidin, 6-MeMPR, 6-methylamino purine riboside, and 8-azaadenosine) which have been examined (Table 2).[44,82,83] These mutants, however, exhibit no cross resistance to the C-purine nucleoside tiazofurin,[44,82] which is not phosphorylated via AK,[90] indicating that the genetic lesion confers resistance to only those C-nucleosides which are substrates for AK.

2.    The Fom[R] or class B mutants, in accordance with their cross-resistance pattern, show greatly reduced phosphorylation of C-nucleosides (viz., [³H]formycin A) but not N-adenosine derivatives (viz. [³H] adenosine or [³H] tubercidin) (Figure 3).[44,82,83]

3.    The cell extracts from the class B mutants show no measurable activity of the enzyme AK, and in this regard they are similar to the class A mutants.[43,44,82,83] In view of the fact that these mutants phosphorylate N-adenosine derivatives, nearly normally in vivo, complete lack of AK activity in their cell extracts is very surprising. However, all attempts to find AK activity in the mutant cell extracts using various conditions (namely preparation of cell extracts by different means such as sonication, detergent solubilization, hypotonic swelling and homogenizing, growth of cells in suspension culture, preparation and assay of AK activity at different temperatures; varying the concentra-

tions of both [³H] adenosine and ATP in the reaction mixture, using substrate other than adenosine and assaying AK activity in presence of high concentrations of salt, urea, and different detergents in the reaction mixture) have so far proven negative.[43,82,83] Likewise, the presence of an inhibitor of AK in cell extracts of these mutants has also been excluded.[43] The lack of AK activity in the Fom$^R$ mutant cell extracts together with the observed reduced phosphorylation of [³H]formycin A, specific cross resistance to C-nucleosides which are substrate for AK, provide strong suggestive evidence that the genetic lesion in these mutants also affects AK but in a novel manner.

4.    In cell hybrids formed between class B mutants and the sensitive cells, the drug-resistance characteristic of the mutants behaves codominantly, i.e., such hybrid cells retain their resistance towards formycin A/formycin B, despite the fact that they contain 50% of AK activity.[43] The genetic and biochemical basis for the codominant behavior of the class B mutants remains unclear at present. However, the codominant behavior of these mutants could not be readily explained if AK serves only the purine salvage pathway role, which under normal growth conditions is a nonessential function. The above observation could be understood if intracellularly AK exists in a complex form with some other essential enzyme(s) that is inhibited by formycin derivatives. The possibility that the Fom$^R$ mutants may contain two independent genetic lesions, one affecting AK and the other leading to codominant behaviour is highly unlikely.[43]

Although at present the precise nature of the biochemical lesion in the Fom$^R$ (class B) mutants and the basis of their observed specificity for C-nucleosides remains unclear, it is of interest that in contrast to various N-adenosine derivatives which normally exist in *anti*-conformation, the C-nucleosides such as formycin A and pyrazofurin are predominantly present in *syn*-conformation.[4,32,33] Because of this difference in their preferred conformations, it is possible that C-nucleosides interact with a certain specific region or domain of AK which is not important in interaction with N-nucleosides but which may be involved in interaction with other enzymes/cellular functions. If the above presumption is correct, then the genetic lesion in the Fom$^R$ mutants may be affecting this specific domain of AK, thus accounting for altered response toward C-nucleosides as well as other unusual characteristics.

The third group (class C) of mutants resistant to purine nucleoside analogs, and affected in AK, have been selected using the inosine analog formycin B, which recent studies indicate is also phosphorylated via AK in mammalian cells.[42] The formycin B-resistant mutants (Fom$^r$ or class C) are obtained in CHO cells at a frequency of about $1 \times 10^{-5}$ in mutagenized cultures.[44] These mutants, like class A mutants, exhibit increased resistance to both N- as well as C-purine nucleoside analogs, but their degree of resistance is much lower in comparison to the class A mutants (Table 2). Cellular uptake studies with the Fom$^r$ mutants show that [³H]adenosine uptake in the mutants was comparable to the WT cells (Figure 3A), but uptake of both [³H]tubercidin and [³H]formycin A was reduced (Figures 3B and C).[44] However, uptake of the latter nucleosides in these mutants was not as severely affected as seen with the class A mutants. Similar to the class A mutants, the Fom$^r$ mutants show recessive behavior in cell hybrids formed with sensitive cells.[44] However, the distinguishing characteristics of these mutants is that in contrast to class A and B mutants which contain virtually no AK activity in their cell extracts, the class C mutants contain substantial amounts (between 60 to 100% of WT activity) of AK activity in cell extracts.[44] (Of all the mutants listed in Table 1, the only other mutants which were reported to contain significant AK activity in cell extracts were those described by McBurney and Whitmore.[72] However, a later study detected no AK activity in such mutants.)[70] Competition studies between [³H]adenosine and the formycin A analog, Bbb-85 (N$^7$-[Δ²-isopentenyl]formycin A),[89] using AK from either WT or the Fom$^r$ mutant cells show that for equivalent competition of [³H]adenosine phosphorylation, much higher concentrations of Bbb-85 are required when

AK from the mutant cells is employed, as compared to the enzyme from the parental cells.[44] These results provide evidence that in comparison to AK from WT cells, the enzyme from the class C mutants show lower affinity for the adenosine analogs to which the mutants exhibit increased resistance.[44] The genetic lesion in the class C mutants thus seems to directly affect AK in a manner that lowers its affinity for adenosine analogs.

Bennett et al.[92] have reported selection of a human epithelial cell mutant resistant to the adenine analog 4-maino-pyrazolo(3,4-d)pyrimidine (APP) which shows multiple biochemical alterations, including reduced activity of AK. In contrast to other types of mutants affected in AK which show stable drug resistance, the drug-resistant phenotype of this mutant partially reverts when grown in nonselective medium. The mutant exhibited high degree of cross resistance (>200-fold) to 6-MeMPR and APP-ribonucleoside but showed comparatively little resistance toward tubercidin, 6-methylpurine riboside, 2-fluoroadenine, etc.[92] The mutant cells showed reduced phosphorylation of 6-MeMPR and in addition, their cell extracts were found to contain enhanced nucleotide dephosphorylating activity. Based on the above characteristics, cellular resistance to purine nucleoside analogs in this particular mutant seems to result from a combination of several factors, including reduced phoshporylation of nucleosides and increased dephosphorylation of nucleotides.[92]

## B. Immunological Studies with the Mutants

As indicated in the previous section, in contrast to the class B and C mutants which are obtained at frequencies comparable to that observed for other types of mutants (viz., resistance to 6-thioguanine, ouabain, etc.), the spontaneous mutant frequency of the class A mutants is unusually high in CHO cells.[19,62,69,70,72,73] The observed high mutant frequency, together with complete loss of AK activity in all class A mutants, raises the question regarding the nature of the genetic lesion responsible for this mutant phenotype. Such a phenotype could conceivably result from either loss, deletion or silencing of the AK gene, as observed for the mutants affected at the adenine phosphoribosyl transferase (*aprt*) and thymidine kinase (*tk*) loci in CHO cells,[93-97] or it could involve a high frequency mutation within the structural gene for AK that leads to complete loss of the enzymic activity. Studies of Eves and Farber[67] indicate that the selection of AK⁻ mutants (Toy$^r$) in mouse CAK cells is frequently associated with the segregation of part or all of one of the chromosomes (i.e., 14) where AK gene is located. In view of the above observations, to gain insight into the nature of the genetic lesion responsible for the different types of mutants, AK from CHO cells has been purified to homogeneity using affinity chromatography and specific antibodies to it have been raised.[84] This antibody pulls out AK activity, and in immunoblots of WT cell extracts it specifically cross reacts with a protein that has the same electrophoretic mobility and relative molecular mass ($\approx$38,000) as purified AK.

Using this antibody, the presence of AK cross reacting material (CRM) in cell extracts of different mutants has been examined by the immunoblotting technique.[84] These studies have been carried out with a large number of independently selected class A mutants (viz. selected for resistance to either toyocamycin, tubercidin, 6-MeMPR, or pyrazofurin), as well as two Fom$^R$ (class B) and Fom$^r$ (class C) mutants. Results of these studies showed that of the 32 class A mutants examined (eight each of Toy$^r$, Tub$^r$, Pyr$^r$, and Mmp$^r$ type), all except one mutant showed the presence of a similar amount of AK antibody cross-reacting protein, as observed in WT cells. Similar results were obtained with the two class B and C mutants, which were examined. The cross-reacting band had identical electrophoretic mobility in different cell lines and except for one mutant which contained reduced amount of CRM its amount was also comparable in different mutants. Similar results have also been observed with a large number of AK⁻ mutants (Tub$^r$ and Mmp$^r$) of HeLa cells.[116] The presence of equivalent amounts of AK CRM of similar molecular mass in the vast majority of the class A mutants strongly indicate that the high frequency of such mutants in CHO cells is not due to an epigenetic or deletion type of events. Instead, these results indicate that such mutants may contain missense types of mutations within the structural gene for AK. The high frequency of the class A mutants may then be due to either the presence of a "mutational hot spot" within the structural gene for AK, or an AK locus specific "mutator gene" in CHO cells.[84] It is of interest that in contrast to the class A mutants of CHO and HeLa cells which contain equivalent amounts of the CRM, the AK⁻ mutants of BHK cells (Ara A-resistant) have been reported to show complete absence of the cross reacting protein.[98]

## C. Cross-Resistance Studies with Mutants Toward Other Purine and Pyrimidine Derivatives

The cross resistance pattern of mutants resistance to specific purine nucleoside analogs toward other purine/pyrimidine derivatives has been examined by several investigators. Based on their reported characteristics, the mutants which have been investigated in this regard are presumably all of the class A type. A summary of the cross resistance data with the AK⁻ mutants is provided in Tables 3 and 4. Since the primary biochemical defect in the mutants examined is a deficiency of the enzyme AK, these mutants are expected to exhibit increased cross resistance to those nucleoside analogs whose cellular toxicity is dependent upon initial phosphorylation via AK. The nucleoside analogs to which the AK mutants have been shown to exhibit cross resistance are listed in Table 3. The presence of a large number of nucleosides differing considerably in structures in this group is consistent with the broad substrate specificity of AK,[99] and many of these analogs are known to be good substrates for AK.[8] On the other hand, with those analogs whose cellular metabolism/toxicity is not dependent upon AK, the AK⁻ mutants are not expected to show any significant cross resistance to them. Some of the purine/pyrimidine derivatives which have been examined in this regard are listed in Table 4. Many of these analogs are known to be phosphorylated via other enzymes viz. 6-thioguanine or 6-mercaptopurine (hypoxanthine guanine phosphoribosyl transferase),[100] 8-azaadenine, or 2-fluoroadenine (APRT),[101] 5-fluorodeoxyuridine (thymidine kinase),[102] etc., and the lack of cross resistance of the AK⁻ mutants to these analogs is in accordance with this expectation. The cross-resistance studies with the AK⁻ mutants thus provide valuable information whether a given nucleoside analog is metabolized via AK or not.

## D. Selection and Characteristics of Second-Step Mutants Resistant to Toyocamycin

As seen above, the vast majority of mutants resistant to purine nucleoside analogs are affected in the phosphorylating enzyme which carries out the first step in their cellular metabolism. However, studies with these mutants do not provide information regarding the cellular reaction(s) which are inhibited by the activated form(s) of the nucleoside analogs. With the view to obtain information in this regard, attempts have been made to select second-step mutants resistant to some of the nucleoside analogs. In our studies with toyocamycin-resistant (Toyʳ) mutants of CHO cells, it was observed that the mutants obtained after a single-step selection in presence of the drug, which lacked AK, were about 400- to 500-fold resistant to the drug (Figure 4).[19,20] However, despite their high degree of resistance to toyocamycin, the Toyʳ mutants are killed at drug concentrations above 200 ng/mℓ (Figure 4A). This observation made it feasible to carry out a second-step selection in presence of higher concentration (400 ng/mℓ, toyocamycin) of the drug to obtain Toyʳᴵᴵ mutants which are about tenfold more resistant to the drug in comparison to the parental Toyʳ cell line (Figure 4A). The Toyʳᴵᴵ mutants were obtained at a frequency of $1 \times 10^{-6}$ in mutagen-treated cells.[20] Similar to the Toyʳ mutants, the drug-resistant phenotype of the Toyʳᴵᴵ mutants was completely stable during prolonged growth in nonselective medium and behaved recessively in cell hybrids formed with sensitive cells.[20]

To find out whether the genetic lesion in the Toyʳᴵᴵ mutants had affected the residual

## Table 3
## CROSS RESISTANCE PATTERNS OF MUTANTS DEFICIENT IN AK TOWARD OTHER PURINE AND PYRIMIDINE NUCLEOSIDE ANALOGS

| Compound | Relative resistance[a] of the AK-mutants | Mutant[b] Characteristics | Ref. |
|---|---|---|---|
| 6-MeMPR | >200 — 400 | Mmp[r], Toy[r], Tub[r], KR[r], Pyr[r] | 6, 19, 20, 44, 60, 62, 71 |
| Tubercidin | >1000 | Mmp[r], Toy[r], Tub[r], Pyr[r], KR[r] | 6, 19, 20, 44, 60, 62 |
| Toyocamycin | >100 | Toy[r], Tub[r], Mmp[r], Pyr[r], KR[r] | 19, 20, 44, 60, 62 |
| Pyrazofurin | >200 | Toy[r], Tub[r], Mmp[r], Pyr[r] | 19, 44, 62, 71 |
| Sangivamycin | >200 | KR[r], Toy[r], Tub[r] | 10, 60, 103 |
| 7-Deazainosine | >10 | Mmp[r], KR[r] | 6, 60 |
| Kinetin-riboside | >60 | KR[r], Pyr[r] | 60, 103 |
| 4-Aminopyrazolo [3,4-d] pyrimidine ribonucleoside | >300 | Mmp[r] | 6 |
| 6-Hydrazinopurine riboside | >80 | Mmp[r] | 6 |
| Purine ribonucleoside | >100 | Mmp[r], KR[r], Toy[r] | 6, 19, 60 |
| 6-Chloropurine riboside | >10 | Mmp[r], Pyr[r] | 6, 60, 71 |
| 2-Chloroadenosine | >10 | Mmp[r] | 6 |
| Adenosine-1-N-oxide | >50 | Mmp[r] | 6 |
| 6-Ethylthiopurine riboside | >100 | Mmp[r] | 6 |
| 6-Benzylthiopurine riboside | >7 | Mmp[r] | 6 |
| N6-($\Delta^2$-Isopentenyl)adenosine | >18 | KR[r] | 60 |
| N6-Isopropyladenosine | >3 | KR[r] | 60 |
| N6-Allyladenosine | >5 | KR[r] | 60 |
| N6-(*cis*-2-C1-Buten-2-yl)-adenosine | >20 | KR[r] | 60 |
| N6-(*trans*-2-C1-Buten-2-yl)-adenosine | >9 | KR[r] | 60 |
| Puromycin aminonucleoside | >2 | KR[r], Toy[r], Pyr[r] | 60, 103 |
| 8-Azaadenosine | >100 | Toy[r] | 44 |
| 6-Methyl aminopurineriboside | >500 | Toy[r], Tub[r], Mmp[r] | 44, 103 |
| Formycin A | >500 | Toy[r], Tub[r], Mmp[r] | 44, 82, 103 |
| Formycin B | 2 | Toy[r], Tub[r], Mmp[r] | 44, 82, 83, 103 |
| N7-Benzyl formycin A | 50 | Toy[r], Tub[r], Mmp[r] | 44, 82, 83, 103 |
| N7-($\Delta^2$-Isopentenyl)formycin A | >1000 | Toy[r], Tub[r], Mmp[r] | 44, 82, 83, 103 |
| 9-Deazaadenosine | >200 | Toy[r], Tub[r], Mmp[r] | 44, 82, 83, 103 |
| Tricyclic nucleoside (TCN) | >100 | Toy[r], Tub[r], Mmp[r] | 20, 103 |
| N6-Ethenoadenosine | >60 | Pyr[r] | 71 |
| Ribavirin | >10 | Toy[r], Pyr[r], Rib[r] | 77, 82, 83, 103 |
| 6-Mercaptopurine riboside | >10 | Toy[r] | 103 |
| 6-Methyl-2′-deoxyadenosine | >100 | Toy[r], Pyr[r] | 103 |
| 6-Methoxypurine riboside | >100 | Toy[r], Pyr[r] | 103 |
| 9-β-D-Xylofuranosyl adenine | >30 | Rib[r] | 77 |
| 9-β-D-Arabinosyladenine | >2 | Pyr[r], Toy[r] | 71, 103 |
| 6-Benzylaminopurine riboside | >10 | Toy[r], Pyr[r] | 103 |
| Bredinin | >10 | Toy[r], Bredinin-R | 103 |
| N-Dimethyladenosine | >200 | Toy[r], Pyr[r] | 103 |
| 2′-Deoxyadenosine | 5 | Toy[r], Pyr[r] | 103 |

[a] Represents the ratio of the equitoxic concentration of the drugs for the mutant (i.e., AK⁻) cells as compared to the parental sensitive cells.

[b] Indicates the specific drug-resistant mutants whose cross resistance has been examined. The abbreviations for drug-resistant mutants are: Mmp[r], resistant to 6-MeMPR; Toy[r], toyocamycin resistant; Tub[r], tubercidin-resistant, Pyr[r], pyrazofurin-resistant; KR[r], resistant to kinetin riboside; Rib[r], ribavirin-resistant.

**Table 4**
**PURINE/PYRIMIDINE DERIVATIVES**
**EXHIBITING NO CROSS RESISTANCE TO AK-**
**MUTANTS[a]**

| Compounds | Mutants examined[b] | Ref. |
|---|---|---|
| 2-Fluoroadenine | Mmp[r] | 6 |
| 4-Aminopyrazole[3,4-d] pyrimidine | Mmp[r] | 6 |
| 6-Mercaptopurine | Mmp[r] | 6 |
| 6-Mercaptopurine ribo-nucleoside | Mmp[r], KR[r] | 6, 60 |
| 5-Fluorodeoxyuridine | Mmp[r], KR[r] | 6, 19, 60 |
| Cytosine arabinoside | Toy[r], Pyr[r] | 103 |
| 8-Azaadenine | Toy[r], Tub[r] | 19, 44 |
| 8-Mercaptopurine arabinoside | Toy[r] | 103 |
| Hypoxanthine-9-β-arabinoside | Toy[r] | 103 |
| 5-Fluorouracil | Toy[r] | 103 |
| 6-Thioguanine | Toy[r], Pyr[r] | 19, 20 |
| 2-Fluoroadenosine | Mmp[r], KR[r] | 6, 60 |
| 6-Thioguanosine | KR[r], Pyr[r] | 19, 60 |
| 6-Thiopurine deoxyribo-nucleoside | KR[r] | 60 |
| 6-Thioguanine deoxyribo-nucleoside | KR[r] | 60 |
| p-Nitrobenzylthioguanosine | KR[r] | 60 |
| 2,6-Diaminopurine deoxy-ribonucleoside | KR[r] | 60 |
| 5-Fluorouridine | KR[r] | 6 |
| Tiazofurin | Toy[r], Tub[r], Mmp[r] | 44, 82 |
| 6-Chloroguanosine | Toy[r] | 103 |
| 6-Chloropurine riboside | Toy[r] | 103 |

[a]  The mutants examined exhibit no significant cross resistance (i.e., <twofold) to the compounds listed in this table.
[b]  Same as in Table 3.

phosphorylating activity, cellular uptake, and phosphorylation of [³H]adenosine and [³H]tubercidin in the mutant cells was studied. Results of these studies showed that cellular uptake and phosphorylation of these nucleosides was occurring to the same extent in the Toy[rII] mutants as seen in the parental Toy[r] cells.[20] These results provide evidence that the genetic lesion in the second-step mutants does not further affect the phosphorylation of adenosine or its analogs.

To characterize the Toy[rII] mutants, their cross resistance toward a number of other 7-deazapurine nucleosides which included tubercidin, sangivamycin, and TCN was determined. Results of these studies for the parental cell lines and two second-step mutants are shown in Figure 4. As can be seen, in contrast to the Toy[r] mutant which showed corresponding increased resistance to all of these analogs, the second-step Toy[rII] mutants showed no further increase in their resistance for tubercidin but they exhibited a further eight- and twofold resistance to sangivamycin and TCN, respectively. The lack of increased resistance of the Toy[rII] mutants to tubercidin further supports the inference that these mutants are not affected in the nucleoside phosphorylation step and that the mechanism of action of tubercidin differs from that of toyocamycin.[20] The observed specificity of the genetic lesion in the Toy[rII] mutants suggests that these may be altered at a specific site that may be inhibited by toyocamycin metabolites. It is of interest in this regard that the nucleoside analogs to which the Toy[rII] mutants exhibit increased resistance (viz., sangivamycin and TCN) produce similar effects on inhibition of cellular macromolecular synthesis as observed with toyocamycin (i.e., primary effect appears to be on RNA synthesis).[20] In contrast, tubercidin, to which the Toy[rII] mutants do not exhibit increased resistance, has more pronounced effect on DNA and protein synthesis in comparison to its effects on RNA synthesis.[20] Further studies with the Toy[rII] mutants could prove very useful in understanding the mechanism of cellular action of this drug.

## E. Revertant Selection

The ability to select either for or against a particular mutant phenotype has proven very useful in genetic analysis, as demonstrated by studies with mutants affected at the HGPRT locus.[104-106] Similar to the HAT selective medium which selects for HGPRT$^+$ cells or AA medium for selection of APRT$^+$ cells,[107] it is possible in principle to select for AK$^+$ cells in medium containing adenosine, alanosine, and uridine (AAU medium).[74] The rationale of this back selection is based on the observation that alanosine, which is an inhibitor of adenylosuccinate synthetase, inhibits *de novo* conversion of IMP to AMP.[108] The WT (i.e., AK$^+$) cells can survive in alanosine containing medium because of their ability to convert exogenously provided adenosine into AMP. However, cells lacking AK should be unable to utilize the exogenous adenosine and, therefore, should not survive in this medium.[74] Since adenosine at high concentrations is toxic to cells due to feedback inhibition of pyrimidine nucleotide biosynthesis,[109] uridine is added to the medium to ameliorate its toxic effects.[109,110]

Chan et al.[74] have reported the use of AAU selective medium to select for hybrid cells with AK$^+$ phenotype. However, the selection of AK$^+$ revertants from AK$^-$ mutant cells has not yet been reported. In our own studies, despite considerable efforts, we have been unable to select an AK$^+$ revertant using this method (unpublished results). The problem appears to be caused by conversion to adenosine into AMP via other metabolic routes (e.g., phosphorolysis of adenosine into adenine and conversion of the latter into AMP via APRT).[70]

## III. USEFULNESS OF AK$^-$ MUTANT SELECTION SYSTEM IN QUANTITATIVE MUTAGENESIS STUDIES

The selection systems for mutants affected at the AK locus also provides a useful genetic marker for quantitative mutagenesis studies in CHO and HeLa cells.[62,65,111] Some of the salient characteristics of this mutant selection system are as follows.

1.  Mutants affected at the AK locus are readily selected using any of a number of nucleoside analogs viz., 6-MeMPR, toyocamycin, tubercidin, pyrazofurin, etc.[62]
2.  All of the mutants obtained show stable high degree of resistance ($>$100-fold) to the selective analogs and they exhibit similar biochemical phenotype (nearly complete loss of AK activity, i.e., AK$^-$ phenotype).[62,65]
3.  Reconstruction experiments using WT and the mutant (i.e., AK$^-$) CHO and HeLa cells show that in both these systems recovery of AK$^-$ mutants during selection is not adversely affected by cell density of the sensitive cells, up to cell concentration of at least $5 \times 10^5$ cells/100 mm diameter dish.
4.  In both CHO as well as HeLa cells, after treatment with mutagens such as ethyl methanesulfonate (EMS) or ultraviolet light, maximum mutagenic response is observed after an expression period of 7 to 8 days.[62,65] This expression period is similar to that observed for mutants affected at the HGPRT locus, which is currently widely used for mutagenesis studies in mammalian cells.[112,113]

5. Upon treatment of CHO or HeLa cells with a number of different physical and chemical mutagens [viz., UV light, ICR-170, EMS, benzo(a)pyrene (BP)], the frequency of AK⁻ mutants in culture was found to increase in a linear dose-dependent manner. In CHO cells, mutagenic responses of a large number of mutagens and anticancer drugs e.g. EMS, ICR-170, BP, chlorambucil, cis-platin, ellipticine, adriamycin, VM26, VP16-213, etc. at the AK and HGPRT loci, have been compared.[62,111] All of the above agents showed a positive mutagenic response at both HGPRT and AK loci and the mutagenic response of the AK locus was comparable with that of the HGPRT locus. Since many of the above drugs/mutagens induce predominantly either frameshifts or chromosome-breakage type of lesions, the AK⁻ mutant selection system is capable of detecting different types of mutagenic agents causing various types of genetic lesions.[62,111]

The selection system for AK⁻ mutants also forms the basis of a cell culture model system for investigating intercellular communication or metabolic cooperation among cells.[64] This is based upon the observation that when Tub^r (AK⁻) mutants of V79 cells are cocultured with increasing numbers of parental V79 (AK⁺) cells in medium containing tubercidin, then due to metabolic cooperation between AK⁺ and AK⁻ cells, a cell density dependent decline in recovery of the resistant cells is observed. This decrease in plating efficiency of the Tub^r cells is attributed to transfer of toxic phosphorylated metabolites from sensitive (i.e., AK⁺) to resistant (i.e., AK⁻) cells and a similar phenomenon has been observed in cocultures of HGPRT⁺/HGPRT⁻ V79 cells.[114] It has been observed that addition of various phorbol ester tumor promoters (e.g. 12-O-tetradecanoylphorbol 13-acetate) which inhibit metabolic cooperation among cells, to the growth medium in these experiments, markedly enhanced the recovery of the Tub^r mutants.[64] A good correlation was observed in these studies between the relative tumor promoting activity of various phorbol esters and the concentrations at which they inhibited metabolic cooperation in the AK⁺/AK⁻ cell system.[64] Thus the selection system for AK⁻ mutants in V79 cells, could be used to examine the effect of tumor promoters, or to screen for those tumor promoters which may act via inhibiting metabolic coopera-tion.[114,115]

## IV. SUMMARY AND PROSPECTS

Studies reviewed in this chapter show that the purine salvage pathway enzyme adenosine kinase is involved in the phosphorylation of a large number of nucleoside analogs differing considerably in their chemical structure. A gross deficiency or alteration in AK, is shown to be the primary and/or major cause of development of resistance in mammalian cells to the pyrrolopyrimidine nucleosides (viz. toyocamycin, tubercidin, sangivamycin, etc.) pyrazolopyrimidine ribosides (viz. formycin A, formycin B, etc.) and a wide variety of other nucleoside analogs. Several kinds of mutants which affect AK in unique ways have been isolated and further studies with these mutants are expected to provide important insight regarding interaction of specific regions of this important enzyme with different structural features of nucleoside analogs. The unusually high spontaneous frequency of AK⁻ mutants in some cell lines (viz. CHO) suggests the presence of certain unique structural features within this gene, a knowledge of which should prove very useful in understanding the mechanism(s) of genetic variation in mammalian cells. The selection system for the AK⁻ mutants also provides a useful genetic marker for quantitative mutagenesis studies in mammalian cells.

# REFERENCES

1. **Bloch, A.,** Chemistry, biology and clinical uses of nucleoside analogs, *Ann. N.Y. Acad. Sci.,* 255, 269, 1975.
2. **Langen, P.,** *Antimetabolite of Nucleic Acid Metabolism,* Gordon and Breach, New York, 1975, 273.
3. **Roy-Burman, P.,** *Analogues of Nucleic Acid Components: Mechanisms of Action,* Springer-Verlag, New York, 1977, 1.
4. **Suhadolnik, R. J.,** Naturally occurring nucleoside and nucleotide antibiotics, *Prog. Nucleic Acid Res. Mol. Biol.,* 22, 193, 1979.
5. **Robins, R. K. and Revankar, G. R.,** Purine analogs and related nucleosides and nucleotides as antitumor agents, *Med. Res. Rev.,* 5, 273, 1985.
6. **Bennett, L. L., Jr., Schnebli, H. P., Vail, M. H., Allan, P. W., and Montgomery, J. A.,** Purine ribonucleoside kinase activity and resistance to some analogs of adenosine, *Mol. Pharmcol.,* 2, 432, 1966.
7. **Lindberg, N., Klenow, H., and Hansen, K.,** Some properties of partially purified mammalian adenosine kinase, *J. Biol. Chem.,* 242, 350, 1967.
8. **Miller, R. L., Adamczyk, D. L., Miller, W. H., Koszalka, G. W., Rideout, J. L., Beacham, L. M., III, Chao, E. Y., Haggerty, J. J., Krenitsky, T. A., and Elion, G. B.,** Adenosine kinase from rabbit liver. II. Substrate and inhibitor specificity, *J. Biol. Chem.,* 254, 2346, 1979.
9. **Chang, C.-H., Brockman, R. W., and Bennett, L. L., Jr.,** Adenosine kinase from L1210 cells. Purification and some properties of the enzyme, *J. Biol. Chem.,* 255, 2366, 1980.
10. **Acs, G. and Reich, E.,** Tubercidin and related pyrrolopyrimidine antibiotics, in *Antiobiotics,* Vol. 1, Gottleib, D. and Shaw, P. D., Eds., Springer-Verlag, New York, 1967, 494.
11. **Suhadolnik, R. J.,** Pyrrolopyrimidine nucleosides, in *Nucleoside Antibiotics,* Wiley-Interscience, New York, 1970, 298.
12. **Ritch, P. S. and Glazer, R. I.,** Pyrrolo(2,3-d)pyrimidine nucleosides, in *Developments in Cancer Chemotherapy,* Glazer, R. I., Ed., CRC Press, Boca Raton, Fla., 1984, 1.
13. **Agarwal, R. P., Sagar, S. M., and Parks, R. E., Jr.,** Adenosine deaminase from human erythrocytes: purification and effects of adenosine analogs, *Biochem. Pharmacol.,* 24, 693, 1978.
14. **Tavitian, A., Uretsky, S. C., and Acs, G.,** The effect of toyocamycin on cellular RNA synthesis, *Biochim. Biophys. Acta,* 179, 50, 1969.
15. **Cohen, M. B. and Glazer, R. I.,** Comparison of the cellular and RNA-dependent effects of sangivamycin and toyocamycin in human colon carcinoma cells, *Mol. Pharmacol.,* 27, 349, 1985.
16. **Bloch, A., Leonard, R. J., and Nichol, C. A.,** On the mode of action of 7-deaza-adenosine (tubercidin), *Biochim. Biophys. Acta,* 138, 10, 1967.
17. **Cohen, M. B. and Glazer, R. I.,** Cytotoxicity and the inhibition of ribosomal RNA processing in human colon carcinoma cells, *Mol. Pharmacol.,* 27, 308, 1985.
18. **Stern, H. J. and Glazer, R. I.,** Inhibition of methylation of nuclear ribonucleic acid in L1210 cells by tubercidin, 8-azaadenosine and formycin, *Biochem. Pharmacol.,* 29, 1459, 1980.
19. **Gupta, R. S. and Siminovitch, L.,** Genetic and biochemical studies with the adenosine analogs toyocamycin and tubercidin: mutation at the adenosine kinase locus in Chinese hamster cells, *Somat. Cell Genet.,* 4, 715, 1978.
20. **Gupta, R. S. and Mehta, K. D.,** Genetic and biochemical studies on mutants of CHO cells resistant to 7-deazapurine nucleosides: differences in the mechanisms of action of toyocamycin and tubercidin, *Biochem. Biophys. Res. Commun.,* 120, 88, 1984.
21. **Ritch, R. S., Glazer, R. I., Pfaffle, P., Hanson, R., Abrams, R., and Anderson, T.,** Phase I clinical trial of sangivamycin, *Proc. Am. Soc. Clin. Oncol.,* 3, 33, 1984.
22. **Ritch, P. S. and Glazer, R. I.,** Preferential incorporation of sangivamycin into ribonucleic acid in Sarcoma 180 cells in vitro, *Biochem. Pharmacol.,* 31, 259, 1982.
23. **Glazer, R. I. and Hartman, K. D.,** In vitro translational activity of messenger RNA following treatment of human colon carcinoma cells with sangivamycin, *Mol. Pharmacol.,* 24, 509, 1983.
24. **Schram, K. H. and Townsend, L. B.,** The synthesis of 6-amino-4-methyl-8-(β-D-ribofuranosyl) (4-H,8-H) pyrrolo-[4,3,2-de] pyrimido (4,5-C) pyridazine, a new tricyclic nucleoside, *Tetrahedron Lett.,* 49, 4757, 1971.
25. **Mittelman, A., Casper, E. S., Godwin, T. A., Cassidy, C., and Young, C. W.,** Phase I study of tricyclic nucleoside phosphate, *Cancer Treat. Rep.,* 67, 159, 1983.
26. **Plagemann, P. G. W.,** Transport, phosphorylation and toxicity of a tricyclic nucleoside in cultured Novikoff rat hepatoma cells and other cell lines and release of its monophosphate by the cells. *J. Nat. Cancer Inst.,* 57, 1283, 1976.
27. **Bennett, L. L., Jr., Smithers, D., Hill, D. L., Rose, L. M., and Alexander, J. A.,** Biochemical properties of the nucleoside of 3-amino-1,5-dihydro-5-methyl,1,4,5,6,8-pentaazaacenaphthylene (NSC-154020), *Biochem. Pharmacol.,* 27, 233, 1978.

28. **Schweinsberg, P. D., Smith, R. G., and Loo, T. L.,** Identification of the metabolites of an antitumor tricyclic nucleoside (NSC-154020), *Biochem. Pharmacol.*, 30, 2521, 1981.
29. **Montgomery, J. A.,** Studies on the biological activity of purine and pyrimidine analogs, *Med. Res. Rev.*, 2, 271, 1982.
30. **Patterson, A. R. P. and Tidd, D. M.,** 6-Thiopurines, in *Antineoplastic and Immunosuppressive Agents*, Sartorelli, D. C. and John, D. G., Eds., Springer-Verlag, New York, 1975, 384.
31. **LePage, G. A.,** Purine antagonists, in *Chemotherapy*, Vol. 5, Becker, F. F., Ed., 1977, 309.
32. **Daves, G. D., Jr. and Cheng, C. C.,** The chemistry and biochemistry of C-nucleosides, *Prog. Med. Chem.*, 13, 304, 1976.
33. **Hacksell, U. and Daves, G. D.,** The chemistry and biochemistry of C-nucleosides and C-arylglycosides, in *Progress in Medicinal Chemistry*, Vol. 22, Ellis, G. P. and West, G. B., Eds., Elsevier, New York, 1985, 1.
34. **Umezawa, H., Sawa, T., Fukagawa, Y., Homma, I., Ishizuka, M., and Takeuchi, T.,** Studies on formycin and formycin B in cells of Ehrlich carcinoma and *E. coli, J. Antibiot.*, Ser. A, 308, 1967.
35. **Glazer, R. I. and Lloyd, L. S.,** Effects of 8-azaadenosine and formycin on cell lethality and the synthesis and methylation of nucleic acids in human colon carcinoma cells in culture, *Biochem. Pharmacol.*, 31, 3207, 1982.
36. **Stoeckler, J. D., Cambor, C., Kuhns, V., Chu, S. H., and Parks, R. E.,** Inhibitors of purine nucleoside phosphorylase, *Biochem. Pharmacol.*, 31, 162, 1982.
37. **Carson, D. A. and Chang, K.-P.,** Phosphorylation and anti-Leishmanial activity of formycin B, *Biochem. Biophys. Res. Commun.*, 100, 1377, 1981.
38. **Nelson, D. J., LaFon, S. W., Jones, T. E., Spector, T., Berens, R. L., and Marr, J. J.,** The metabolism of formycin B in *Leishmania donovani, Biochem. Biophys. Res. Commun.*, 108, 349, 1982.
39. **Rainey, P. and Santi, D. V.,** Metabolism and mechanism of action of formycin B in Leishmania, *Proc. Natl. Acad. Sci. U.S.A.*, 80, 288, 1983.
40. **Berman, J. D., Rainey, P., and Santi, D. V.,** Metabolism of formycin B by Leishmania amastigotes in vitro. Comparative metabolism in infected and uninfected human macrophages, *J. Exp. Med.*, 158, 1983.
41. **Spector, T., Jones, R. E., LaFon, S. W., Nelson, D. J., Berens, R. L., and Marr, J. J.,** Monophosphates of formycin B and allopurinol riboside. Interactions with Leishmanial and mammalian succino-AMP synthetase and GMP reductase, *Biochem. Pharmacol.*, 33, 1611, 1984.
42. **Mehta, K. D. and Gupta, R. S.,** Involvement of adenosine kinase in the phosphorylation of formycin B in CHO cells, *Biochem. Biophys. Res. Commun.*, 130, 910, 1985.
43. **Mehta, K. D. and Gupta, R. S.,** Formycin B resistant mutants of Chinese hamster ovary cells: a novel genetic and biochemical phenotype affecting adenosine kinase, *Mol. Cell. Biol.*, 3, 1468, 1983.
44. **Mehta, K. D. and Gupta, R. S.,** Novel mutants of CHO cells resistant to adenosine analogs and containing biochemically altered form of adenosine kinase in cell extracts, *Som. Cell. Mol. Genet.*, 12, 21, 1986.
45. **LaFon, S. W., Cohn, N. K., and Nelson, D. J.,** Metabolism of inosine analogs, allopurinol riboside and formycin B in mouse L cells, *Fed. Proc.*, 42, 2006, 1983.
46. **Cadman, E.,** Pyrazofurin, in *Antibiotics*, Vol. 6, Hahn, F. E., Ed., Springer-Verlag, Berlin, 1983, 153.
47. **Plagemann, P. G. W. and Behrens, M.,** Inhibition of de novo pyrimidine nucleotide and DNA synthesis and growth of cultured Novikoff rat hepatoma cells and other cell lines by pyrazofurin. *Cancer Res.*, 36, 380, 1976.
48. **Dix, D. E., Lehman, C. P., Jakubowski, A., Moyer, J. D., and Handschumacher, R. E.,** Pyrazofurin metabolism, enzyme inhibition, and resistance in L5178Y cells, *Cancer Res.*, 39, 4485, 1979.
49. **Lim, M. I. and Klein, R. S.,** Synthesis of 9-deazaadenosine, a new cytolytic C-nucleoside isostere of adenosine, *Tetrahedron Lett.*, 22, 25, 1981.
50. **Glazer, R. I., Hartman, K. D., and Knode, M. C.,** 9-Deazaadenosine. Cytocidal activity and effects on nucleic acids and protein synthesis in human colon carcinoma cells in culture, *Mol. Pharmacol.*, 24, 309, 1983.
51. **Chu, M. Y., Zuckerman, L. B., Sato, S., Crabtree, G. W., Bogden, A. E., Lim, M.-I., and Klein, R. S.,** 9-Deazaadenosine — a new potent antitumor agent, *Biochem. Pharmacol.*, 33, 1229, 1984.
52. **Brockmann, R. W.,** Mechanism of resistance, in *Handbook of Experimental Pharmacology*, Sartorelli, A. C. and John, D. G., Eds., Springer-Verlag, New York, 1979, 352.
53. **Henderson, J. F.,** Analogs of purine and purine nucleosides: biological and biochemical effects, in *Horizons in Biochemistry and Biophysics*, Vol. 4, Quagliariello, E., Palmieri, F., and Singer, T. P., Eds., Addison-Wesley, Reading, Penn., 1984, 130.
54. **Tidd, A. M.,** Antipurines, in *Handbook of Experimental Pharmacology*, Vol. 72, Fox, B. W. and Fox, M., Eds., Springer-Verlag, Berlin, 1984, 445.
55. **Henderson, J. F. and Brockman, R. W.,** Biochemical mechanisms of drug resistance in cancer chemotherapy, in *Pharmacological Basis of Cancer Chemotherapy*, Williams and Wilkins, Baltimore, 1975, 629.

56. **Hakala, M. T.,** Enzyme changes in resistant tissues, in *Drug Resistance and Selectivity: Biochemical and Cellular Basis,* Mihich, E., Ed., Academic Press, New York, 1973, 263.

57. **Caldwell, I. C., Henderson, J. F., and Paterson, A. R. P.,** Resistance to purine ribonucleoside analogues in an ascites tumor, *Can. J. Biochem.,* 45, 735, 1967.

58. **Ho, D. H. W., Luce, J. K., and Frei, E., III,** Distribution of purine ribonucleoside kinase and selective toxicity of 6-methylthiopyurine ribonucleoside, *Biochem. Pharmacol.,* 17, 1025, 1968.

59. **Lomax, C. A. and Henderson, J. F.,** Phosphorylation of adenosine and deoxyadenosine in Ehrlich ascites carcinoma cells resistant to 6-(methylmercapto)purine ribonucleoside, *Can. J. Biochem.,* 50, 423, 1971.

60. **Divekar, A. Y., Fleysher, M. H., Slocum, H. K., Kenny, L. N., and Hakala, M. T.,** Changes in sarcoma 180 cells associated with drug-induced resistance to adenosine analogs, *Cancer Res.,* 32, 2530, 1972.

61. **Chan, T.-S., Ishii, K., Long, C., and Green, H.,** Purine excretion by mammalian cells deficient in adenosine kinase, *J. Cell. Physiol.,* 81, 315, 1973.

62. **Gupta, R. S. and Singh, B.,** Quantitative mutagenesis at the adenosine kinase locus in Chinese hamster ovary cells. Development and characteristics of the selection system, *Mutation Res.,* 113, 441, 1983.

63. **Thacker, J.,** Resistance to methyl mercaptopurine riboside in cultured hamster cells, *Mutation Res.,* 74, 37, 1979.

64. **Gupta, R. S., Singh, B., and Stetsko, D. K.,** Inhibition of metabolic cooperation by phorbol esters in a cell culture system based on adenosine kinase deficient mutants of V79 cells, *Carcinogenesis,* 6, 1359, 1985.

65. **Murray, W. and Gupta, R. S.,** Mutants of HeLa cells resistant to the adenosine analogs toyocamycin, tubercidin and 6-methylmercaptopurine riboside: a potential genetic marker for quantitative mutagenesis studies in human cells, *Can. J. Genet. Cytol.,* 576, 1984.

66. **Debatisse, M. and Buttin, G.,** The control of cell proliferation by preformed purines: a genetic study. I. Isolation and preliminary characterization of Chinese hamster lines with single or multiple defects in purine "salvage" pathways, *Som. Cell Genet.,* 3, 497, 1977.

67. **Eves, E. M. and Farber, R. A.,** Chromosome segregation is frequently associated with the expression of recessive mutations in mouse cells, *Proc. Natl. Acad. Sci. U.S.A.,* 78, 1768, 1981.

68. **Gupta, R. S. and Hodgson, M.,** Genetic markers in mouse teratocarcinoma cells. Selection and partial characterization of mutants resistant to toyocamycin, DRB and podophyllotoxin, *Exp. Cell Res.,* 132, 496, 1981.

69. **Rabin, M. S. and Gottesman, M. M.,** High frequency of mutation to tubercidin resistance in CHO cells, *Som. Cell Genet.,* 5, 571, 1979.

70. **Plagemann, P. G. W. and Wohlhueter, R. M.,** Adenosine metabolism in wild-type and enzyme-deficient variants of Chinese hamster ovary and Novikoff rat hepatoma cells, *J. Cell. Physiol.,* 116, 236, 1983.

71. **Suttle, D. P., Harkrader, R. J., and Jackson, R. C.,** Pyrazofurin-resistant hepatoma cells deficient in adenosine kinase, *Eur. J. Cancer,* 17, 43, 1984.

72. **McBurney, M. W. and Whitmore, G. F.,** Mutants of Chinese hamster cells resistant to adenosine, *J. Cell. Physiol.,* 85, 87, 1974.

73. **Koyama, H. and Tsuji, M.,** Genetic and biochemical studies on the activation and cytotoxic mechanism of bredinin, a potent inhibitor of purine biosynthesis in mammalian cells, *Biochem. Pharmacol.,* 32, 3547, 1983.

74. **Chan, T.-S., Creagan, R. P. and Reardon, M. P.,** Adenosine kinase as a new selective marker in somatic cell genetics: isolation of adenosine kinase-deficient mouse cell lines and human-mouse hybrid cell lines containing adenosine kinase, *Som. Cell Genet.,* 4, 1, 1978.

75. **Chan, V. L. and Juranka, P.,** Isolation and preliminary characterization of 9-β-D-arabinofuranosyladenine-resistant mutants of baby hamster cells, *Som. Cell Genet.,* 7, 147, 1981.

76. **Cass, C. E., Selner, M., and Phillips, J. R.,** Resistance to 9-β-D-arabinofuranosyladenine in cultured leukemia L1210 cells, *Cancer Res.,* 43, 4791, 1983.

77. **Harris, B. A., Saunders, P. P., and Plunkett, W.,** Metabolism of 9-β-D-xylofuranosyladenine by the Chinese hamster ovary cells, *Mol. Pharmacol.,* 20, 200, 1981.

78. **Cohen, A., Ullman, B., and Martin, D. W., Jr.,** Characterization of a mutant mouse lymphoma cell with deficient transport of purine and pyrimidine nucleosides, *J. Biol. Chem.,* 254, 112, 1979.

79. **Suttle, D. P. and Stark, G. R.,** Coordinate overproduction of orotate phosphoribosyltransferase and orotidine-5'-phosphate-decarboxylase in hamster cells resistant to pyrazofurin and 6-azauridine, *J. Biol. Chem.,* 254, 4602, 1979.

80. **Levinson, B. B., Ullman, B., and Martin, D. W., Jr.,** Pyrimidine pathway variants of cultured mouse lymphoma cells with altered levels of both orotate phosphoribosyl transferase and orotidylate decarboxylase, *J. Biol. Chem.,* 254, 4396, 1979.

81. **Fernandez-Mejia, C., Debatisse, M., and Buttin, G.,** Adenosine-resistant Chinese hamster fibroblast variants with hyperactive adenosine-deaminase: An analysis of the protection against exogenous adenosine afforded by increased activity of the deamination pathway, *J. Cell. Physiol.,* 120, 321, 1984.

82. **Mehta, K. D. and Gupta, R. S.,** Chinese hamster ovary cell mutants specifically affected in the phosphorylation of C-purine nucleosides, *Can. J. Biochem. Cell Biol.,* 63, 10-44, 1985.
83. **Gupta, R. S. and Mehta, K. D.,** Genetic and biochemical characteristics of three different types of mutants of mammalian cells affected in adenosine kinase, in *Purine and Pyrimidine Metabolism in Man,* Vol. 5, Part B, Nyhan, W. L., Thompson, L. F., and Watts, R. W. E., Eds., Plenum Press, New York, 1986, 595.
84. **Gupta, R. S. and Mehta, K. D.,** Immunological studies with different classes of mutants affected at the adenosine kinase locus in CHO cells, *Som. Cell. Mol. Genet.,* 12, 265, 1986.
85. **Dhar, V., Searle, B. M., and Athwal, R. S.,** Transfer of Chinese hamster chromosome 1 to mouse cells and regional assignment of 7 genes: a combination of gene transfer and microcell fusion, *Som. Cell. Mol. Genet.,* 10, 547, 1984.
86. **Siminovitch, L.,** On the nature of hereditable variation in cultured somatic cells, *Cell,* 7, 1, 1976.
87. **Gupta, R. S., Chan, D. H. Y., and Siminovitch, L.,** Evidence obtained by segregation analysis for functional hemizygosity at the Emt$^r$ locus in CHO cells, *Cell,* 14, 1007, 1978.
88. **Campbell, C. E. and Worton, R. G.,** Evidence obtained by induced mutation frequency analysis for functional hemizygosity at the *emt* locus in CHO cells, *Som. Cell Genet.,* 5, 51, 1979.
89. **Robins, M. J. and Trip, E. M.,** Sugar-modified N$^6$-(3-methyl-2-butenyl) adenosine derivatives, N$^6$-benzyl analogs and cytokinine-related nucleosides containing sulfur or formycin, *Biochemistry,* 12, 2179, 1973.
90. **Saunders, P. P., Kuttan, R., Lai, M. M., and Robins, R. K.,** Action of 2-β-D-ribofuranosylthiazole-4-carboxamide (tiazofurin) in Chinese hamster ovary and variant cell lines, *Mol. Pharmacol.,* 23, 534, 1983.
91. **Prusimer, P., Brennan, T., and Sunderalingam, M.,** Crystal structure and molecular conformation of formycin monohydrates. Possible origin of the anomalous circular dichroic spectra in formycin mono- and polynucleotides, *Biochemistry,* 12, 1196, 1973.
92. **Bennett, L. L., Jr., Allan, P. W., Smithers, D., and Vail, M. H.,** Resistance to 4-aminopyrazolo-(3,4-d)pyrimidine, *Biochem. Pharmacol.,* 18, 725, 1969.
93. **Bradley, W. E. C.,** Reversible inactivation of autosomal alleles in Chinese hamster cells, *J. Cell. Physiol.,* 101, 325, 1979.
94. **Bradley, W. E. C. and Letovanec, D.,** High-frequency nonrandom mutational event at the adenine phosphoribosyltransferase (*aprt*) locus of sib-selected CHO variants heterozygous for *aprt, Som. Cell Genet.,* 8, 51, 1982.
95. **Simon, A. E. and Taylor, M. W.,** High-frequency mutation at the adenine phosphoribosyl transferase locus in Chinese hamster ovary cells due to deletion of the gene, *Proc. Natl. Acad. Sci. U.S.A.,* 80, 810, 1983.
96. **Simon, A. E., Taylor, M. W., Bradley, W. E. C., and Thompson, L. H.,** Model involving gene inactivation in the generation of autosomal recessive mutants in mammalian cells in culture, *Mol. Cell. Biol.,* 2, 1126, 1982.
97. **Adair, G. M., Stallings, R. L., Nairn, R. S., and Siciliano, M. J.,** High-frequency structural gene deletion as the basis for functional hemizygosity of the adenine phosphoribosyltransferase locus in Chinese hamster ovary cells, *Proc. Natl. Acad. Sci. U.S.A.,* 80, 5961, 1983.
98. **Juranka, P. and Chan, V.-L.,** Analysis of adenosine kinase mutants of baby hamster kidney cells using affinity purified antibody, *J. Biol. Chem.,* 260, 7738, 1985.
99. **Bennett, L. L., Jr. and Hill, D. L.,** Structural requirement for activity of nucleosides as substrates for adenosine kinase: orientation of substituents on the pentafuranosyl ring, *Mol. Pharmacol.,* 11, 803, 1975.
100. **Morrow, J.,** Cellular resistance to guanine and hypoxanthine analogs, in *Drug Resistance in Mammalian Cells,* Gupta, R. S., Ed., CRC Press, Boca Raton, Fla., 1987,
101. **Taylor, M. J.,** Cellular resistance to adenine analogs, in *Drug Resistance in Mammalian Cells,* Gupta, R. S., Ed., CRC Press, Boca Raton, Fla., 1987,
102. **Kaufman, E.,** Cellular resistance to various halogenated pyrimidine derivatives, in *Drug Resistance in Mammalian Cells,* Gupta, R. S., Ed., CRC Press, Boca Raton, Fla., 1987,
103. **Gupta, R. S. and Mehta, K. D.,** unpublished results.
104. **Szybalski, W., Szybalska, E. H., and Ragni, G.,** Genetic studies with human cell lines, *Nat. Cancer Inst. Monogr.,* 7, 75, 1962.
105. **Littlefield, J. W.,** Selection of hybrids from matings of fibroblasts *in vitro* and their presumed recombinants, *Science,* 145, 709, 1964.
106. **Caskey, C. T. and Kruh, G. D.,** The HPRT locus, *Cell,* 16, 1, 1979.
107. **Kusano, T., Long, C., and Green, H.,** A new reduced human-mouse somatic cell hybrid containing the human gene for adenine phosphoribosyl transferase, *Proc. Natl. Acad. Sci. U.S.A.,* 68, 82, 1971.
108. **Graff, J. C. and Plagemann, P. G. W.,** Alanosine toxicity in Novikoff rat hepatoma cells due to inhibition of the conversion of inosine monophosphate to adenosine monophosphate, *Cancer Res.,* 36, 1428, 1976.
109. **Ishii, K. and Green, H.,** Lethality of adenosine for cultured mammalian cells by interference with pyrimidine biosynthesis, *J. Cell Sci.,* 13, 429, 1973.

110. **Gupta, R. S.,** A novel synergistic effect of alanosine and guanine on adenine nucleotide synthesis in mammalian cells: alanosine as a useful probe for investigating purine nucleotide metabolism, *J. Cell. Physiol.,* 104, 241, 1980.

111. **Singh, B. and Gupta, R. S.,** Comparison of the mutagenic responses of 12 anticancer drugs at the hypoxanthine-guanine phosphoribosyltransferase and adenosine kinase loci in Chinese hamster ovary cells, *Environ. Mutations,* 5, 271, 1983.

112. **O'Neill, J. P., Couch, D. B., Machanoff, R., San Sebastian, J. R., Brimer, P. A., and Hsie, A. W.,** A quantitative assay of mutation induction at the hypoxanthine-guanine phosphoribosyltransferase locus in Chinese hamster ovary cells (CHO/HGPRT system); utilization with a variety of mutagenic agents, *Mutation Res.,* 45, 103, 1977.

113. **Gupta, R. S.,** Genetic markers for quantitative mutagenesis studies in CHO cells: applications to mutagen screening studies, in *Handbook of Mutagenicity Test Procedures,* Kilbey, B. J., Legator, M., Nichols, W., and Ramel, C., Eds., Elsevier, New York, 1984, 291.

114. **Yotti, L. P., Chang, C. C., and Trosko, J. E.,** Elimination of metabolic cooperation in Chinese hamster cells by a tumor promoter, *Science,* 206, 1089, 1979.

115. **Trosko, J. E., Chang, C. C., and Medcalf, A.,** Mechanism of tumor promotion: Potential role of intercellular communication, *Cancer Invest.,* 1, 511, 1983.

116. **Gupta, R. S. and Murray, W.,** unpublished results.

Chapter 8

## ADENINE ANALOGS

**M. W. Taylor and A. Sahota**

## TABLE OF CONTENTS

I.      Introduction ................................................................ 112

II.     Adenine Metabolism ....................................................... 112

III.    Adenine Toxicity .......................................................... 113

IV.    Adenine Analogs and Their Mechanisms of Action ........................... 114
      A.     2,6-Diaminopurine (DAP) and 8-Azaadenine (AA) ..................... 117
      B.     Halogenated Adenines ................................................ 118
      C.     4-Aminopyrazolo(3,4-d)Pyrimidine .................................... 118
      D.     Bredenin and its Derivatives ........................................ 119
      E.     2-Aminopurine and 6-N-Hydroxylaminopurine ......................... 119

V.     Collateral Sensitivity ...................................................... 119

VI.    Selection of Mutants Resistant to Adenine Analogs .......................... 120

VII.   Concluding Remarks ....................................................... 120

References .................................................................... 121

# I. INTRODUCTION

This chapter will confine itself to resistance of cultured mammalian cells to adenine analogs. The main topics discussed are (1) metabolism and toxicity of adenine; (2) metabolism, toxicity, and mechanisms of action of adenine analogs; (3) mechanisms of resistance to these compounds; (4) the selection of drug resistant mutants; and (5) collateral sensitivity. We will not discuss analogs of adenine nucleosides or nucleotides, or other agents that affect adenine metabolism. Some of these compounds are described elsewhere in this volume.

# II. ADENINE METABOLISM

Although adenine is the most widely distributed purine in nature, it does not occur as the free base but is found mainly in nucleic acids and nucleotides. Free adenine is not an intermediate in the biosynthesis or degradation of adenine nucleotides and it is not known to have any cellular functions. Unlike hypoxanthine and guanine, no significant pathway for the formation of adenine via purine nucleoside phosphorylase (EC 2.4.2.1) has been demonstrated in mammalian or human cells.[1-4] The most likely source of endogenous adenine appears to be 5′-methylthioadenosine, a by-product of polyamine synthesis.[5,6]

The metabolism of exogenous adenine has been studied extensively in mammalian cells.[7] At low concentration ($<10$ μ$M$) adenine is rapidly converted into AMP by adenine phosphoribosyltransferase (APRT, E.C. 2.4.2.7) in the presence of 5-phosphoribosyl-1-pyrophosphate (PRPP) (salvage synthesis), but at higher concentrations a large percentage of the adenine remains unmetabolized.[3] Nucleotide synthesis at higher concentrations appears to be limited by the availability of PRPP.[8]

In prokaryotes and lower eukaryotes, adenine can be deaminated to hypoxanthine by adenine aminohydrolase (E.C. 3.5.4.2), but this enzyme has not been demonstrated in higher eukaryotes.[9] At high concentrations, adenine is oxidized by xanthine oxidase (E.C. 1.3.2.3.) to 2,8-dihydroxyadenine, an adenine metabolite characterized by extremely low solubility.[10] Thus, under normal conditions the only enzyme likely to be involved in adenine metabolism is APRT. This enzyme has been extensively purified from many mammalian tissues, and Km values of 1 μ$M$ for adenine and 5 μ$M$ for PRPP have been reported.[11,12] In addition to adenine, many adenine analogs are substrates for APRT.

In addition to salvage synthesis from adenine, AMP is also formed by a *de novo* pathway. Most cell types possess both the *de novo* and salvage pathways, and there is a close interaction between the two. Mammalian erythrocytes and platelets lack the ability to synthesize purine ribonucleotides *de novo*, and are thus dependent on the salvage pathway for their nucleotide requirements.[13] The *de novo* pathway can also be blocked by purine antimetabolites such as azaserine, alanosine, or aminopterin, making the cells dependent on the salvage pathway.[14] This is of great experimental value and is the basis of selection for revertants at the APRT and hypoxanthine-guanine phosphoribosyltransferase (HGPRT, E.C. 2.4.2.8) loci in cultured cells.

Transport of adenine into mammalian cells does not appear to be linked to its conversion to AMP.[16] Zylka and Plagemann[17] showed that in cultured Novikoff cells, adenine at low concentrations was transported by a carrier-mediated process, but at higher concentrations adenine gained entry by simple diffusion. Evidence was also presented that the transport system of adenine was different from that for hypoxanthine and guanine. Witney and Taylor[18] demonstrated that adenine is transported by facilitated diffusion in cultured Chinese hamster fibroblasts. Studies with mutants with partial or negligible APRT activity showed that adenine did not accumulate against a concentration gradient. These studies suggest that adenine is transported as the free base and is subsequently phosphoribosylated by APRT.

The regulation of adenine metabolism has been studied extensively at the nucleotide level, for it is principally at this level that adenine participates in intermediary metabolism. The factors or mechanisms which may potentially regulate adenine metabolism have been reviewed[11,15] and will not be discussed here.

## III. ADENINE TOXICITY

The first observation of purine toxicity was made by Wilson[19] who showed that adenine was toxic to Drosophila larvae. Since then there has been extensive research into the phenomenon of adenine toxicity.[7] Adenine toxicity, as measured by inhibition of cell growth, has been observed in a variety of cell types from human and other mammalian sources. Various parameters have been used as indicators of cell growth, including cell number, protein content, and microscopic examination of monolayers. In some cases, cell viability has also been studied by colony formation techniques. Growth of lymphocyte cultures is usually assayed by measuring thymidine uptake following blastogenesis.

Three studies have compared adenine toxicity in parental sensitive cell lines, and in cell lines resistant to adenine analogs. Blair and Hall[20] used mouse L-cells and a 2,6-diaminopurine resistant L-cell line. (See later for a discussion of 2,6-diaminopurine resistance.) The relative APRT activity in the two lines was 253 and 0.6 U, respectively. However, the uptake of adenine by intact cells was only seven- to ninefold higher in the parental than in the mutant cell lines. The concentration of 2,6-diaminopurine required for 50% inhibition was related to APRT activity. This was 9.0 $\mu M$ for the parental, and 471 $\mu M$ for the mutant cell line. Similar results were found with 8-azaadenine. Thus these analogs must be converted into nucleotides to exert their toxic effects. In contrast, the inhibitory dose for adenine for the parental and mutant lines was 148 and 202 $\mu M$, respectively. This would suggest that adenine itself was toxic, and that conversion to a nucleotide was not required for toxicity.

Debatisse and Buttin[21,22] studied 8-azaadenine resistant Chinese hamster lung fibroblast lines lacking detectable APRT activity. The mutants incorporated about 1% of the labeled adenine compared to control cells. In studies parallel to these[20], 0.3 m$M$ adenine inhibited cell growth completely in the parental lines as did 1 m$M$ adenine in the mutant lines. Unfortunately no other concentrations of adenine were tested, leaving open the question as to whether adenine itself was the toxic agent.

Hershfield et al.[23] studied adenosine kinase (E.C. 2.7.1.20) and APRT mutants of the W1-L2 line of human lymphoblasts. Despite high levels of resistance to 6-methylthioinosine (2 $\mu M$) or 2,6-diaminopurine (20 $\mu M$), both cell lines were as sensitive as parental cells to adenosine or adenine. Adenine toxicity was unaltered in lymphoblasts which had lost >99% of their APRT activity, suggesting that the base itself was toxic. As a possible explanation of their results, the authors suggested that interaction between adenine and purine receptors on the cell surface may mediate the toxic effect on the cell. Adenosine is much more toxic than adenine, and most studies on toxicity have been done with this nucleoside.[7]

It is generally assumed that adenine is not directly toxic but that a nucleotide byproduct is the source of cell death or growth inhibition.[7] In support of this, Green and Martin[24] described an adenine-resistant human fibroblast, which they concluded had altered regulation of PRPP synthetase (E.C. 2.7.6.1). Debatisse and Buttin[22] showed that adenine inhibited PRPP synthesis in Chinese hamster fibroblasts. Snyder et al.[8] showed lowered PPRP concentrations in cultured human lymphoblasts grown in toxic levels of adenine. However, similar findings have been reported for hypoxanthine, a nontoxic purine.

It is now generally accepted that the nucleotides AMP and GMP affect PPRP levels by feedback inhibition.[15] If inhibition of PRPP synthesis by feedback from adenine nucleotides was the reason for adenine toxicity with a resulting imbalance in nucleotide pools, addition of pyrimidines might be expected to overcome this effect. However, addition of uridine did not alter adenine toxicity. Other studies[25] have provided evidence that adenine toxicity mediated by nucleotides may be affected by conversion of adenine to guanine nucleotides, since coformycin and deoxycoformycin enhanced the toxic effect of adenine. Coformycin inhibits both adenosine deaminase (E.C. 3.5.4.4) and adenylate deaminase (E.C. 3.5.4.6) in Chinese hamster lung cells.[25] That adenine toxicity in *E. coli* is the result of an imbalance in guanine nucleotide pools has also been reported.[26]

The finding that adenine toxicity occurs in the absence of APRT might be due to an alternate pathway for conversion of adenine to nucleotides. In the yeast *Saccharomyces cerevisae* such a pathway has been found, namely, adenine aminohydrolase.[27] This enzyme is inducible and only found if the yeast is grown in high adenine concentrations. The recent reports of Turker and Martin[28] and Turker et al.,[29] showing "pseudorevertants" of APRT deficient cells can best be explained by an alternative pathway for adenine utilization, since adenine uptake occurred in these 2,6-diaminopurine resistant cells in the absence of detectable APRT activity.

## IV. ADENINE ANALOGS AND THEIR MECHANISMS OF ACTION

All drug resistance to adenine analogs in mammalian cells appears to be a result of the loss or defect of the purine salvage enzyme APRT. All available evidence suggests that this is the only enzyme in mammalian cells that can utilize free adenine as a substrate. This enzyme can also use adenine analogs as substrates (often, however, with much higher $K_i$ values). Table 1 gives the $K_i$ values for various purine analogs for monkey APRT[30] and Figure 1 the structures of some of these compounds. Once converted by APRT to a nucleotide, these analogs are often toxic, and may affect other enzymes of the salvage or *de novo* pathway. Krenitsky et al.[30] carried out an extensive study of the binding kinetics of Rhesus monkey liver APRT to purine analogs. In these studies, adenine was bound 40 times better than the most effective analog. The apparent Km for adenine (1 $\mu M$ at 0.25 m$M$ PRPP) was only slightly higher than the $K_i$. Replacement of one of the amino hydrogens by an amino or hydroxyl group, gave compounds that still bound the enzyme fairly well. Methylation, dimethylation, or alkylation of the 6-amino group resulted in a 100-fold or more decrease in binding (Table 1). Other 6-substituted purines, e.g., chloro-, cyano-, carboxy-, carboxamido-, and hydroxy- were even more poorly bound by the enzyme.

Adenine derivatives substituted at position 2 with chloro-, amino, methylamino-, dimethylamino-, thio-, or methyl-derivatives also showed weak binding to APRT. Methylation of the purine ring of adenine typically diminished enzyme binding, although substitutions at position 8 were less deleterious to binding than other substitutions.

Interestingly enough, the analogs most frequently used to select for resistant cells, 2,6-diaminopurine and 8-azaadenine bind the enzyme very poorly ($K_i$ of >1 m$M$). Krenitsky et al.[30] suggest that enzymes have two types of specificity: the effectiveness with which a potential substrate is bound to the active site of the enzyme, and the rate at which the substrate undergoes reaction once binding has occurred. 2,6-Diaminopurine binds very poorly, but once bound reacts rapidly. Thus in order to predict whether a particular adenine analog may be useful in selecting mutants, one must not only examine binding, but also the rate of ribonucleotide formation. A comparison of the rate of nucleotide formation from some purines is presented in Table 2.

A point of continuing discussion is whether adenine analogs must be converted to nucleotide derivatives in order to function as toxic compounds in the cell, either by inhibiting *de novo* purine biosynthesis or by some other mechanism. Le Page and Jones[31] found in a variety of tumors that nucleotide formation and inhibitory activity were related. Others[32,33] have shown that purine analogs were inactive in cells lacking the ability to convert them to nucleotides. However, as discussed above under adenine toxicity, it has been reported[15] that drug nucleotide synthesis may not be necessary for its inhibitory effects on *de novo* purine

## Table 1
## INHIBITION CONSTANTS OF PURINES AND PURINE ANALOGS OF MONKEY ADENINE PHOSPHORIBOSYLTRANSFERASE

| Inhibitor | 6-Purine substituent | 2-Purine substituent | $K_i \times 10^3$ at 38°C and pH 7.7 |
|---|---|---|---|
| Purine | H | H | 0.46 |
| Adenine | $NH_2$ | H | 0.00069[a] |
| 6-Methylaminopurine | $NHCH_3$ | H | 0.091 |
| 6-Ethylaminopurine | $NHC_2H_5$ | H | 0.19 |
| 6-n-Propylaminopurine | $NHC_3H_7$ | H | 0.13 |
| 6-n-Butylaminopurine | $NHC_4H_9$ | H | 0.59 |
| 6-n-Pentylaminopurine | $NHC_5H_n$ | H | >1 |
| 6-Dimethylaminopurine | $N(CH_3)_2$ | H | >1 |
| 6-Anilinopurine | $NHC_6H_5$ | H | >1 |
| 6-Benzylaminopurine | $NHCH–C_6H_5$ | H | >1 |
| 6-β-Phenylethylaminopurine | $NHC_2H_4–C_6H_5$ | H | >1 |
| 6-Isopropylaminopurine | $NHCH(CH_3)_2$ | H | >1 |
| 6-Isopentylaminopurine | $NHC_2H_4CH(CH_3)_2$ | H | >1 |
| 6-Isopentenylaminopurine | $NHC_2H_4C–(CH_3)=CH_2$ | H | >1 |
| 6-N-Hydroxylaminopurine | NHOH | H | 0.045 |
| 6-Hydrazinopurine | $NHNH_2$ | H | 0.47 |
| 6-β-Aminoethylaminopurine | $NHC_2H_4NH_2$ | H | 0.53 |
| 6-β-Dimethylaminoethylaminopurine | $NHC_2H_4N(CH_3)_2$ | H | >1 |
| 6-p-Aminphenylpurine | $C_6H_4NH_2(p)$ | H | >1 |
| 6-Methylpurine | $CH_3$ | H | 0.58 |
| 6-Cyanopurine | C=N | H | >1 |
| Purine-6-aldoxine | CH=NOH | H | 0.055 |
| 6-Purinecarboxylic acid | COOH | H | >1 |
| 6-Purinecarboxamide | $CONH_2$ | H | >1 |
| 6-Purinecarbohydrazide | $CONHNH_2$ | H | >1 |
| 6-Purinethiocarboxamide | $CSNH_2$ | H | >1 |
| 6-Purinecarboxamidine | $C(=NH)NH_2$ | H | >1 |
| 6-Chloropurine | Cl | H | >1 |
| Hypoxanthine | $OH^b$ | H | >1 |
| 6-Methoxypurine | $OCH_3$ | H | >1 |
| 6-Mercaptopurine | SH | H | >1 |
| 6-Methylthiopurine | $SCH_3$ | H | >1 |
| 2-Aminopurine | H | $NH_2$ | >1 |
| 2,6-Diaminopurine | $NH_2$ | $NH_2$ | >1 |
| 2-Methylamino-6-aminopurine | $NH_2$ | $NHCH_2$ | >1 |
| 2-Dimethylamino-6-aminopurine | $NH_2$ | $N(CH_3)$ | >1 |
| 2-Methyl-6-aminopurine | $NH_2$ | $CH_3$ | 0.82 |
| Isoguanine | $NH_2$ | OH | >1 |
| Guanine | OH | $NH_2$ | >1 |
| 2-Amino-6-methylthiopurine | $SCH_3$ | $NH_2$ | >1 |
| Xanthine | OH | OH | >1 |
| 2-Chloro-6-aminopurine | $NH_2$ | Cl | >1 |
| 2-Fluoro-6-aminopurine | $NH_2$ | F | 0.028 |
| 2-Mercapto-6-aminopurine | $NH_2$ | SH | 0.53 |
| 2-Methylthio-6-purine | $NH_2$ | $SCH_3$ | 0.26 |
| 3-Methyl-6-aminopurine | $NH_2$ | II 3-$CH_3$ | >1 |
| 6-Amino-7-methylpurine | $NH_2$ | II 7-$CH_3$ | 0.35 |
| 6-Amino-8-methylpurine | $NH_2$ | II 8-$CH_3$ | 0.053 |
| 6-Amino-8-hydroxypurine | $NH_2$ | II 8-OH | 0.64 |
| 6-Amino-8-mercaptopurine | $NH_2$ | II 8-SH | 0.14 |
| 6-Amino-8-m-nitrophenylpurine | $NH_2$ | II 8-$C_6H_4NO_2(m)$ | 0.074 |
| 6-Amino-9-methylpurine | $NH_2$ | II 9-$CH_3$ | 0.43 |
| 6-Amino-9-(tetrahydro-2′-furyl)purine | $NH_2$ | II 9-$C_4H_7O$ | 0.80 |
| Adenosine | $NH_2$ | II 9-$C_5H_8O_4$ | >1 |

## Table 1 (continued)
### INHIBITION CONSTANTS OF PURINES AND PURINE ANALOGS OF MONKEY ADENINE PHOSPHORIBOSYLTRANSFERASE

[a]   This value was determined by measuring the inhibition of the conversion of $^{14}$C-adenine to $^{14}$C-AMP by nonradioactive adenine.

[b]   Although some of the compounds listed exist primarily in the oxo or thio form the substituent is designated −OH or −SH, respectively, to indicate the availability of a proton.

(Reproduced from Krenitsky, T. A., Neil, S. M., Elion, G. B., and Hitchings, G. H., *J. Biol. Chem.*, 244, 4779, 1969. With permission from the copyright owner.)

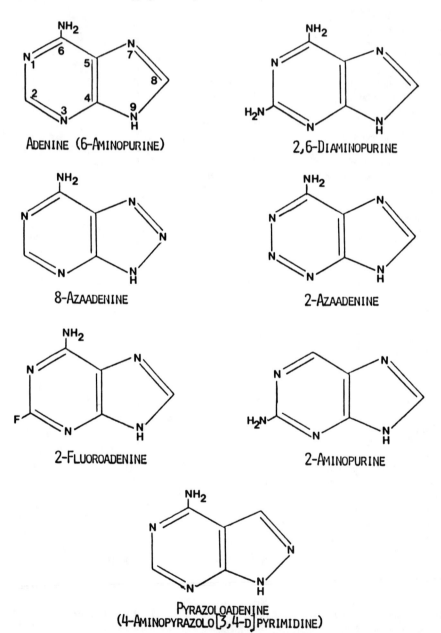

FIGURE 1.   Structure of adenine and some of its analogs.

**Table 2**
**RATES OF NUCLEOTIDE FORMATION FROM**
**PURINES AND PURINE ANALOGUES CATALYZED BY**
**ENZYME PREPARATION FROM RHESUS MONKEY**
**LIVER**

| [14]C-base | Ribonucleotide formed | |
|---|---|---|
| | Observed rates at 0.025 m$M$ [14]C-base and 1 m$M$ PP-ri-bose-P | Estimated[a] rate at saturating levels of [14]C-base and 1 m$M$ PP-ribose-P |
| | **µmol/min/mg protein** | |
| Adenine | 50 | 51 |
| 2,6-Diaminopurine | 0.43 | 31 |
| 4-Aminopyrazolo(3,4-d)pyrimidine | 0.57 | 1.2 |
| 5-Aminoimidazole-4-carboxamide | 0.83 | 20 |
| Hypoxanthine | 0.22 | 35 |
| Uracil | 0.06 | |

[a]  Maximal velocities were calculated from the equation

$$V = v\left(\frac{Km}{S} + 1\right)$$

$K_m$ was assumed equal to $K_i$ (Table 1). The $K_i$ values for 2,6-diaminopurine and hypoxanthine were 1.8 and 4.0 m$M$, respectively.
Reproduced from Krenitskey, T. A., Neil, S. M., Elion, G. B., and Hitchings, G. H., *J. Biol. Chem.*, 244, 4779, 1969. With permission.

**Table 3**
**ADENINE ANALOGS USED IN STUDIES**
**OF DRUG RESISTANT MAMMALIAN**
**CELLS**

| Inhibitor | Mode of action |
|---|---|
| 2,6-Diaminopurine | Lose of APRT |
| 8-Azaadenine | Loss of APRT |
| 2-Fluoroadenine | Loss of APRT |
| 4-Carbamoylimazolium-5-olate | Loss of APRT |
| Pyrazoloadenine | Loss of APRT |
| 2-Aminopurine | Mutagenic |

synthesis. There appears to be three possible sites of action of adenine (and guanine) analogs which block *de novo* purine biosynthesis. These three are PRPP utilization, PRPP synthesis, and PRPP amidotransferase (E.C. 2.4.2.14). These have been discussed fully elsewhere.[11,15] Table 3 lists those adenine analogs that have been used as drug resistant markers in mammalian cells, and Figure 1 their structure. These analogs are discussed in the following.

**A. 2,6-Diaminopurine (DAP) and 8-Azaadenine (AA)**
DAP was shown in 1955 to inhibit the incorporation of glycine-[14]C into nucleic acid purines.[34] It has also been found to inhibit aminoimidazole carboxamide accumulation in *E.*

*coli*[35] and phosphoribosyl formylglycinamide synthesis in Ehrlich ascites tumor cells and HEp-2 cells.[36] Henderson and Khoo[37] observed that DAP decreased PRPP concentrations in Ehrlich ascites tumor cells (2.6% of control). Thus, the available evidence suggests that the ribonucleotide of DAP inhibits purine biosynthesis through utilization of PRPP. It is possible that the toxic effects of DAP are by more than one mechanism. DAP is deaminated to guanine by adenosine deaminase, and in addition is oxidized to 8-hydroxy-2,6-diaminopurine by xanthine oxidase.[38] DAP inhibits the reproduction of polio virus by mechanisms not understood.[39]

Resistance to DAP and AA appears in all cases to involve a loss or defect of APRT activity. Thus resistance arises from an inability of cells to phosphoribosylate the analogs to cytotoxic monophosphates. Cells resistant to one analog show cross resistance to the other. Complete APRT deficiency has been noted in a number of human families.[44-47] Cells from such individuals, in culture, are resistant to DAP and AA.

The most detailed study of a mammalian APRT system at the genetic level has been in the Chinese hamster ovary (CHO) cell. Most resistant mutants arise as point mutations, although first step mutants often arise through deletion.[14] Mutants resistant to low levels of the drugs are either hemizygous or true heterozygotes.[40-42] Second step resistant mutants, or mutants resistant to high concentrations of the drugs, are usually homozygotes.[43]

A large number of studies have been done with DAP resistant mouse cells. These include cells of unknown origin resistant to DAP,[48] 3T6 cells,[49] mouse teratocarcinoma,[50,29] Ehrlich ascites carcinoma,[51,52] L-cells,[53] and L5178Y cells.[54] Although the majority of such resistant strains show little or no APRT activity, we have recently isolated mutants of L5178Y resistant to DAP, which have normal levels of APRT activity. Conversely, Turker and Martin,[28] and Turker et al.[29] have reported DAP resistant cells, lacking APRT activity, that are still able to take up adenine. These lines have been termed pseudorevertants.

## B. Halogenated Adenines

Montgomery[55] has reported the preparation of a series of related fluoropurines. Both 2-fluoroadenine (FA) and 2-fluoroadenosine are highly toxic to cells in culture. The $ID_{50}$ for FA using HEp-2 cells was 0.03 $\mu M$ (compared to 100 $\mu M$ for adenine), and 10 $\mu M$ for chloroadenine. APRT-HEp-2 cells were >2000 more resistant than parental cells. An adenosine kinase mutant was as sensitive as wild-type cells, indicating again that APRT was the enzyme necessary for the conversion of the base to a toxic nucleotide. However, halogenated di- and triphosphates are not incorporated into nucleic acids. 2-Fluoroadenosine 5'-triphosphate has been reported to inhibit RNA polymerase, and perhaps be incorporated into RNA.[56] It also may cause feedback inhibition of *de novo* purine biosynthesis. The halogenated compounds, although cytotoxic *in vitro*, do not have any selective cytotoxicity for neoplastic cells.

## C. 4-Aminopyrazolo(3,4-d)Pyrimidine

4-Amino-pyrazolopyrimidine (pyrazoloadenine), an analog of adenine, has been studied in a number of laboratories. This compound is converted into the nucleotide in mammalian tissues.[57] Pyrazoloadenine inhibits incorporation of radioactive precursors into nucleic acids[58-60] and also inhibits the first enzyme of purine synthesis *de novo*. The mechanism of the cytostatic action of the drug is unknown, since pyrazolohypoxanthine causes feedback inhibition, but has no cytostatic effect.[57] The cytostatic activity of pyrazoloadenine can be increased by guanine, but it is abolished by adenine. A HEp-2 cell line resistant to this drug has been isolated.[61]

Pyrazoloadenine can be deaminated to a hypoxanthine derivative by adenosine deaminase.[62] Both compounds are inhibitors of xanthine oxidase. Pyrazoloadenine inhibits the growth of a number of cell lines (Hela and adenocarcinoma) in tissue culture.[57] In mice about 50% of a dose of pyrazoloadenine is excreted in the urine within 24 hr after administration.[57] It is not used clinically as an anticancer agent because of high toxicity.[57]

### D. Bredinin and its Derivatives

Mouse mammary tumor FM3A cells resistant to 4-carbamoylimidazolium-5-olate (Clo), the aglycone of the nucleoside antibiotic bredinin (4-carbamoyl-1-β-D-ribofuranosylimidazolium-5-olate), are cross resistant to DAP.[63,64] Clo[r] lines were 27- to 40-fold more resistant to DAP than wild-type cells. These resistant cells completely lack APRT activity. It would appear that Clo is phosphoribosylated by APRT to an active cytotoxic nucleotide, which then inhibits IMP dehydrogenase (E.C. 1.2.1.14) and blocks *de novo* synthesis of guanine nucleotides.

Another antitumor agent of the same class, 5-carbamoyl-1H-imidozol-4-yl-piperonylate, is rapidly deacylated in cell cultures to 4-carbamoylimidazolium-5-olate.[65] This compound inhibits growth of L5178Y cells, and as mentioned above, is metabolized by APRT. It was originally thought that bredinin itself may function as an antibiotic in the same fashion, since the toxicity of the aglycone of bredinin was reduced by adenine. It was suggested[63] that the aglycone was converted to bredinin by APRT. However, the mechanism of bredinin resistance is not through APRT, but rather through adenosine kinase. Bredinin resistant mutants have less than 3% of normal levels of adenosine kinase activity.[66]

### E. 2-Aminopurine and 6-N-Hydroxylaminopurine

Unlike other adenine analogs, 2-aminopurine is highly mutagenic to bacteria and phage by incorporation into DNA and resulting mismatching of base pairs during DNA replication. 2-Aminopurine-2-deoxyriboside inhibits DNA synthesis, and also adenosine deaminase.[57]

It has been proposed that 2-aminopurine and cytosine base pair by hydrogen bonding, resulting in an A:T → G:C error of replication, and a C:G. → A:T error of incorporation.[57] 2-Aminopurine can induce chromosome aberration and aneuploidy in murine sarcoma cells.[67] Barrett[68] has also reported that 2-aminopurine is weakly mutagenic in Syrian hamster embryo cells. In contrast, 6-N-hydroxylaminopurine is less potent a mutagen in prokaryotes, but is more mutagenic in eukaryotic systems.

## V. COLLATERAL SENSITIVITY

Cells resistant to one drug may show greater sensitivity, compared with the parent cells, to another drug. In other words, the parent cells are less sensitive to the second drug than the resistant cells. This phenomenon is known as collateral sensitivity.[69] Many examples of collateral sensitivity to chemotherapeutic agents, including purine analogs, have been described in cultured mammalian cells.[70-72]

Collateral sensitivity in cells resistant to adenine analogs was first observed by Morris,[73] although the importance of this observation was not commented upon. Pig kidney cells resistant to DAP were cross resistant to purine and 6-methylpurine, but they showed somewhat increased sensitivity to mercaptopurines compared with the parent cells. Both cell types were equally resistant to hydroxypurines.

In a more recent study,[74] it was shown that 6-mercaptopurine resistant sublines of P388 and L1210 cultured leukemic cells were 5 to 10 times more sensitive than the parental cells to 4-carbamoylimidazolium-5-olate. As mentioned earlier, this compound is a substrate for APRT. The biochemical basis for the increased sensitivity was explained in terms of the interrelationship between the *de novo* and salvage pathways. The 6-mercaptopurine resistant cells, deficient in HGPRT, are unable to synthesize GMP by the salvage pathway. They are, therefore, dependent on the *de novo* pathway for this nucleotide. The nucleotide of 4-carbamoylimidazolium-5-olate is an inhibitor of IMP dehydrogenase,[65] a key enzyme in the conversion of IMP to GMP. Inhibition of IMP dehydrogenase in resistant cells by this nucleotide further restricts the supply of GMP formed by the *de novo* pathway. The parent cells are less affected by 4-carbamoylimidazolium-5-olate as they are able to form GMP by both the salvage and *de novo* pathways. However, the inhibition of IMP dehydrogenase by this compound has not been demonstrated in intact cells, so its mechanism of action must await further studies.

## VI. SELECTION OF MUTANTS RESISTANT TO ADENINE ANALOGS

Heterozygote mutants at the APRT locus (partially resistant) are normally selected in low levels of the analogs (usually DAP or AA), whereas homozygotes require high levels of the analogs for selection. Such homozygotes can grow on analog levels as high as 500 $\mu$g/m$\ell$. Adair et al.[75] have reported the selection of heterozygous CHO-C10A cells at 4.5 to 5.0 $\mu$g/m$\ell$ AA. Below this level, large numbers of background clones developed. For the selection of homozygotes these workers used 80 $\mu$g/m$\ell$ AA. Using the parental cell line the spontaneous mutation frequency to AA resistance (80 $\mu$g/m$\ell$) was $<3.0 \times 10^{-7}$, and the induced frequency (100 to 125 $\mu$g/m$\ell$ ethyl methanesulfonate, 16 to 18 hr exposure), $9.6 \times 10^{-6}$ per cell generation. Using a heterozygote, the spontaneous and induced frequencies were $3.7 \times 10^{-5}$ and $6.6 \times 10^{-4}$ per cell generation, respectively.

Dickerman and Tischfield[76] have studied the effect of metabolic cooperation on the recovery of adenine analog resistant mutants. Metabolic cooperation leads to the supression of the mutant phenotype of enzyme deficient cells by contact with normal cells.[77] Thus in selecting mutants in certain cell lines, cell density is important. CHO-K1 cells are very sensitive to adenine analogs. However at concentrations above $10^5$ cells per 100 mm dish, there is a steady decline in the recovery of DAP resistant cells in the presence of DAP and even more so in the presence of FA. Not only did metabolic cooperation occur, but cell death from FA toxicity led to the release of a toxic by-product into the media.[76]

Thompson et al.[78] studied the conditions for efficient detection of AA resistant CHO cells. Unlike the case of thioguanine resistance, where a long recovery period appears necessary for expression of the mutant phenotype, 3 days recovery after mutagenesis was sufficient for selection of the mutant phenotype.

DAP or AA resistance is a recessive phenotype as shown by studies with human-mouse somatic cell hybrids. This is the predicted result, since the presence of APRT activity on one allele would lead to the production of a toxic analog intermediate. Kusano et al.[49] have reported the selection of mouse 3T6 cells (3T6-DF8) resistant to high levels of DAP and FA by serially cultivating the cells in increasing quantities of the analog. 3T6 cells were cultured initially in 2.6 $\mu$g/m$\ell$ DAP, and progressively grown in increasing amounts until 100 $\mu$g/m$\ell$ DAP. These researchers report that these cells were initially sensitive to 0.1 $\mu$g/m$\ell$ FA, but with growth in increasing amounts of FA, adapt to 25 $\mu$g/m$\ell$ FA.

Revertants at the APRT locus can be selected using a variation of the standard HAT (hypoxanthine, aminopterin, thymidine) selection procedure. This is done by growing the cells in the presence of alanosine and adenine (AA medium).[49] Alanosine inhibits the endogenous synthesis of AMP from IMP, so only cells with functional APRT can grow on adenine.

## VII. CONCLUDING REMARKS

The use of adenine analogs to select mutants of mammalian cells has proved to be of great value for the study of mutation in somatic cells. The ease of selection of both forward and reverse mutants makes this an ideal system for studying mutagenesis and mechanism of mutation. Since resistance to adenine analogs appears to be the result of modification of

APRT, comparative studies of different mutants will facilitate the analysis of APRT at both the protein and gene level.

# REFERENCES

1. **Zimmerman, T. P., Gersten, N. B., Ross, A. F., and Miech, R. P.,** Adenine as a substrate for purine nucleoside phosphorylase, *Can. J. Biochem.,* 49, 1050, 1971.
2. **Snyder, F. F. and Henderson, J. F.,** Alternative pathways of deoxyadenosine and adenosine metabolism, *J. Biol. Chem.,* 248, 5899, 1973.
3. **Dean, B. M., Perrett, D., Simmonds, H. A., Sahota, A., and Van Acker, K. J.,** Adenine and adenosine metabolism in intact erythrocytes deficient in adenosine monophosphate-pyrophosphate phosphoribosyltransferase: a study of two families, *Clin. Sci. Mol. Med.,* 55, 407, 1978.
4. **Sahota, A., Simmonds, H. A., Potter, C. F., Watson, J. G., Hugh-Jones, K., and Perrett, D.,** Adenosine and deoxyadenosine metabolism in the erythrocytes of a patient with adenosine deaminase deficiency, in *Advances in Experimental Medicine and Biology,* Vol. 122A, Rapado, A., Watts, R. W. E., and De Bruyn, C. H. M. M., Eds., Plenum Press, New York 1980, 397.
5. **Kamatani, N. and Carson, D. A.,** Dependence of adenine production upon polyamine synthesis in cultured human lymphoblasts, *Biochem. Biophys. Acta,* 675, 344, 1981.
6. **Sahota, A., Webster, D. R., Potter, C. F., Simmonds, H. A., Rodgers, A. V., and Gibson, T.,** Methylthioadenosine phosphorylase activity in human erythrocytes, *Clin. Chem. Acta,* 128, 283, 1983.
7. **Henderson, J. F. and Scott, F. W.,** Inhibition of animal and invertebrate cell growth by naturally occurring purine bases and ribonucleosides, *Pharmacol. Ther.,* 8, 539, 1980.
8. **Snyder, F. F., Hershfield, M. S., and Seegmiller, J. E.,** Cytotoxic and metabolic effects of adenosine and adenine on human lymphoblasts, *Cancer Res.,* 38, 2357, 1978.
9. **Zielke, C. L. and Suelter, C. H.,** Purine, purine nucleoside, and purine nucleotide aminohydrolases, *The Enzymes,* Vol. 5, 3rd ed., Boyer, P. D., Ed., Academic Press, New York, 1971, 47.
10. **Simmonds, H. A., Van Acker, K. J., Cameron, J. S., and Snedden, W.,** The identification of 2,8-dihydroxyadenine, a new compound of urinary stones, *Biochem. J.,* 157, 485, 1976.
11. **Holmes, E. W., Jr.,** Regulation of purine biosynthesis *de novo,* In *Uric Acid,* Kelley, W. N. and Weiner, I. M., Eds., Springer-Verlag, Berlin, 21, 1978.
12. **Raivio, K. O. and Seegmiller, J. E.,** The role of phosphoribosyltransferases in purine metabolism, *Curr. Topics Enzyme Regul.,* 2, 201, 1970.
13. **Murray, A. W.,** The biological significance of purine salvage, *Annu. Rev. Biochem.,* 40, 811-826, 1971.
14. **Taylor, M. W., Simon, A. E., and Kothari, R. M.,** The APRT system, in *Molecular Cell Genetics,* Gottesman, M. M., Ed., John Wiley, New York, 1985, 311.
15. **Henderson, J. F.,** Regulation of purine biosynthesis, *American Chemical Society Monograph 170,* Washington, D.C., 1972.
16. **Sirotnak, F. M., Chello, P. L., and Brockman, R. W.,** Potential for the exploitation of transport systems in anticancer drug design, in *Methods in Cancer Research,* Vol. 16, DeVita, V. T., Jr. and Busch, H., Eds., Academic Press, New York, 1979, 381.
17. **Zylka, J. M. and Plagemann, P. G. W.,** Purine and pyrimidine transport by cultured Novikoff cells, *J. Biol. Chem.,* 250, 5766, 1975.
18. **Witney, F. R. and Taylor, M. W.,** Role of adenine phosphoribosyltransferase in adenine uptake in wild type and APRT⁻ mutants of CHO, *Biochem. Genet.,* 16, 917, 1978.
19. **Wilson, L. P.,** Tolerance of larvae of Drosophila for nucleic acid components: adenine, *Growth,* 6, 1, 1942.
20. **Blair, D. G. R., Peesker, S. J., and Cross, D. C.,** Toxicity of adenine and of purine analogs to 2,6-diaminopurine sensitive and resistant L-strain mouse cells, *Can. J. Microbiol.,* 16, 775, 1970.
21. **Debatisse, M. and Buttin, G.,** The control of cell proliferation by preformed purines: a genetic study. I. Isolation and preliminary characterization of Chinese hamster lines with single or multiple defects in purine "salvage" pathways, *Somat. Cell Genet.,* 3, 497, 1977.
22. **Debatisse, M. and Buttin, G.,** The control of cell proliferation by preformed purines: a genetic study. II. Pleiotrophic manifestation and mechanism of a control exerted on adenylic purines or PRPP synthesis, *Somat. Cell Genet.,* 3, 513, 1977.
23. **Hershfield, M. S., Snyder, F., and Seegmiller, J. E.,** Adenine and adenosine are toxic to human lymphoblast mutants defective in purine salvage enzymes, *Science,* 197, 1284, 1977.

24. **Green, C. D. and Martin, D. W., Jr.,** Characterization of a feedback-resistant phosphoribosylpyrophosphate synthetase from cultured, mutagenized hepatoma cells that overproduce purines, *Proc. Natl. Acad. Sci. U.S.A.,* 70, 3698, 1973.

25. **Henderson, J. F., Brox, L., Zombor, G., Hunting, D., and Lomax, C. A.,** Specificity of adenosine deaminase inhibition, *Biochem. Pharmacol,*. 26, 1967, 1977.

26. **Levine, R. A. and Taylor, M. W.,** The mechanism of adenine toxicity in *E. coli, J. Bacteriol.,* 149, 1041, 1982.

27. **Woods, R. A., Roberts, D. G., Stein, D. S., and Filpula, D.,** Adenine phosphoribosyltransferase mutants in *Saccharomyces cerevisiae, J. Gen. Microbiol.,* 130, 2629, 1984.

28. **Turker, M. S. and Martin, G. M.,** Induction of adenine salvage in mouse cell lines deficient in adenine phosphoribosyltransferase, *Mol. Cell. Biol.,* 5, 2662, 1985.

29. **Turker, M. S., Tischfield, J. A., Rabinovitch, P., Stambrook, P. J., Trill, J. J., Smith, A. C., Ogburn, C. E., and Martin, G. M.,** Differentiation alters the unstable expression of adenine phosphoribosyltransferase in mouse teratocarcinoma cells, *J. Exp. Pathol.,* 2, 299, 1986.

30. **Krenitsky, T. A., Neil, S. M., Elion, G. B., and Hitchings, G. H.,** Adenine phosphoribosyltransferase from monkey liver: specificities and properties, *J. Biol. Chem.,* 244, 4779, 1969.

31. **Le Page, G. A. and Jones, M. A.,** Purinethiols as feedback inhibitors of purine synthesis in ascites tumor cells, *Cancer Res.,* 21, 642, 1961.

32. **Brockman, R. W. and Chumley, S.,** Inhibition of formylglycinamide ribonucleotide synthesis in neoplastic cells by purine analogs, *Biochim. Biophys. Acta,* 95, 365, 1965.

33. **Caldwell, S. C., Henderson, J. F., and Patterson, A. R. P.,** Resistance to purine nucleoside analogues in an ascites tumor, *Can. J. Biochem.,* 45, 735, 1967.

34. **Le Page, G. A. and Greenlees, J. L.,** Investigation of disease system for cancer chemotherapy screening: incorporation of glycine-2-C$^{14}$ into ascites tumor cell purines as a biological test system, *Cancer Res.,* 15, Suppl. 3, 102, 1955.

35. **Gots, J. S. and Gollub, E. G.,** Purine analogs as feedback inhibitors, *Proc. Soc. Exp. Biol. Med.,* 101, 641, 1959.

36. **Henderson, J. F.,** Feedback inhibition of purine biosynthesis in ascites tumor cells by purine analogues, *Biochem. Pharmacol.,* 12, 551, 1963.

37. **Henderson, J. F. and Khoo, M. K. Y.,** On the mechanism of feedback inhibition of purine biosynthesis *de novo* in Ehrlich ascites tumor cells *in vitro, J. Biol. Chem.,* 240, 3107, 1965.

38. **Wyngaarden, J. B.,** 2,6-Diaminopurine as substrate and inhibitor of xanthine oxidase, *J. Biol. Chem.,* 224, 453, 1953.

39. **Munyon, W.,** Inhibition of poliovirus by 2,6-diaminopurine, *Virology,* 22, 15, 1964.

40. **Jones, G. E. and Sargent, P. A.,** Mutants of cultured Chinese hamster cells deficient in adenine phosphoribosyltransferase, *Cell,* 2, 43, 1974.

41. **Chasin, L. A.,** Mutations affecting adenine phosphoribosyltransferase activity in Chinese hamster cells, *Cell,* 2, 37, 1974.

42. **Simon, A. E. and Taylor, M. W.,** High frequency mutation of the adenine phosphoribosyltransferase locus in CHO cells is due to deletion of the gene, *Proc. Natl. Acad. Sci. U.S.A.,* 80, 810, 1983.

43. **Simon, A. E., Taylor, M. W., and Bradley, W. E. C.,** Mechanism of mutation of the aprt locus in Chinese hamster ovary cells: analysis of heterozygotes and hemizygotes, *Mol. Cell Biol.,* 3, 1703, 1983.

44. **Kelley, W. N., Levy, R. I., Rosenbloom, F. M., Henderson, J. F., and Seegmiller, J. E.,** Adenine phosphoribosyltransferase deficiency: A previously undescribed genetic defect in man, *J. Clin. Invest.,* 17, 1968, 2281.

45. **Fox, I. H., Meade, J. C., and Kelley, W. N.,** Adenine phosphoribosyltransferase deficiency in man: report of a second family, *Am. J. Med.,* 55, 614, 1973.

46. **Van Acker, K. J., Simmonds, H. A., Potter, C. F., and Sahota, A.,** Inheritance of adenine Phosphoribosyltransferase (APRT) deficiency, in *Advances in Experimental Medicine and Biology,* Vol. 122B, Rapado, A., Watts, R. W. E., and DeBruyn, C. H. M. M., Eds., Plenum Press, New York, 1980, 349.

47. **Simmonds, H. A. and Van Acker, K. J.,** Adenine phosphoribosyltransferase deficiency, in *The Metabolic Basis of Inherited Disease,* 5th ed., Stanbury, J. B., Wyngaarden, J. B., Fredrickson, D. S., Goldstein, J. L., and Brown, M. S., Eds., McGraw-Hill, New York, 1983, chap. 52.

48. **Atkins, J. H. and Gartler, S. M.,** Development of a nonselective technique for studying 2,6-diaminopurine resistance in an established murine cell line, *Genetics,* 60, 781, 1968.

49. **Kusano, T., Long, C., and Green, H.,** A new reduced human mouse somatic cell hybrid containing the human gene for adenine phosphoribosyltransferase, *Proc. Natl. Acad. Sci., U.S.A.,* 68, 82, 1971.

50. **Reuser, A. J. J. and Mintz, B.,** Mouse teratocarcinoma mutant clones deficient in adenine phosphoribosyltranferase and developmentally pluripotent, *Somat. Cell Genet.,* 5, 781, 1979.

51. **Hori, M. and Henderson, J. F.,** Purification and properties of adenylate pyrophosphorylase from Ehrlich ascites tumor cells, *J. Biol. Chem.,* 251, 1406, 1966.

52. **Murray, A. W.,** Studies on the nature of the regulation by purine nucleotides of adenine phosphoribosyltranferase from Ehrlich ascites tumor cells, *Biochem. J.,* 103, 271, 1967.
53. **Tischfield, J. A., Trill, J. J., Lee, Y. I., Coy, K., and Taylor, M. W.,** Genetic instability at the adenine phosphoribosyltransferase locus in mouse L-cells, *J. Mol. Cell Biol.,* 2, 250, 1982.
54. **Paeratakul, U. and Taylor, M. W.,** Isolation and characterization of mutants at the APRT locus in the L5178Y TK$^+$/TK$^-$ mouse lymphoma cell line, *Mutation Res.,* 160, 61, 1986.
55. **Montgomery, J. A.,** Studies on the biologic activities of purine and pyrimidine analogs, *Med. Res. Rev.,* 2, 271, 1982.
56. **Shiguera, H. T., Boxer, G. E., Sampson, L. D., and Melon, M. L.,** Metabolism of fluoroadenosine by Ehrlich ascites cells, *Arch. Biochem. Biophys.,* 111, 713, 1965.
57. **Langen, P.,** *Antimetabolites of Nucleic Acid Metabolism,* Gordon Research, New York, 1975.
58. **Bennett, L. L., Jr., Smithes, D., Teague, C., Baker, H. T., and Stutts, P.,** Some effects of 4-aminopyrazalo(3-4-d)pyrimidine on purine metabolism, *Biochem. Pharmacol.,* 11, 81, 1962.
59. **Booth, B. A. and Sartorelli, A. C.,** 4-Aminopyrazalo(3-4-d)pyrimidine: an inhibitor of the synthesis of purines and proteins in Ehrlich ascites cells, *J. Biol. Chem.,* 236, 203, 1961.
60. **Henderon, J. F. and Junga, J. G.,** Effect of purine antagonists on the metabolism of other purine antagonists, *Can. Res.,* 24, 173, 1961.
61. **Bennett, L. L., Jr., Allan, A. W., Smithes, D., and Vail, M. H.,** Resistance to 4-aminopyrazalo(3,4,-d)pyrimidine, *Biochem. Pharmacol.,* 18, 725, 1969.
62. **Fiegelson, P. and Davidson, J. D.,** The metabolism of pyrazolo(3,4-3)pyrimidines by the rat, *Cancer Res.,* 18, 226, 1958.
63. **Sakaguchi, K., Tsujino, M., Mizuno, K., Hayano, K., and Ishida, N.,** Effect of Bredinin and its aglycone on L5178Y cells, *J. Antibiot.,* 28, 798, 1975.
64. **Koyama, H. and Kodama, H.,** Adenine phosphoribosyltransferase deficiency in cultured mouse mammary tumor FM3A cells resistant to 4-carbamoylimidazolium-5-olate, *Cancer Res.,* 42, 4210, 1982.
65. **Fukui, M., Inaba, M., Tsukagoshi, S., and Sakurai, Y.,** New anti-tumor imidazole derivative, 5-carbamoyl-1-H-imidazol-4-yl piperonylate, as an inhibitor of purine synthesis and its activation by adenine phosphoribosyltranferase, *Cancer Res.,* 42, 1098, 1983.
66. **Koyama, H. and Tsuji, M.,** Genetic and biochemical studies on the activation and cytotoxic mechanism of bredinin, a potent inhibitor of purine biosynthesis in mammalian cells, *Biochem. Pharmacol.,* 32, 3547, 1983.
67. **Tsutsui, T., Maizumi, H., and Barrett, J. C.,** Induction by modified purines (2-aminopurines and 6-N-hydroxylaminopurine) of chromosome aberrations and aneuploidy in Syrian hamster embryo cells, *Mutation Res.,* 148, 107, 1985.
68. **Barrett, J. C.,** Induction of gene mutations in cell transformation of mammalian cells by modified purines: 2-aminopurine and 6-N-hydroxylamino purine, *Proc. Natl. Acad. Sci. U.S.A.,* 78, 5685, 1981.
69. **Szybalski, W. and Bryson, V.,** Genetic resistance of microbial cross resistance to toxic agents. 1. Cross resistance of *Escherichia coli* to fifteen antibiotics, *J. Bacteriol.,* 64, 489, 1952.
70. **Hutchison, D. J.,** Cross resistance and collateral sensitivity studies in cancer chemotherapy, in *Advances in Cancer Research,* Vol. 7, Haddow, A. and Weinhouse, S., Eds., Academic Press, New York, 235, 1963.
71. **Hutchison, D. J. and Schmid, F. A.,** Cross resistance and collateral sensitivity, in *Drug Resistance and Sensitivity,* Mihich, E., Ed., Academic Press, New York, 73, 1973.
72. **Hutchison, D. J.,** Studies on cross resistance and collateral sensitivity (1962-1964), *Cancer Res.,* 25, 1581, 1985.
73. **Morris, M.,** Specificity and cross reactions in a strain of pig kidney cells resistant to 2,6-diaminopurine, *Exp. Cell Res.,* 21, 439, 1960.
74. **Inaba, M., Fukui, M., Yoshida, N., Tsukagoshi, S., and Sakurai, Y.,** Collateral sensitivity of 6-mercaptopurine resistant sublines of P388 and L1210 leukemia to the new purine antagnonists, 5-carbamoyl-1H-imidazol-4-yl-piperonylate and 4-carbamoylimidazolium-5-olate, *Cancer Res.,* 42, 1103, 1982.
75. **Adair, G. M., Carver, J. H., and Wandres, D. L.,** Mutagenicity testing in mammalian cells. 1. Derivatives of a Chinese hamster ovary cell line heterozygous for the adenine phosphoribosyltransferase and thymidine kinase locus, *Mutation Res.,* 72, 187, 1980.
76. **Dickerman, L. H. and Tischfield, J. A.,** Comparative effects of adenine analogs upon metabolic cooperation between Chinese hamster cells with different levels of adenine phosphoribosyltransferase activity, *Mutation Res.,* 49, 83, 1978.
77. **Van Zeeland, A. A., Van Diggeen, M. C. E., and Simons, J. W. I. M.,** The role of metabolic cooperation in selection of hypoxanthine guanine phosphoribosyltransferase (HGPRT) deficient mutants from diploid mammalian cell strains, *Mutation Res.,* 14, 355, 1972.
78. **Thompson, L. H., Fong, S., and Brookman, K.,** Validation of conditions for efficient detection of HPRT and APRT mutations in suspension cultured CHO cells, *Mutation Res.,* 74, 91, 1980.

Chapter 9

# 9-β-D-ARABINOFURANOSYLADENINE AND 9-β-D-ARABINOFURANOSYL-2-FLUOROADENINE

**Carol E. Cass**

## TABLE OF CONTENTS

I.    Introduction ................................................................. 126

II.   Cellular and Molecular Pharmacology ........................................ 127
      A.    Transport ............................................................. 129
      B.    Metabolism ............................................................ 130
      C.    Inhibition of DNA synthesis ........................................... 131
      D.    Incorporation in Nucleic Acids ........................................ 133
      E.    Inhibition of S-Adenosylhomocysteine Hydrolase ........................ 133

III.  Resistance ................................................................. 134
      A.    Alterations in Uptake and Metabolism .................................. 134
      B.    DNA Synthesis ......................................................... 135

IV.   Summary .................................................................... 137

Acknowledgment ................................................................. 137

References ..................................................................... 137

# I. INTRODUCTION

AraA (Figure 1, structure I) was initially synthesized as a potential antitumor agent,[1,2] and, although its activity in human cancer patients has been disappointing, araA has established activity against systemic herpesvirus infections in humans.[3,4] AraA was the first systemically active antiviral agent to be licensed in the U.S. for use in man[5] and, while it is gradually being replaced by acyclovir,[6-8] araA remains the drug of choice for a variety of systemic infections involving DNA viruses.[3,4] The antiviral activity of araA has been considered in several recent reviews.[3-5,9-11]

Shortly after araA was synthesized,[1,2] it was shown to be a potent inhibitor of DNA synthesis in *Escherichia coli*,[12] and biological activity was demonstrated in vivo against transplantable tumors in mice[13-15] and in vitro against herpes simplex and vaccinia virus[16,17] and against cultured murine fibroblasts.[18] However, the activity of araA in these experimental systems was seriously limited by low solubility ($\leq 0.0018\ M$[19]) and rapid inactivation by adenosine deaminase to 9-β-D-arabinofuranosylhypoxanthine (araH).[12,13-15,18,20,21]

The problem of solubility, which limits dosages that can be administered systemically, has been approached through use of the 5'-monophosphate of araA (Figure 1, structure II), which is highly soluble, as a prodrug of araA. AraAMP is equally as effective as araA against herpes simplex virus in cell cultures[22] and laboratory animals[23,24] and, similarly, araAMP and araA exhibit comparable antitumor activity in therapy of mice bearing the L1210 leukemia.[25] Pharmacokinetic studies in humans have shown that administration of araAMP provides sustained levels of araA in body fluids for longer periods than can be obtained by administration of araA,[26,27] indicating that the 5'-monophosphate can be used in humans as a prodrug of araA.

Inactivation of araA by deamination can be prevented by simultaneous administration of potent inhibitors of adenosine deaminase, such as coformycin (Figure 2, structure I), deoxycoformycin (Figure 2, structure II) and EHNA (Figure 3). Coformycin[28,29] and deoxycoformycin[30,31] are natural products that bind tightly to adenosine deaminase ($K_i$ values, $10^{-10}$ and $10^{-12}\ M$, respectively), resulting in ''pseudo-irreversible'' inhibition of the enzyme.[32-35] EHNA (Figure 3), a synthetic compound,[36] is also a tight-binding inhibitor ($K_i$ values, about $10^{-9}\ M$) but its interaction with adenosine deaminase is reversible.[35,37] Deoxycoformycin and EHNA have been shown to enhance the activity of araA by preventing adenosine deaminase-dependent conversion to araH in a variety of in vivo and in vitro experimental systems,[5,9,38] and deoxycoformycin has been the subject of a number of clinical investigations, alone[39-41] and in combination with araA.[42-45] The immunosuppressive activity of deoxycoformycin[41] has limited its value in combination therapy with araA. The pharmacology and biological activity of the inhibitors of adenosine deaminase have been reviewed in detail.[46]

Although it is well established that araH does not exhibit activity against cultured cells or transplantable tumors,[38] a number of investigators have reported that araH exhibits antiviral activity.[5,9] However, the antiviral activity of araH is much less than that of araA, particularly when compared to araA in the presence of an inhibitor of adenosine deaminase.[9] Adenosine deaminase activity is high in many cells and tissues and in the serum supplements used in cell culture growth media, and rapid conversion of araA to araH takes place, frequently resulting in the complete degradation of araA. When araA is administered as a single agent, cells and tissues are, in effect, subjected to simultaneous exposures to araA and araH, with the relative concentrations of the two agents continuously changing. Until the potent inhibitors of adenosine deaminase (coformycin, deoxycoformycin, and EHNA) became available,[28-31,36] it was not possible to experimentally separate the pharmacological effects of araA and araH. Enhanced araA activity in the presence of inhibitors of adenosine deaminase has been observed in most experimental systems, including virally infected cultured cells,[5,9,38] and there has been little, if any, interest in the possible antiviral activity of araH.

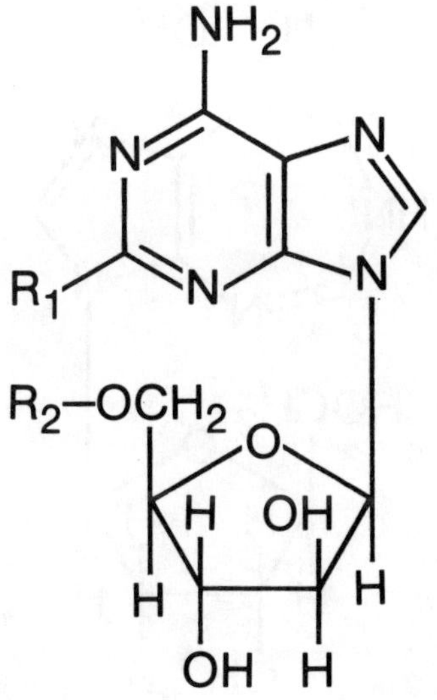


**I,** $R_1 = H$
$R_2 = H$

**II,** $R_1 = H$
$R_2 = PO_3^{=}$

**III,** $R_1 = F$
$R_2 = H$

**IV,** $R_1 = F$
$R_2 = PO_3^{=}$

FIGURE 1. Chemical structure of araA and araA derivatives. I, 9-β-D-arabinofuranosyladenine (araA); II, 9-β-D-arabinofuranosyladenine 5′-monophosphate (araAMP); III, 9-β-D-arabinofuranosyl-2-fluoroadenine (2-F-araA); IV, 9-β-D-arabinofuranosyl-2-fluoroadenine 5′-monophosphate (2-F-araAMP).

2-F-AraA (Figure 1, structure III), a congener of araA, was synthesized by Montgomery[47,48] in a search for biologically active analogs of adenosine that are resistant to deamination. 2-F-AraA was shown to be effective in therapy of mice bearing the L1210 leukemia,[49] and subsequent studies in a variety of experimental systems have demonstrated that 2-F-araA equals or exceeds the activity of araA in combination with deoxycoformycin either in vivo against transplantable tumors of mice[50,51] or in vitro against cultured cells.[52,53] Like araA, 2-F-araA is relatively insoluble, and 2-F-araAMP, the 5′-monophosphate of 2-F-araA (Figure 1, structure IV), was developed as a prodrug for in vivo administration.[50] Based on promising results of phase I studies, which indicated that the dose-limiting toxicity was moderate myelosuppression,[54,55] 2-F-araAMP was advanced to phase II studies.[56] Although objective responses were observed in leukemic patients who received the highest doses of 2-F-araAMP, delayed toxicity to the central nervous system, resulting in progressive neurologic deterioration and death, was observed in the majority of patients. Thus, the future of 2-F-araAMP in cancer therapy is uncertain.

## II. CELLULAR AND MOLECULAR PHARMACOLOGY

Considerable information is available concerning the biochemical mechanisms of action

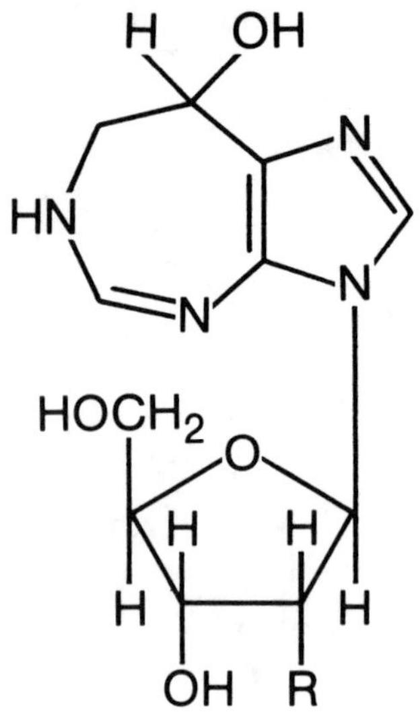

I,  R = OH

II,  R = H

FIGURE 2.    Chemical structure of coformycin and deoxycoformycin.  I, (R)-3-(β-D-*erythro*-pentafuranosyl)-3,6,7,8,-tetrahydroimidazo[4,5-d][1,3]diazepin-8-ol (coformycin); II, (R)-3-(2-deoxy-β-D-*erythro*-pentafuranosyl)-3,6,7,8-tetrahydroimidazo[4,5-d][1,3]diazepin-8-ol (deoxycoformycin).

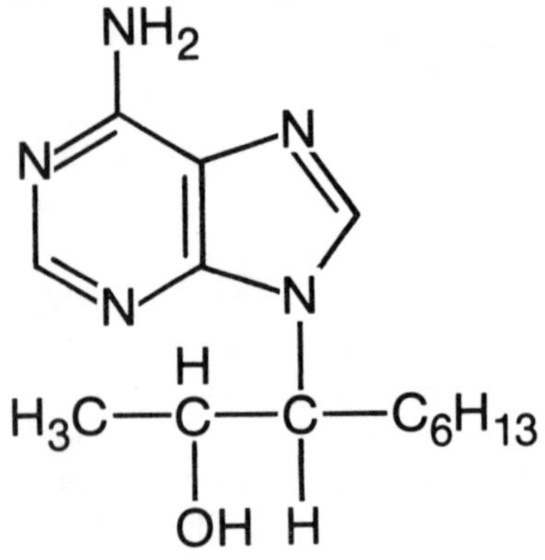

FIGURE 3.    Chemical structure of *erythro*-9-(2-hydroxy-3-nonyl)adenine (EHNA).

of araA and 2-F-araA. The reader is referred to the review articles by Cohen[57] and Suhadolnik[58] for discussion of the early literature and to the articles by Shannon and Schabel,[5] North and Cohen,[9] and Cass[38] for discussion of the literature up to 1979. In addition, the monograph edited by Pavan-Langston et al.[59] deals with preclinical studies of the antiviral effects of araA. The information in this section is limited primarily to more recent reports, particularly those biochemical and pharmacological studies in mammalian cells that are relevant to an understanding of the basis of resistance to araA and its derivatives.

## A. Transport

Uptake of nucleosides by mammalian cells is a complex process that consists of passage across the plasma membrane by passive diffusion and mediated transport, followed by intracellular metabolism. Phosphorylation, which is the principal fate of the physiologic nucleosides and many cytotoxic nucleosides, effectively traps influent nucleosides inside cells because of the low permeability of the plasma membrane toward nucleotides. Since most nucleosides are hydrophilic molecules, entry by passive diffusion is minimal, and nucleoside-specific transporters in the plasma membrane are required for cellular uptake. In many cell types, the transport step is a reversible process and, because it is often more rapid than the subsequent metabolic steps, analysis of transport kinetics requires rapid-assay technology that provides initial rates of cellular uptake of radiolabeled permeant. The most thoroughly characterized nucleoside transport systems are the equilibrative transporters of human erythrocytes and a few cultured cell types, which accept both purine and pyrimidine nucleosides as permeants and are sensitive to inhibition by S-substituted thiopurine nucleosides. A number of comprehensive reviews are available,[60-66] including articles that deal specifically with methods of measurement of nucleoside transport,[64] adenosine transport in cultured cells and erythrocytes,[65] and transport of nucleoside drugs.[66]

Early studies with human and mouse erythrocytes, in which cellular uptake of araA was reduced in the presence of tight-binding inhibitors of nucleoside transport, provided evidence that influx of araA in erythrocytes occurs via "facilitated diffusion", much like that of adenosine and deoxyadenosine.[67,68] Reduced accumulation of araA was observed in a transport-deficient mutant ($AE_1$) of murine S49 lymphoma cells,[69] indicating that araA is also a substrate for the broadly specific, equilibrative transporter of S49 lymphoma cells. The involvement of nucleoside transport in araA cytotoxicity is uncertain since the transport-defective mutant ($AE_1$) and the transport-competent parent (S49) were equally sensitive to the antiproliferative effects of araA during continuous exposures.[69] In a detailed kinetic study of transport of adenosine and adenosine analogs by mouse leukemia L1210 cells,[70,71] the ability of araA to compete for entry with adenosine ($K_i$, 67.8 ± μ$M$) was demonstrated, indicating high affinity transport of araA in this cell type. L1210 cells, which apparently possess multiple nucleoside transport systems, have recently been shown to exhibit concentrative ($Na^+$-dependent) transport of formycin B, a nonmetabolized analog of adenosine.[72] L1210 cells apparently are capable of both equilibrative and concentrative transport of adenosine and adenosine analogs, including araA. The relative importance of equilibrative and concentrative transport in the manifestation of araA cytotoxicity in L1210 leukemia cells has not yet been determined.

Transport of 2-F-araA was the subject of two recent studies that were conducted in L1210 leukemia cells[70,73] and in proliferative intestinal epithelia cells of mice.[73] Analysis of initial rates of uptake of $^3$H-2-F-araA indicated the presence of two transport systems in L1210 cells, with high and low affinities for 2-F-araA, and of a single transport system in intestinal epithelia cells, with low affinity for 2-F-araA. $K_m$ values in L1210 cells were 68 ± 14 and 326 ± 48 μ$M$ and in epithelial cells were 317 ± 44 μ$M$.[73] Results of reciprocal inhibition studies with 2-F-araA and adenosine suggested that 2-F-araA enters L1210 cells and intestinal epithelia cells by the same routes as does adenosine. Furthermore, 2-F-araA accumulation was nonconcentrative when transport was analyzed in mutant L1210 cells that lacked deoxycytidine kinase activity and were thus incapable of phosphorylating 2-F-araA,[70] suggesting that the primary route of entry at cytotoxic concentrations (<200 μ$M$) is via the equilibrative transporter. Cellular uptake of 2-F-araA was significantly greater in L1210 cells than in epithelia cells, apparently because of the combined effects of the two transport systems and the high level of nucleoside kinase activity in L1210 cells. Apparently, the selective activity of 2-F-araA in the treatment of mice bearing the L1210 leukemia is due to higher rates of transport and phosphorylation in drug-sensitive tumor tissues than in drug-limiting host tissues.

## B. Metabolism

The metabolism of araA has been studied extensively, and most cells and tissues are capable of both phosphorylating and deaminating araA, with conversion either to the biologically active triphosphate (araATP) or to the biologically inactive derivative, araH.[5,9,38] Conversion of araA to araATP requires the action of nucleoside kinases(s) as the first step, and at least three different kinases appear to be capable of phosphorylating araA, depending on experimental conditions. Characterization of the substrate specificities of enzyme preparations from L1210 cells and rabbit liver showed that deoxycytidine kinase[74] and purine deoxyribonucleoside kinase,[75] but not adenosine kinase,[76-78] readily accept araA as a substrate. However, identification of the enzyme defects in several araA-resistant mammalian cell lines (see Section III.A), including a mutant derived from the L1210 leukemia, have established that adenosine kinase must be involved, at least in some cell types, in the intracellular conversion of araA to araAMP.[79-83] The current view, based largely on results from studies with resistant cell lines (see Section III.A), is that araA is phosphorylated primarily by deoxycytidine kinase and adenosine kinase. $K_m$ values of 2.1 and 3.5 m$M$, respectively, were reported for araA phosphorylation by deoxycytidine kinase and adenosine kinase, purified by DEAE-cellulose chromatography from cultured human lymphoblastoid CCRF-CEM cells.[81] Ratios of $V_{max}$ values to $K_m$ values for phosphorylation of deoxycytidine and araA by deoxycytidine kinase were, respectively, $2.7 \times 10^3$ and 9, and for phosphorylation of adenosine and araA by adenosine kinase were, respectively, $2.4 \times 10^5$ and 3. Thus, relative to the physiologic nucleosides, araA is a poor substrate for both enzymes, particularly for adenosine kinase.[81] Nevertheless, exposure of drug-sensitive human and murine leukemia cells to araA results in substantial accumulation of intracellular araATP,[84] particularly when exposures are conducted in the presence of inhibitors of adenosine deaminase.[53,81,85,86] The phosphorylation of araAMP and araADP is presumably catalyzed, respectively, by adenylate kinase and nucleoside-diphosphate kinase, although there have not been detailed studies of production of araA nucleotides with the purified enzymes.[38,57]

Unlike the nucleoside kinases, adenosine deaminase readily accepts araA as a substrate. The $K_m$ values for adenosine deaminase preparations from human erythrocytes and calf intestinal mucosa were, respectively, for adenosine 25 and 37 μ$M$ and for araA 100 and 77 to 140 μ$M$, and, when $V_{max}$ values for adenosine deamination were normalized to 100, the relative values for araA deamination by the erythrocytic and intestinal enzymes were, respectively, 47 and 18 to 25.[87] Using adenosine as substrate, the apparent $K_i$ values for inhibition of adenosine deaminase from human erythrocytes by deoxycoformycin, coformycin, and EHNA were, respectively, $2.5 \times 10^{-12}$, $1 \times 10^{-11}$ and $1.6 \times 10^{-9} M$.[35] The apparent $K_i$ for inhibition by deoxycoformycin of deamination of araA by adenosine deaminase of murine tissues was estimated to be $2 \times 10^{-11} M$,[88] which is only an order of magnitude less than the value obtained for inhibition of deamination of adenosine by the erythrocytic deaminase.[35]

The metabolic fate of 2-F-araA differs from that of araA. Studies with a subline of leukemia L1210 cells that are resistant to 1-β-D-arabinosyl-cytosine (araC) have established that conversion of 2-F-araA to the 5'-monophosphate is catalyzed primarily by deoxycytidine kinase.[50] $K_m$ values of 0.2 to 4 μ$M$ were obtained for preparations of cytoplasmic deoxycytidine kinase from L1210 leukemia cells,[50] calf thymus,[74] cultured human lymphoblastoid CCRF-CEM cells,[81] and human leukemic blast cells[89] using deoxycytidine as the substrate, and values of 213 to 500 μ$M$ were obtained with the same preparations using 2-F-araA as the substrate.[50,74,81,89] In at least two of these studies,[81,89] the maximal velocities of 2-F-araA phosphorylation were significantly greater than those of deoxycytidine phosphorylation. 2-F-araA was not a substrate for the mitochondrial deoxycytidine kinase of human leukemic blast cells.[89] The enzymes responsible for phosphorylating 2-F-araAMP and 2-F-araADP have not been identified.

2-F-araA is a poor substrate for adenosine deaminase,[47-51] and has been proposed as a deaminase-insensitive alternative to araA for use in anticancer and antiviral therapy.[49,50] Inhibitors of adenosine deaminase (deoxycoformycin, EHNA) did not potentiate the growth-inhibitory effects of 2-F-araA against cultured human lymphoblastoid CCRF-CEM cells[52,53] or L1210 leukemia cells,[90] indicating little, if any, deamination of 2-F-araA in these cell types. Although the initial expectation was that 2-F-araA would not be deaminated when utilized in vivo as a therapeutic agent, recent studies of the metabolic disposition of radiolabeled 2-F-araA in dogs, mice, and monkeys have shown significant excretion of the deamination product, particularly in dogs.[91,92] Production of 9-β-D-arabinofuranosyl-2-fluo-rohypoxanthine (2-F-araH), as well as 2-fluoroadenine and its 5'-triphosphate, were sub-sequently reported in studies with P388 leukemia cells.[93] The relative importance of these metabolites in 2-F-araA toxicity is unknown. Derivatives of 2-fluoroadenine are highly active both in vivo and in vitro,[47,51,90] whereas 2-F-araH did not exhibit antitumor activity or gross toxicity when administered to mice bearing the L1210 leukemia.[92]

Phosphorylation of araA and 2-F-araA to their respective 5'-triphosphates is required for biological activity,[50,81] and a number of studies[49,53-81,85,86,93-96] have examined the production of araA and 2-F-araA nucleotides by intact cells after in vivo or in vitro exposures to drug. In murine leukemia cells,[49,94] hamster cells,[85] and cultured human lymphoblastoid cells,[53,81,95] the intracellular levels of either araATP or 2-F-araATP, which greatly exceeded extracellular concentrations, were dose-dependent over a broad range of concentrations. Intracellular exposure to araATP has been correlated with cytotoxicity and inhibition of DNA synthesis in Chinese hamster ovary (CHO) cells.[86,96] In human lymphoblastoid CCRF-CEM cells, the time courses of accumulation of araATP and 2-F-araATP differed substantially in that araATP levels reached an equilibrium after 2-hr exposures whereas 2-F-araATP levels were still increasing after 5-hr exposures.[53] Although the presence of an inhibitor of adenosine de-aminase (deoxycoformycin) increased net accumulation of araA nucleotides in CHO cells exposed to araA,[96] the rate of disappearance,[85] which followed first-order decay kinetics was unaffected. The $T_{1/2}$ values for loss of araATP from CHO cells were 1.7 and 1.6 hr, respectively, after 3-hr exposures to araA alone or to araA and deoxycoformycin.[85] Similar $t_{1/2}$ values (2.8 and 2.9 hr) were reported for loss of 2-F-araATP from P388 leukemia cells after intraperitoneal administration of low and high doses of 2-F-araA to tumor-bearing mice.[94] The $t_{1/2}$ values for loss of araATP and 2-F-araATP from cultured human lympho-blastoid CCRF-CEM cells were substantially different, 12.9 to 15.3 and 2.5 to 4.7 hr, respectively, after 2-hr exposures to araA and deoxycoformycin or to 2-F-araA.[53] Of interest is the recent report of differences in decay kinetics of araATP in uninfected and herpes simplex virus-infected cells;[97] $t_{1/2}$ values of 3.2 and 9.3 hr, respectively, were observed in uninfected and infected human KB cells, suggesting viral-dependent changes in degradation of araATP that contribute to the selective action of araA.

## C. Inhibition of DNA Synthesis

Although both araA and 2-F-araA apparently exhibit multiple biochemical sites of action, the predominant effect in drug-sensitive cells is inhibition of replication of DNA, through the combined effects of inhibition of enzymes of DNA synthesis[89,98-102] and inhibition of production of precursors required for DNA synthesis.[89,101,103,104] The role of inhibition of the DNA polymerases in lethality of araA and 2-F-araA is controversial, and results of several recent studies suggest that incorporation of araAMP and 2-F-araAMP into DNA may be of greater importance in cytotoxicity (see Section II.D).

The effects of araATP on DNA polymerases $\alpha$, $\beta$, and $\gamma$ and terminal deoxynucleotidyltransferase have been examined in a group of human leukemia cell lines in a detailed kinetic study that attempted to identify potential sites of action of araA.[98] AraATP inhibition of DNA polymerases $\alpha$ and $\beta$ was competitive with respect to dATP, and similar $K_i$ values (0.2 to 0.4 and 0.3 to 0.6 $\mu M$, respectively) were obtained for both enzymes, suggesting that araATP binds to polymerases $\alpha$ and $\beta$ with similar affinities. AraATP had no effect on polymerase $\gamma$. Inhibition of terminal deoxynucleotidyltransferase by araATP was competitive with respect to each of the 4 substrates (dATP, dGTP, dCTP, or dTTP), and $K_i$ values of 0.4 to 0.7 $\mu M$ were obtained. In a separate study, which examined the kinetics of araATP inhibition of DNA polymerases from murine tumor cells,[100] polymerases $\alpha$ and $\gamma$ were more sensitive to araATP than polymerase $\beta$, and $K_i$ values depended greatly on the template primer. Consistent with the view that araATP inhibits replicative DNA synthesis (polymerase $\alpha$) are results from a kinetic study conducted *in situ* in which araATP was a competitive inhibitor ($K_i$, 0.6 $\mu M$) with respect to dATP of the DNA-replication complex in permeabilized murine leukemia P815 cells.[102]

The relative abilities of araATP and 2-F-araATP to inhibit DNA polymerases $\alpha$ and $\beta$ have been determined with preparations obtained from leukemia L1210 cells.[101] Polymerase $\alpha$ was equally sensitive to araATP and 2-F-araATP ($K_i$ values, 11 $\mu M$), and polymerase $\beta$ was relatively insensitive to both compounds since the concentrations of araATP and 2-F-araATP that gave 50% inhibition of enzyme activity were >200 $\mu M$. In cultured HeLa cells,[89] 2-F-araATP was a competitive inhibitor ($K_i$, 1.2 $\mu M$) with respect to dATP of polymerase $\alpha$ whereas polymerase $\beta$ was relatively insensitive.

AraATP and 2-F-araATP also inhibit ribonucleotide reductase.[89,101-104] In an early work,[103] araATP inhibited reduction of the four ribonucleotides in crude extracts of a rat tumor to the same extent, leading to the conclusion that araATP inhibits ribonucleotide reductase by the same mechanism as dATP. A different conclusion was reached in a recent study,[104] which employed a more highly purified preparation (free of nucleotide phosphatase and nucleoside diphosphate kinase activity) from cultured human leukemia Molt-4F cells. AraATP was a competitive inhibitor with respect to either ATP or GTP for reduction, respectively, of CDP ($K_i$, 15 $\mu M$) or ADP ($K_i$, 4 $\mu M$), whereas it was a relatively weak inhibitor of UDP reduction. A similar pattern of inhibition was observed in studies with 2-F-araATP,[101,104] which was a more potent inhibitor of ribonucleotide reductase than araATP in preparations from mouse L1210 leukemia cells,[101] human HEp-2 cells,[101] and human HeLa cells.[104] The inhibition of ADP reduction by araATP and 2-F-araATP is "self-potentiating" in that inhibition of one target enzyme potentiates inhibition of a second target enzyme.[104] Reduced intracellular levels of dATP, caused by inhibition of ribonucleotide reduction, increases the susceptibility of DNA synthesis to inhibition by araATP or 2-F-araATP since both nucleotides inhibit DNA polymerase $\alpha$ competitively with respect to dATP.[89,98,100-102]

The sensitivity of viral DNA polymerases to araATP has been extensively studied (for reviews, see References 5 and 9) and will only be mentioned briefly here. Exposure of herpesvirus-infected cells to araA results in selective inhibition of viral replication and viral DNA synthesis, suggesting that viral DNA polymerase is more sensitive to inhibition by araATP than one or more of the cellular polymerases. A number of biochemical studies[105-109] directed toward identifying the mechanism of action of araA have provided evidence that viral DNA polymerase is the ultimate target, although other possibilities have been proposed.[5,9,97] Analysis of the biochemical basis of araA resistance in mutants of herpes simplex virus[110,111] (see Section III.B) also indicates that DNA polymerase is the site of action of araATP. There is relatively little information concerning the sensitivity of viral DNA synthesis to 2-F-araATP. In one study,[89] 2-F-araA inhibited replication of herpes simplex virus types 1 and 2 only at concentrations that were toxic to the host cells, indicating an absence of selective action against viral DNA synthesis.

## D. Incorporation in Nucleic Acids

Although incorporation of araA and 2-F-araA nucleotides into nucleic acids of cellular and viral origin has been reported by a number of investigators,[84,107,109,112-120] the role of incorporation in cytotoxicity and antiviral activity remains controversial. Results of two recent studies with cultured cell lines[119,120] have suggested a causative relationship between incorporation of araA and 2-F-araA into DNA and cytotoxicity, apparently related to the ability of the arabinonucleotides to terminate elongation of DNA chains. Incorporation of 2-F-araA into RNA has been reported and may also contribute to cytotoxicty,[120] whereas incorporation of araA into RNA is insignificant.[119]

AraA residues are incorporated into internucleotide linkages[84,113-115,118] and at the 3'-termini of DNA chains,[112] and the relative importance of these sites of incorporation has been debated.[109,116,117,119] An early study,[112] which examined incorporation of araATP into DNA of isolated rat liver nuclei, clearly established that araAMP incorporation at the 3'-terminus of growing DNA chains prevented or greatly reduced further chain elongation. However, the amounts of araAMP present in internucleotide linkages greatly exceeded the amounts found at 3'-termini,[84,113-115,118] and the chain terminating activity of araA was considered to be minimal. More recent studies with partially purified preparations of DNA polymerases of herpes simplex virus[109,116] and mammalian cells[117] have provided strong evidence for the notion that DNA synthesis is inhibited in araA-treated cells because of the presence of 3'-terminal araAMP residues. The presence of araAMP at 3'-termini caused a reduction, but did not completely inhibit, the rate of chain elongation;[109,117] the extent of inhibition of DNA synthesis was related to the amount of 3'-terminal araAMP;[117] and araAMP could not replace dATP in supporting in vitro DNA synthesis.[109] The earlier observations of low levels of 3'-terminal araAMP, relative to araA residues in internucleotide linkages, were attributed to their removal during isolation procedures by the 3'- to -5' exonuclease associated with mammalian and viral DNA polymerases.[109,117]

Incorporation of araA and 2-F-araA residues into DNA has been related to loss of clonogenicity in cultured cells.[119,120] A linear relationship was shown between clonogenic survival of cultured L1210 cells and incorporation of araA into DNA.[119] Furthermore, exposure of cells to increasing concentrations of araA resulted in an increased proportion of araA residues at the 3'-terminus of DNA and greater inhibition of DNA synthesis. A different result was obtained when a similar study was conducted with 2-F-araA and cultured human leukemia HL-60 cells.[120] In contrast to araA, 2-F-araA was incorporated into both RNA and DNA. A correlation was observed between clonogenic survival of HL-60 cells and incorporation of 2-F-araA into both RNA and DNA, raising the possibility of significantly different cytotoxicity profiles of araA and 2-F-araA.

## E. Inhibition of S-Adenosylhomocysteine Hydrolase

S-Adenosylhomocysteine (SAH) hydrolase catalyzes the reversible hydrolysis of SAH to adenosine and L-homocysteine.[121] SAH is a potent feedback inhibitor of methyltransferase reactions and has been proposed as a potential target of cytotoxic agents.[122] AraA inactivates SAH hydrolase from a variety of cells and tissues,[101,123-128] and studies with intact cells have established that intracellular levels of SAH are elevated during treatment with araA and deoxycoformycin.[128,130-133] Inactivation of SAH hydrolase and elevated intracellular SAH has also been observed in leukemic lymphoblasts of a patient treated with araA and deoxycoformycin.[44] $K_i$ values of 24, 5, and 19 $\mu M$ have been obtained, respectively, for araA-dependent inactivation of SAH hydrolase activity in extracts of cultured human lymphoblastoid WI-L2 cells,[123] mouse liver,[125] and leukemia L1210 cells.[101] In contrast, a $K_i$ value of 122 $\mu M$ was obtained for 2-F-araA-dependent inactivation of SAH hydrolase activity in L1210 cell extracts,[101] indicating that the substitution of a fluorine at position 2 of adenine significantly decreases the capacity of araA to bind to SAH hydrolase. The importance of inactivation of SAH hydrolase in cytotoxicity is uncertain since cell lines that are incapable of phosphorylation of araA and 2-F-araA (see Section III.A) are highly resistant to these nucleosides.[50,80-83] Furthermore, 2-F-araA exhibits the same degree of activity as araA (when the latter is protected from deamination by deoxycoformycin) against cultured cell lines[52,53] and transplantable tumors of mice.[49,50] In support of the view that inactivation of SAH hydrolase contributes to araA cytotoxicity under certain conditions is the observation of reduced growth rates and decreased SAH levels in araA-treated mutants of CCRF-CEM cells that were unable to phosphorylate araA because of reduced adenosine and deoxyctidine kinase activities,[134] although a separate study with a similar double mutant failed to demonstrate a relationship between SAH inactivation by araA and toxicity.[135]

## III. RESISTANCE

Development of resistance to araA has been observed in transplantable tumors, cultured cell lines and herpes simplex virus type 1. As is apparent from the discussion in Section II, characterization of biochemical mechanisms of resistance has contributed importantly to understanding of the metabolism and cytotoxic actions of araA and 2-F-araA. This section describes characteristics of particular resistant variants. The discussion deals first with biochemical alterations that affect drug uptake and metabolism, resulting in decreased levels of araA- or 2-F-araA-nucleotides, and second with alterations that decrease the sensitivity of DNA synthesis to araATP and 2-F-araATP. The discussion has been limited primarily to resistant cell lines that were selected for resistance to araA, usually in the presence of an inhibitor of adenosine deaminase. In a few instances, cell lines selected for resistance to other nucleoside analogs have been included because analysis of cross-resistance to araA or 2-F-araA has been useful in identification of biochemical determinants of cytotoxicity. Because altered sensitivity of adenosine deaminase to deoxycoformycin could give rise to an apparent resistance to araA when the two agents are administered in combination, resistance to deoxycoformycin is considered as well. Although the primary emphasis is on mammalian cells, a limited discussion of viral resistance, resulting from changes in the sensitivity of viral DNA polymerase to araATP, is also presented.

### A. Alterations in Uptake and Metabolism

A detailed series of studies[79,80,83,136] of araA resistance in baby hamster kidney (BHK) cells has demonstrated that mutations affecting the activity of adenosine kinase are the most common cause of resistance in this cell type. Of the three classes of araA-resistance mutants obtained, two involved alterations in adenosine kinase activity, which led to either an absence of adenosine kinase (Class I mutants) or to an altered enzyme (Class III mutants), and the third involved alterations in ribonucleotide reductase activity (Class II mutants). The existence of adenosine-kinase deficient cells, which comprised the major class of araA-resistant mutants,[80] provided evidence that (1) phosphorylation of araA is required for cytotoxicity and (2) adenosine kinase, which had previously been thought to be relatively unimportant in phosphorylation of araA,[76-78] is a key enzyme in the bioactivation of araA in intact cells. Subsequent studies of araA resistance in cultured human lymphoblastoid CCRF-CEM cells[81] and mouse leukemia L1210 cells[82] have confirmed these conclusions.

AraA-resistant BHK mutants were selected by a single-step procedure in which cells were exposed to cytotoxic levels of araA in the presence of an inhibitor of adenosine deaminase (EHNA).[79,80] The spontaneous mutation rate for development of araA resistance was $1.1 \times 10^{-7}$ mutations per cell per division, and mutagenesis with ethylmethane sulfonate significantly increased mutation frequencies.[80] Although the majority of the mutant clones lacked detectable adenosine kinase activity, a small number were unusually sensitive to adenosine cytotoxicity,[80] apparently resulting from production of a structurally altered enzyme since the catalytic properties of adenosine kinase of Class III mutants differed from those of parental cells.[136] Polyclonal antibodies have been raised against adenosine kinase preparations of parental BHK cells,[83] and the immunoreactivity of extracts from mutant cells indicated that Class I mutants lack detectable adenosine kinase polypeptides, whereas Class III mutants exhibit reduced levels of adenosine kinase polypeptides of similar electrophoretic mobilities as the wild-type enzyme. The latter observation led to the conclusion that Class III mutants arose by point mutations in the structural gene for adenosine kinase. Analysis of the araA sensitivity of cell hybrids made by fusing parental BHK cells with adenosine-kinase deficient mutants demonstrated that the resistant phenotype is recessive,[137] leading to the conclusion in a later work[83] that there is a single active gene for adenosine kinase in BHK cells.

Adenosine kinase has also been implicated in araA resistance in cultured mouse leukemia L1210 cells and human CCRF-CEM cells. AraA-resistant L1210 cells,[82] which were obtained after five cycles of exposure to araA and deoxycoformycin, were cross resistant to cordycepin, methylmercaptopurine ribonucleoside (MMPR) and tubercidin but not to araC or 2-F-araA, and the levels of resistance to the adenosine analogs were greater (40- to 170-fold) than resistance to araA (8-fold). The resistant phenotype was shown to be due to loss of adenosine kinase activity, which apparently contributes to phosphorylation of araA by intact L1210 cells, even though araA had previously been shown to be a poor substrate for the isolated enzyme of this cell type.[78] Continued accumulation of araA nucleotides by araA-resistant L1210 cells was attributed to the action of deoxycytidine kinase and/or purine deoxyribonucleoside kinase. Characterization of araA resistance in CCRF-CEM cells has established that deoxycytidine kinase is involved in bioactivation of araA.[52,81] A variant line of CCRF-CEM cells resistant to araC and deficient in deoxycytidine kinase activity was also partially resistant (threefold) to araA,[52] and a second mutant, obtained after three cycles of selection in the presence of araA and deoxycoformycin, was deficient in adenosine kinase activity and strongly resistant (100-fold) to araA.[81] AraATP formation in intact cells was moderately reduced (about 50%) in the deoxycytidine kinase-deficient mutant and greatly reduced (>95%) in the deoxycytidine/adenosine kinase-deficient mutant, indicating that both enzymes are involved in bioactivation of araA.[81] AraA resistance, possibly due to reduced adenosine kinase activity, has also been described in a line of mouse cells that are deficient in adenosine deaminase activity.[138]

Although alterations in bioactivation of araA most commonly lead to resistance, changes in catabolic enzymes (e.g., adenosine deaminase) could also give rise to araA resistance. Overproduction of adenosine deaminase by genetic amplification has been reported in mouse cells selected for resistance to adenosine in the presence of deoxycoformycin,[139] and, although sensitivity to araA was not reported, such cells would be expected to also be resistant to araA. Overproduction of adenosine deaminase has also been reported in rat hepatoma cells,[140-145] mouse L cells,[144] and CHO cells.[144] Deoxycoformycin resistance was obtained by forcing adenosine-kinase deficient mutants to use adenosine as the sole carbon source by deamination to inosine and phosphorolysis to ribose-1-P. Stepwise exposure of rat hepatoma cells to increasing concentrations of deoxycoformycin resulted in progressively higher levels of adenosine deaminase activity,[140] reaching levels up to 2000-fold greater than those found in the parental cells.[143] The kinetic properties of adenosine deaminase in the resistant and parental hepatoma cells were identical,[141] and resistance was accompanied by increased gene copy number[143,144] and increased levels of adenosine deaminase mRNA.[142,143] Genetic amplification was also demonstrated in mouse L cells but not in CHO cells,[144] which apparently overproduce adenosine deaminase by a mechanism other than increased gene copy number.

## B. DNA Synthesis

Perturbation of DNA synthesis, by inhibition of DNA polymerase(s)[89,98-102] and ribonucleotide reductase[89,101,103,104] or by incorporation into 3' termini of DNA chains,[112,117,119,120] is the major biochemical effect of araATP and 2-F-araATP. Resistance to these agents could arise if structural changes in replicative enzymes or ribonucleotide reductase resulted in reduced affinities for araATP and/or 2-F-araATP. Alterations in metabolism of precursor nucleotides, if they resulted in increased intracellular nucleotide pool sizes, could also lead to resistance since araATP and 2-F-araATP are competitive inhibitors of both DNA polymerase(s) and ribonucleotide reductase. Altered DNA polymerase was proposed as the basis of araA resistance in a transplantable mouse tumor,[146] and alterations in the regulation of ribonucleotide reductase by effector nucleotides have been reported in several cell lines that were selected for araA resistance or that exhibit cross-resistance to araA.[80,137,147-153] Mutations in viral DNA polymerase have been well documented in araA-resistant herpes simplex virus.[110,111,154-157] Although none have been reported, genetic changes leading to increased activity of enzymes capable of excising 3'-terminal araAMP and/or 2-F-araAMP would also confer resistance by removing the block to chain elongation presented by the arabinonucleotides.

The evidence for altered DNA polymerase in araA-resistant cells consists of a demonstration of altered sensitivity of DNA polymerase activity to araATP in crude extracts of drug-sensitive and drug-resistant mouse tumor cells[146] and thus is only suggestive. Partially purified DNA polymerase $\alpha$ from cultured Chinese hamster V79 cells selected for resistance to aphidicolin[150] exhibits altered kinetic properties, indicating that resistance can arise through structural changes in the replicative polymerase. Altered DNA polymerase is the basis of araA resistance in a series of mutants of herpes simplex virus.[110,111,156,157] Mutants, which were selected for resistance to araA, were cross resistant to phosphonoacetic acid (an inhibitor of the viral polymerase), and the mutant polymerase exhibited an altered $K_i$ for inhibition by araATP.[110] Several of the araA resistant mutations have recently been mapped within the DNA polymerase locus of the viral genome.[111,156]

Alterations in the activity of ribonucleotide reductase have been implicated in resistance to araA in a number of cell lines obtained by selection in the presence of araA and an inhibitor of adenosine deaminase.[80,148,151,153] Cross resistance to araA has also been shown in mutants resistant to aphidicolin, a specific inhibitor of DNA polymerase $\alpha$, by virtue of altered ribonucleotide reductase.[147-149,153] Although the phenotypic characteristics of these mutants differ, particularly with respect to cross resistance to other inhibitors, the common feature appears to be increased pools of deoxyribonucleotides. Two mechanisms have been identified: increased levels of ribonucleotide reductase activity[148] and alterations in feedback inhibition of ribonucleotide reductase by effector deoxyribonucleotides.[80,147,149,151] One class of araA-resistant mutants of mouse FM3A[148] cells were cross resistant to aphidicolin, excess thymidine and hydroxyurea and exhibited ribonucleotide reductase levels that were two- to fivefold greater than the parental sensitive cells, raising the possibility of genetic amplification. The sensitivity of partially purified mutant enzyme to inhibition of CDP reduction by dATP was similar to that of the wild-type enzyme. In contrast, CDP reduction by the other class of araA-resistant FM3A mutants[147] was relatively insensitive to dATP, indicating production of a structurally altered enzyme with decreased sensitivity to feedback inhibition by dATP. The characteristics of araA-resistant CCRF-CEM cells[151] also suggested altered ribonucleotide reductase with respect to feedback inhibition by dATP. The resistant clones were cross resistant to deoxyadenosine and excess thymidine and exhibited two- to eightfold increases in the levels of all four deoxyribnucleotide triphosphates under normal growth conditions. The resistant clones exhibited a tenfold decrease, relative to wild-type cells, in the sensitivity of CDP reduction to dATP, apparently reflecting a structural change in the mutant ribonucleotide reductase. Altered sensitivity of mutant ribonucleotide reductase to inhibition by araATP has not been reported, and, in at least one study,[151] CDP reduction by extracts of wild-type and mutant cells was equally sensitive to inhibition by araATP.

## IV. SUMMARY

AraA and 2-F-araA have multiple and complex biochemical effects, making evaluation of relationships between biochemical effects and cytotoxicity difficult. Studies with resistant cells have established that phosphorylation occurs by different routes for araA and 2-F-araA and, for both drugs, is essential for cytotoxicity. Adenosine kinase and deoxycytidine kinase activate araA in intact cells, although araA is a poor substrate for the purified enzymes. Deoxycytidine kinase phosphorylates 2-F-araA. Resistance resulting from decreased bioactivation is more likely to occur with 2-F-araA, which is phosphorylated by a single kinase, then with araA, which is phosphorylated by multiple kinases. Combination therapy with araA and the tight-binding inhibitors of adenosine deaminase may select for resistance due to increased levels of adenosine deaminase by genetic amplification. AraA is a potent inhibitor of SAH hydrolase, yet cells that are incapable of phosphorylating araA are frequently highly resistant. 2-F-araA, which is equitoxic with araA against a number of cell types, is a weak inhibitor of SAH hydrolase. Thus, although inhibition of SAH hydrolase does not appear to be an important cytotoxic mechanism for araA or 2-F-araA in cultured cells and transplantable tumors, inhibition of SAH hydrolase may result in toxicity in some cells and tissues, particularly during prolonged exposures to high levels of araA in the presence of an inhibitor of adenosine deaminase. Inhibition of DNA synthesis by araATP and 2-F-araATP results from inhibition of replicative DNA polymerase ($\alpha$), from depletion of deoxyribonucleotide triphosphates by inhibition of ribonucleotide reductase, and from slowing of chain elongation because of incorporation at $3'$-terminal ends. Incorporation of araAMP and 2-F-araAMP, which results in inhibition of DNA synthesis, has been correlated with cytotoxicity and may be more significant in cell death than inhibition of DNA polymerase(s). An important mechanism of resistance is altered sensitivity of ribonucleotide reductase to feedback inhibition by dATP, resulting in increased levels of deoxyribonucleotide triphosphates, which, in turn, decrease the sensitivity of DNA synthesis to inhibition by araATP. Resistance to araA in viral systems arises through mutations in viral DNA polymerase, confirming the proposed role of selective inhibition of DNA synthesis in the antiviral action of araA. The significance of these resistance mechanisms in in vivo use of araA and 2-F-araA in chemotherapy of disease remains to be determined.

## ACKNOWLEDGMENT

CEC is a Senior Research Scientist of the National Cancer Institute of Canada.

## REFERENCES

1. **Lee, W. W., Benitez, A., Goodman, L., and Baker, B. R.,** Potential anticancer agents. XL. Synthesis of the β-anomer of 9-(D-arabinofuranosyl)-adenine, *J. Am. Chem. Soc.,* 82, 2648, 1960.
2. **Reist, E. J., Benitez, A., Goodman, L., Baker, B. R., and Lee, W. W.,** Potential anticancer agents. LXXVI. Synthesis of purine nucleosides of β-D-arabinofuranose, *J. Org. Chem.,* 27, 3274, 1962.
3. **Hirsch, M. S. and Schooley, R. T.,** Treatment of herpesvirus infections (first of two parts), *N. Engl. J. Med.,* 309, 963, 1983.
4. **Hirsch, M. S. and Schooley, R. T.,** Treatment of herpesvirus infections (second of two parts), *N. Engl. Med.,* 309, 1034, 1983.
5. **Shannon, W. M. and Schabel, F. M., Jr.,** Antiviral agents as adjuncts in cancer chemotherapy, *Pharmacol. Ther.,* 11, 263, 1980.
6. **Skoldenberg, B. and Forsgren, M.,** Acyclovir versus vidarabine in herpes simplex encephalitis, *Scand. J. Infect. Dis. Suppl.,* 47, 89, 1985.

7. **Shepp, D. H., Dandliker, P. S., and Meyers, J. D.,** Treatment of varicella-zoster virus infection in severely immunocompromised patients. A randomized comparison of acyclovir and vidarabine, *N. Engl. J. Med.*, 314, 208, 1986.
8. **Whitley, R. J., Alford, C. A., Hirsch, M. S., Schooley, R. T., Luby, J. P., Aoki, F. Y., Hanley, D., Nahmias, A. J., and Soong, S.-J.,** Vidarabine versus acyclovir therapy in herpes simplex encephalitis, *N. Engl. J. Med.*, 314, 144, 1986.
9. **North, T. W. and Cohen, S. S.,** Aranucleosides and aranucleotides in viral chemotherapy, in *The International Encyclopedia of Pharmacology and Therapeutics: Viral Chemotherapy (Part I),* Shugar, D., Ed., Pergamon Press, Oxford, 1984, 303.
10. **Whitley, R., Alford, C., Hess, F., and Buchanan, R.,** Vidarabine: a preliminary review of its pharmacological properties and therapeutic use, *Drugs,* 20, 267, 1980.
11. **Park, N. H. and Pavan-Langston, D.,** Purines, in *Chemotherapy of Viral Infections,* Came, P. E. and Caliguiri, L. A., Eds., Springer-Verlag, Berlin, 1982, 117.
12. **Hubert-Habart, M. and Cohen, S. S.,** The toxicity of 9-β-D-arabinofuranosyladenine to purine-requiring *Escherichia coli, Biochem. Biophys. Acta,* 59, 468, 1962.
13. **Brink, J. J. and LePage, G. A.,** Metabolic effects of 9-D-arabinosylpurines in ascites tumor cells, *Cancer Res.,* 24, 312, 1964.
14. **Brink, J. J. and LePage, G. A.,** Metabolism and distribution of 9-β-D-arabinofuranosyladenine in mouse tissues, *Cancer Res.,* 24, 1024, 1964.
15. **Brink, J. J. and LePage, G. A.,** 9-β-D-Arabinofuranosyladenine as an inhibitor of metabolism in normal and neoplastic cells, *Can. J. Biochem.,* 43, 1, 1965.
16. **Privat de Garilhe, M. and De Rudder, J.,** Effet de deux nucleosides de l'arabinose sur la multiplication des virus de l'herpes et de la vaccine en culture cellulaire, *C. R. Acad. Sci. D (Paris),* 259, 2725, 1964.
17. **Schabel, F. M.,** The antiviral activity of 9-β-D-arabinofuranosyladenine (ara-A), *Chemotherapy,* 13, 321, 1968.
18. **Doering, A., Keller, J., and Cohen, S. S.,** Some effects of D-arabinosyl nucleosides on polymer synthesis in mouse fibroblasts, *Cancer Res.,* 26, 2444, 1966.
19. **Repta, A. J., Rawson, B. J., Shatter, R. D., Sloan, K. R., Bodor, N., and Higuchi, T.,** Rational development of a soluble prodrug of a cytotoxic nucleoside: preparation and properties of arabinosyladenine 5'-formate, *J. Pharm. Sci.,* 64, 392, 1975.
20. **Cory, J. G. and Suhadolnik, R. J.,** Structural requirements of nucleosides for binding by adenosine deaminase, *Biochemistry,* 4, 1729, 1965.
21. **Frederiksen, S.,** Specificity of adenosine deaminase toward adenosine and 2'-deoxyadenosine analogues, *Arch. Biochem. Biophys.,* 113, 383, 1966.
22. **Shannon, W. M.,** Adenine arabinoside: antiviral activity *in vitro,* in *Adenine Arabinoside: An Antiviral Agent,* Pavan-Langston, D., Buchanan, R. A., and Alford, C. A., Jr., Eds., Raven Press, New York, 1975, 1.
23. **Sidwell, R. W., Allen, L. B., Huffman, J. H., Khwaja, T. A., Tolman, R. L., and Robins, R. K.,** Anti-DNA virus activity of the 5'-nucleotide and 3',5'-cyclic nucleotide of 9-β-D-arabinofuranosyladenine, *Chemotherapy,* 19, 325, 1973.
24. **Kern, E. R., Richards, J. T., Overall, J. C., Jr., and Glasgow, L. A.,** Alteration of mortality and pathogenesis of three experimental *Herpesvirus hominis* infections of mice with adenine arabinoside 5'-monophosphate, adenine arabinoside, and phosphonoacetic acid, *Antimicrob. Agents Chemother.,* 13, 53, 1978.
25. **LePage, G. A., Worth, L. S., and Kimball, A. P.,** Enhancement of the antitumor activity of arabinofuranosyladenine by 2'-deoxycoformycin, *Cancer Res.,* 36, 1481, 1976.
26. **LePage, G. A., Lin, T.-T., Orth, R. E., and Gottlieb, J. A.,** 5'-Nucleotides as potential formulations for administering nucleoside analogs in man, *Cancer Res.,* 32, 2441, 1972.
27. **LePage, G. A., Naik, S. R., Katakkar, S. B., and Kahliq, A.,** 9-β-D-Arabinofuranosyladenine 5'-phosphate metabolism and excretion in humans, *Cancer Res.,* 35, 3036, 1975.
28. **Sawa, T., Fukagawa, Y., Homma, I., Takeuchi, T., and Umezawa, H.,** Mode of inhibition of coformycin on adenosine deaminase, *J. Antibiot. Ser. A,* 20, 227, 1967.
29. **Nakamura, H., Koyama, G., Iitaka, Y., Ohno, M., Yagisawa, N., Kondo, S., Maeda, K., and Umezawa, H.,** Structure of coformycin, an unusual nucleoside of microbial origin, *J. Am. Chem. Soc.,* 96, 4327, 1974.
30. **Woo, P. W. K., Dion, H. W., Lange, S. M., Dahl, L. F., and Durham, L. J.,** A novel adenosine and ara-A deaminase inhibitor (R)-3-(2-deoxy-β-D-*erythro*-pentofuranosyl)-3,6,7,8-tetrahydroimidazo[4,5d][1,3]diazepin-8-ol, *J. Heterocyl. Chem.,* 11, 641, 1974.
31. **Dion, H. D., Woo, P. W. K., and Ryder, A.,** Isolation and properties of a vidarabine deaminase inhibitor, co-vidarabine, *Ann. N.Y. Acad. Sci.,* 284, 21, 1977.
32. **Cha, S.,** Tight-binding inhibitors. I. Kinetic behavior, *Biochem. Pharmacol.,* 24, 2187, 1975.

33. **Cha, S., Agarwal, R. P., and Parks, R. E., Jr.**, Tight-binding inhibitors. II. Non-steady state nature of inhibition of milk xanthine oxidase by allopurinol and alloxanthine and of human erythrocytic adenosine deaminase by coformycin, *Biochem. Pharmacol.*, 24, 2187, 1975.

34. **Cha, S.**, Tight-binding inhibitors. III. A new approach for the determination of competition between tight-binding inhibitors and substrate-inhibition of adenosine deaminase by coformycin, *Biochem. Pharmacol.*, 25, 2695, 1976.

35. **Agarwal, R. P., Spector, T., and Parks, R. E., Jr.**, Tight-binding inhibitors. IV. Inhibition of adenosine deaminase by various inhibitors, *Biochem. Pharmacol.*, 26, 359, 1977.

36. **Schaeffer, H. J. and Schwender, C. F.**, Enzyme inhibitions. 26. Bridging hydrophobic regions on adenosine deaminase with some 9-(2-hydroxy-3-alky)adenines, *J. Med. Chem.*, 17, 6, 1974.

37. **Lapi, L. and Cohen, S.**, Toxicities of adenosine and 2'-deoxyadenosine in L cells treated with inhibitors of adenosine deaminase, *Biochem. Pharmacol.*, 26, 71, 1977.

38. **Cass, C. E.**, 9-β-D-Arabinofuranosyladenine (araA), in *Antibiotics V/2*, Hahn, F. E., Ed., Springer-Verlag, Berlin, 85, 1979.

39. **Major, P. P., Agarwal, R. P., and Kufe, D. W.**, Clinical pharmacology of deoxycoformycin, *Blood*, 58, 91, 1981.

40. **Poplack, D. G., Sallan, S. E., Rivera, G., Holcenberg, J., Murphy, S. B., Blatt, J., Lipton, J. M., Venner, P., Glaubiger, D. L., Ungerleider, R., and Johns, D.**, Phase I study of 2'-deoxycoformycin in acute lymphoblastic leukemia, *Cancer Res.*, 41, 3343, 1981.

41. **Grever, M. R., Siaw, M. F. E., Jacob, W. F., Neidhart, J. W., Miser, J. S., Coleman, M. S., Hutton, J. J., and Balcerzak, S. P.**, The biochemical and clinical consequences of 2'-deoxycoformycin in refractory lymphoproliferative malignancy, *Blood*, 57, 406, 1981.

42. **Agarwal, R. P., Blatt, J., Miser, J., Sallan, S., Lipton, J. M., Reaman, G. H., Holcenberg, J., and Poplack, D. G.**, Clinical pharmacology of 9-β-D-arabinofuranosyladenine in combination with 2'-deoxy-coformycin, *Cancer Res.*, 42, 3884, 1982.

43. **Gray, D. P., Grever, M. R., Siaw, M. F. E., Coleman, M. S., and Balcerzak, S. P.**, 2'-Deoxyco-formycin (dCF) and 9-β-D-arabinofuranosyladenine (ara-A) in the treatment of refractory acute myeloyctic leukemia, *Cancer Treat. Rep.*, 66, 253, 1982.

44. **Hershfield, M. S., Kredich, N. M., Koller, C. A., Mitchell, B. S., Kurtzberg, J., Kinney, T. R., and Falletta, J. M.**, S-Adenosylhomocysteine catabolism and basis for acquired resistance during treatment of T-cell acute lymphoblastic leukemia with 2'-deoxycoformycin alone and in combination with 9-β-D-arabinofuranosyladenine, *Cancer Res.*, 43, 3451, 1983.

45. **Plunkett, W., Nowak, B., Feun, L. G., Benjamin, R. S., Keating, M. and Freirich, E. J.**, Modulation of arabinosyladenine metabolism by 2'-deoxycoformycin in the therapy of human acute leukemia, *Adv. Expt. Med. Biol.*, 165, 345, 1984.

46. **Glazer, R. I.**, Adenosine deaminase inhibitors: their role in chemotherapy and immunosuppression, *Cancer Chemother. Pharmacol.*, 4, 227, 1980.

47. **Montgomery, J. A. and Hewson, K.**, Nucleosides of 2-fluoroadenine, *J. Med. Chem.*, 12, 498, 1969.

48. **Montgomery, J. A., Clayton, S. D., and Shortnacy, A. T.**, An improved synthesis for the preparation of 9-β-D-arabinofuranosyl-2-fluoroadenine, *J. Heterocycl. Chem.*, 16, 157, 1979.

49. **Brockman, R. W., Schabel, F. M., Jr., and Montgomery, J. A.**, Biologic activity of 9-β-D-arabino-furanosyl-2-fluoroadenine, a metabolically stable analog of 9-β-D-arabinofuranosyladenine, *Biochem. Phar-macol.*, 26, 2193, 1977.

50. **Brockman, R. W., Cheng, Y.-C., Schabel, F. M., Jr., and Montgomery, J. A.**, Metabolism and chemotherapeutic activity of 9-β-D-arabinofuranosyl-2-fluoroadenine against murine leukemia L1210 and evidence for its phosphorylation by deoxycytidine kinase, *Cancer Res.*, 40, 3610, 1980.

51. **Montgomery, J. A.**, Has the well gone dry? The first Cain Memorial Award Lecture, *Cancer Res.*, 42, 3911, 1982.

52. **Dow, L. W., Bell, D. E., Poulakos, L., and Fridland, A.**, Differences in metabolism and cytotoxicity between 9-β-D-arabinofuranosyladenine and 9-β-D-arabinofuranosyl-2-fluoroadenine in human leukemic lymphoblasts, *Cancer Res.*, 40, 1405, 1980.

53. **Plunkett, W., Chubb, S., Alexander, L., and Montgomery, J. A.**, Comparison of the toxicity and metabolism of 9-β-arabinofuranosyl-2-fluoroadenine and 9-β-arabinofuranosyladenine in human lymphob-lastoid cells, *Cancer Res.*, 40, 2349, 1980.

54. **Hutton, J. J., Von Hoff, D. D., Kuhn, J., Phillips, J., Hersh, M., and Clark, G.**, Phase I clinical investigation of 9-β-D-arabinofuranosyl-2-fluoroadenine 5'-monophosphate (NSC 312887), a new purine antimetabolite, *Cancer Res.*, 44, 4183, 1984.

55. **Boldt, D. H., Von Hoff, D. D., Kuhn, J. G., and Hersh, M.**, Effects on human peripheral lymphocytes of *in vivo* administration of 9-β-D-arabinofuranosyl-2-fluoroadenine-5'-monophosphate (NSC 312887), a new purine antimetabolite, *Cancer Res.*, 44, 4661, 1984.

56. **Warrell, R. P., Jr. and Berman, E.**, Phase I and II study of fludarabine phosphate in leukemia: therapeutic efficacy with delayed central nervous system toxicity, *J. Clin. Oncol.*, 4, 74, 1986.

57. **Cohen, S. S.,** The lethality of aranucleotides, *Med. Biol.,* 54, 299, 1976.
58. **Suhadolnik, R. M.,** Spongosine and arabinosyl nucleosides, in *Nucleoside Antibiotics,* Suhadolnik, R. J., Ed., John Wiley and Sons, New York, 1970, 123.
59. **Pavan-Langston, D., Buchanan, R. A., and Alford, C. A., Jr., Eds.,** *Adenine Arabinoside: An Antiviral Agent,* Raven Press, New York, 1974.
60. **Plagemann, P. G. W. and Wohlhueter, R. M.,** Permeation of nucleosides, nucleic acid bases and nucleotides in animal cells, *Curr. Topics Memb. Transport,* 14, 225, 1980.
61. **Wohlhueter, R. M. and Plagemann, P. G. W.,** The roles of transport and phosphorylation in nutrient uptake in cultured animal cells, *Int. Rev. Cytol.,* 64, 171, 1980.
62. **Paterson, A. R. P., Kolassa, N., and Cass, C. E.,** Transport of nucleoside drugs in animal cells, *Pharmacol. Ther.,* 12, 515, 1981.
63. **Young, J. D. and Jarvis, S. M.,** Nucleoside transport in animal cells, *Biosci. Rep.,* 3, 309, 1983.
64. **Paterson, A. R. P., Harley, E. R., and Cass, C. E.,** Measurement of inhibition of membrane transport of adenosine, in *Methods in Pharmacology,* Vol. 6, Paton, E. D., Ed., Plenun Publishing, New York, 1985, 165.
65. **Cass, C. E., Belt, J. A., and Paterson, A. R. P.,** Adenosine transport in cultured cells and erythrocytes, in *Prog. Clin. Biol. Res.,* 230, 13, 1987.
66. **Paterson, A. R. P. and Cass, C. E.,** Transport of nucleoside drugs in animal cells, in *Membrane Transport of Antineoplastic Agents,* Goldman, I. D., Ed., Pergamon Press, 1986, 309.
67. **Cass, C. E. and Paterson, A. R. P.,** Mediated transport of nucelosides by human erythrocytes. Specificity toward purine nucleosides as permeants, *Biochem. Biophys. Acta,* 291, 734, 1973.
68. **Cass, C. E. and Paterson, A. R. P.,** Inhibition by nitrobenzylthioinosine of uptake of adenosine, 2'-deoxyadenosine and 9-β-D-arabinofuranosyladenine by human and mouse erythrocytes, *Biochem. Pharmacol.,* 24, 1989, 1975.
69. **Cass, C. E., Kolassa, N., Uehara, Y., Dahlig-Harley, E. R., and Paterson, A. R. P.,** Absence of binding sites for the transport inhibitor nitrobenzylthioinosine on nucleoside transport-deficient mouse lymphoma cells, *Biochem. Biophys. Acta,* 649, 769, 1981.
70. **Sirotnak, F. M., Chello, P. L., Dorick, D. M., and Montgomery, J. A.,** Specificity of systems mediating transport of adenosine, 9-β-D-arabinofuranosyl-2-fluoroadenine, and other purine nucleoside analogues in L1210 cells, *Cancer Res.,* 43, 104, 1983.
71. **Chello, P. L., Sirotnak, F. M., Dorick, D. M., Yang, D.-H., and Montgomery, J. A.,** Initial rate kinetics and evidence for duality of mediated transport of adenosine, related purine nucleosides, and nucleoside analogues in L1210 cells, *Cancer Res.,* 43, 97, 1983.
72. **Dagnino, L. and Paterson, A. R. P.,** Concentrative transport of nucleosides in L1210 leukemia cells, *Proc. Am. Assoc. Cancer Res.,* 28, 15, 1987.
73. **Barrueco, J. R., Jacobsen, D. M., Chang, C.-H., Brockman, R. W., and Sirotnak, F. M.,** Proposed mechanism of therapeutic selectivity for 9-β-D-arabinofuranosyl-2-fluoroadenine against murine leukemia based upon lower capacities for transport and phosphorylation in proliferative intestinal epithelium compared to tumor cells, *Cancer Res.,* 47, 700, 1987.
74. **Krenitsky, T. A., Tuttle, J. V., Koszalka, J. V., Chen, G. W., Chen, I. S., Beacham, L. M., Rideout, J. L., and Elion, G. B.,** Deoxycytidine kinase from calf thymus, *J. Biol. Chem.,* 251, 4055, 1976.
75. **Chang, C.-H., Brockman, R. W., and Bennet, L. L., Jr.,** Purification and some properties of a deoxyribonucleoside kinase from L1210 cells, *Cancer Res.,* 42, 3033, 1982.
76. **Miller, R. L., Adamczyk, D. L., and Miller, W. H.,** Adenosine kinase from rabbit liver. I. Purification by affinity chromatography and properties, *J. Biol. Chem.,* 254, 2339, 1979.
77. **Miller, R. L., Adamczyk, D. L., Miller, W. H., Koszalka, G. W., Rideout, J. L., Beacham, L. M., Chao, E. Y., Haggerty, J. J., Krenitsky, T. A., and Elion, G. B.,** Adenosine kinase from rabbit liver. II. Substrate and inhibitor specificity, *J. Biol. Chem.,* 254, 2346, 1979.
78. **Chang, C.-H., Brockman, R. W., and Bennett, L. L., Jr.,** Adenosine kinase from L1210 cells, *J. Biol. Chem.,* 255, 2366, 1980.
79. **Juranka, P. and Chan, V.-L.,** Relative cytotoxicity of 9-β-D-arabinofuranosyladenine and 9-β-D-arabinofuranosyladenine 5'-monophosphate, *Cancer Res.,* 40, 4123, 1980.
80. **Chan, V.-L. and Juranka, P.,** Isolation and preliminary characterization of 9-β-D-arabinofuranosyladenine-resistant mutants of baby hamster cells, *Somat. Cell. Genet.,* 7, 147, 1981.
81. **Verhoef, V., Sarup, J., and Fridland, A.,** Identification of the mechanism of activation of 9-β-D-arabinofuranosyladenine in human lymphoid cells using mutants deficient in nucleoside kinases, *Cancer Res.,* 41, 4478, 1981.
82. **Cass, C. E., Selner, M., and Phillips, J. R.,** Resistance to 9-β-D-arabinofuranosyladenine in cultured leukemia L1210 cells, *Cancer Res.,* 43, 4791, 1983.
83. **Juranka, P. and Chan, V.-L.,** Analysis of adenosine kinase mutants of baby hamster kidney cells using affinity-purified antibody, *J. Biol. Chem.,* 260, 7738, 1985.

84. **Plunkett, W. and Cohen, S. S.,** Metabolism of 9-β-D-arabinofuranosyladenine by mouse fibroblasts, *Cancer Res.,* 35, 415, 1975.
85. **Shewach, D. S. and Plunkett, W.,** Effect of 2'-deoxycoformycin on the biologic half-life of 9-β-D-arabinofuranosyladenine 5'-triphosphate in CHO cells, *Biochem. Pharmacol.,* 28, 2401, 1979.
86. **Shewach, D. S. and Plunkett, W.,** Correlation of cytotoxicity with total intracellular exposure to 9-β-D-arabinofuranosyladenine 5'-triphosphate, *Cancer Res.,* 42, 3637, 1982.
87. **Agarwal, R. P., Sagar, S. M., and Parks, R. E., Jr.,** Adenosine deaminase from human erythrocytes: purification and effects of adenosine analogs, *Biochem. Pharmacol.,* 24, 693, 1975.
88. **Lee, S. H., Caron, N., and Kimball, A. P.,** Therapeutic effects of 9-β-D-arabinofuranosyladenine and 2'-deoxycoformycin combinations on intracerebral leukemia L1210, *Cancer Res.,* 37, 1953, 1977.
89. **Tseng, W.-C., Derse, D., Cheng, Y.-C., Brockman, R. W., and Bennett, L. L.,** *In vitro* biological activity of 9-β-D-arabinofuranosyl-2-fluoroadenine and the biochemical actions of its triphosphate on DNA polymerases and ribonucleotide reductase from HeLa cells, *Mol. Pharmacol.,* 21, 474, 1982.
90. **Sato, A., Montgomery, J. A., and Cory, J. G.,** Synergistic inhibition of leukemia L1210 cell growth *in vitro* by combinations of 2-fluoroadenine nucleosides and hydroxyurea or 2,3-dihydro-1H-pyrazole[2,3-a]imidazole, *Cancer Res.,* 44, 3286, 1984.
91. **El Dareer, S. M., Struck, R. F., Tillery, K. F., Rose, L. M., Brockman, R. W., Montgomery, J. A., and Hill, D. L.,** Disposition of 9-β-D-arabinofuranosyl-2-fluoroadenine in mice, dogs, and monkeys, *Drug Metab. Dispos.,* 8, 60, 1980.
92. **Struck, R. F., Shortnacy, A. T., Kirk, M. C., Thorpe, M. C., Brockman, R. W., Hill, D. L., El Dareer, S. M., and Montgomery, J. A.,** Identification of metabolites of 9-β-D-arabinofuranosyl-2-fluoroadenine, an antitumor and antiviral agent, *Biochem. Pharmacol.,* 31, 1975, 1982.
93. **Avramis, V. I. and Plunkett, W.,** 2-Fluoro-ATP: a toxic metabolite of 9-β-D-arabinosyl-2-fluoroadenine, *Biochem. Biophys. Res. Commun.,* 113, 35, 1983.
94. **Avramis, V. I. and Plunkett, W.,** Metabolism and therapeutic efficacy of 9-β-D-arabinofuranosyl-2-fluoroadenine against murine leukemia P388, *Cancer Res.,* 42, 2587, 1982.
95. **Verhoef, V. and Fridland, A.,** Metabolic basis of arabinonucleoside selectivity for human leukemic T- and B-lymphoblasts, *Cancer Res.,* 45, 3646, 1985.
96. **Shewach, D. S. and Plunkett, W.,** Cellular retention of 9-β-arabinofuranosyladenine 5'-triphosphate and the pattern of recovery of DNA synthesis of Chinese hamster ovary cells, *Cancer Res.,* 46, 1581, 1986.
97. **Schwartz, P. M., Novack, J., Shipman, C., Jr., and Rach, J. C.,** Metabolism of arabinosyladenine in herpes simplex virus-infected and uninfected cells, *Biochem. Pharmacol.,* 33, 2431, 1984.
98. **Dicioccio, R. A. and Srivastava, B. I. S.,** Kinetics of inhibition of deoxynucleotide-poymerizing enzyme activities from normal and leukemic human cells by 9-β-D-arabinofuranosyladenine 5'-triphosphate and 1-β-D-arabinofuranosylcytosine 5'-triphosphate, *Eur. J. Biochem.,* 79, 411, 1977.
99. **Okura, A. and Yoshida, S.,** Differential inhibition of DNA polymerases of calf thymus by 9-β-D-arabinofuranosyladenine 5'-triphosphate, *J. Biochem. (Tokyo),* 84, 727, 1978.
100. **Ono, K., Ohashi, A., Yamamoto, A., Matsukage, A., Takahasi, T., Saneyoshi, M., and Ueda, T.,** Inhibitory effects of 9-β-D-arabinofuranosylguanine 5'-triphosphate and 9-β-D-arabinofuranosyladenine 5'-triphosphate and on DNA polymerases from murine cells and oncornavirus, *Cancer Res.,* 39, 4673, 1979.
101. **White, E. L., Shaddix, S. C., Brockman, R. W., and Bennet, L. L., Jr.,** Comparison of the actions of 9-β-D-arabinofuranosyl-2-fluoroadenine and 9-β-D-arabinofuranosyladenine on target enzymes from mouse tumor cells, *Cancer Res.,* 42, 2260, 1982.
102. **Geurtsen, W., Zahn, R. K., Maidhof, A., Schmidseder, R., and Muller, W. E. G.,** Inhibition of DNA synthesis in permeabilized mouse P815 mast cells by arabinofuranosyladenine 5'-triphosphate, *Chemotherapy,* 27, 61, 1981.
103. **Moore, E. C. and Cohen, S. S.,** Effects of arabinonucleotides on ribonucleotide reduction by an enzyme from rat tumor, *J. Biol. Chem.,* 242, 2116, 1967.
104. **Chang, C.-H. and Cheng, Y.-C.,** Effects of deoxyadenosine triphosphate and 9-β-D-arabinofuranosyladenine 5'-triphosphate on human ribonucleotide reductase from Molt-4F cells and the concept of "self-potentiation", *Cancer Res.,* 40, 3555, 1980.
105. **Bennett, L. L., Jr., Shannon, W. M., Allen, P. W., and Arnett, G.,** Studies on the biochemical basis for the antiviral activity of some nucleoside analogs, *Ann. N.Y. Acad. Sci.,* 255, 345, 1975.
106. **Shipman, C., Jr., Smith, S. H., Carlson, R. H., and Drach, J. C.,** Antiviral activity of arabinosyladenine and arabinosylhypoxanthine in herpes simplex virus-infected KB cells: selective inhibition of viral deoxyribonucleic acid synthesis in synchronized suspension cultures, *Antimicrob. Agents Chemother.,* 9, 120, 1976.
107. **Muller, W. E. G., Zahn, R. K., Bittlingmaier, K., and Falke, D.,** Inhibition of herpesvirus DNA synthesis by 9-β-D-arabinofuranosyladenine in cellular and cell-free systems, *Ann. N.Y. Acad. Sci.,* 284, 34, 1977.
108. **Ostrander, M. and Cheng, Y.-C.,** Properties of herpes simplex virus type 1 and type 2 DNA polymerase, *Biochim. Biophys. Acta,* 609, 232, 1980.

109. **Derse, D. and Cheng, Y. C.,** Herpes simplex virus type I DNA polymerase: kinetic properties of the associated 3'-5' exonuclease and its role in araAMP incorporation, *J. Biol. Chem.,* 256, 8525, 1984.

110. **Coen, D. M., Furman, P. A., Gelep, P. T., and Schaffer, P. A.,** Mutations in the herpes simplex virus DNA polymerase gene can confer resistance to 9-β-D-arabinofuranosyladenine, *J. Virol.,* 41, 909, 1982.

111. **Fleming, H. E., Jr. and Coen, D. M.,** Herpes simplex virus mutants resistant to arabinosyladenine in the presence of deoxycoformycin, *Antimicrob. Agents Chemother.,* 26, 382, 1984.

112. **Wagar, M. A., Burgoyne, L. A., and Atkinson, M. R.,** Deoxyribonucleic acid synthesis in mammalian nuclei: incorporation of deoxyribonucleotides and chain-terminating nucleotide analogues, *Biochem. J.,* 121, 803, 1971.

113. **Plunkett, W., Lapi, L., Ortiz, P. J., and Cohen, S. S.,** Penetration of mouse fibroblasts by the 5'-phosphate of 9-β-D-arabinofuranosyladenine and incorporation of the nucleotide into DNA, *Proc. Natl. Acad. Sci.,* 71, 73, 1974.

114. **Cohen, S. S. and Plunkett, W.,** The utilization of nucleotides by animal cells, *Ann. N.Y. Acad. Sci.,* 255, 269, 1975.

115. **Muller, W. E. G., Rohde, H. J., Beyer, R., Madhof, A., Lachmann, M., Taschner, H., and Zahn, R. K.,** Mode of action of 9-β-D-arabinofuranosyladenine on the synthesis of DNA, RNA, and protein *in vivo* and *in vitro, Cancer Res.,* 35, 2160, 1975.

116. **Muller, W. E. G., Zahn, R. K., Beyer, R., and Falke, D.,** 9-β-D-Arabinofuranosyladenine as a tool to study herpes simplex virus DNA replication *in vitro, Virology,* 76, 787, 1977.

117. **Tsang Lee, M. Y. W., Byrnes, J. J., Downey, K. M., and So, A. G.,** Mechanism of inhibition of deoxyribonucleic acid synthesis by 1-β-D-arabinofuranosyladenosine triphosphate and its potentiation by 6-mercaptopurine ribonucleoside 5'-monophosphate, *Biochem.,* 19, 215, 1980.

118. **Pelling, J. C., Drach, J. C., and Shipman, C., Jr.,** Internucleotide incorporation of arabinosyladenine into herpes simplex virus and mammalian cell DNA, *Virology,* 109, 323, 1981.

119. **Kufe, D. W., Major, P. P., Munroe, D., Egan, M., and Herrick, D.,** Relationship between incorporation of 9-β-D-arabinofuranosyladenine in L1210 DNA and cytotoxicity, *Cancer Res.,* 43, 2000, 1983.

120. **Spriggs, D., Robbins, G., Mitchell, T., and Kufe, D.,** Incorporation of 9-β-D-arabinofuranosyl-2-fluoroadenine into HL-60 cellular RNA and DNA, *Biochem. Pharmacol.,* 35, 247, 1986.

121. **Richards, H. H., Chiang, P. K., and Cantoni, G. L.,** Adenosylhomocysteine hydrolase. Crystallization of the purified enzyme and its properties, *J. Biol. Chem.,* 253, 4476, 1978.

122. **Borchadt, R. T.,** S-Adenosyl-L-methionine-dependent macromolecule methyltransferases: potential targets for the design of chemotherapeutic agents, *J. Med. Chem.,* 23, 347, 1980.

123. **Hershfield, M. S.,** Apparent suicide inactivation of human lymphoblast S-adenosyl-homocysteine hydrolase by 2'-deoxyadenosine and adenine arabinoside, *J. Biol. Chem.,* 254, 22, 1979.

124. **Helland, S. and Ueland, P. M.,** The relation between the functions of 9-β-D-arabinofuranosyladenine as inactivator and substrate of S-adenosylhomocysteine hydrolase, *J. Pharmacol. Ther.,* 218, 758, 1981.

125. **Helland, S. and Ueland, P. M.,** Interaction of 9-β-D-arabinofuranosyladenine, 9-β-D-arabinofuranosyladenine 5'-triphosphate with S-adenosylhomocysteinase, *Cancer Res.,* 41, 673, 1981.

126. **Guranowski, A., Montgomery, J. A., Cantoni, G. L., and Chiang, P. K.,** Adenosine analogues as substrates and inhibitors of S-adenosylhomocysteine hydrolase, *Biochem.,* 20, 110, 1981.

127. **Chiang, P. K., Guranowski, A., and Segall, J. E.,** Irreversible inhibition of S-adenosylhomocysteine hydrolase by nucleoside analogs, *Arch. Biochem. Biophys.,* 207, 175, 1981.

128. **Cass, C. E., Selner, M., Ferguson, P. J., and Phillips, J. R.,** Effects of 2'-deoxyadenosine, 9-β-D-arabinofuranosyladenine, and related compounds on S-adenosyl-L-homocysteine hydrolase activity in synchronous and asynchronous cultured cells, *Cancer Res.,* 42, 4991, 1982.

129. **Helland, S. and Ueland, P. M.,** S-Adenosylhomocysteine and S-adenosylhomocysteine hydrolase in various tissues of mice given injections of 9-β-D-arabinofuranosyladenine, *Cancer Res.,* 43, 1847, 1983.

130. **Zimmerman, T. P., Wolberg, G., Duncan, G. S., and Elion, G. B.,** Adenosine analogues as substrates and inhibitors of S-adenosylhomocysteine hydrolase in intact lymphocytes, *Biochem.,* 19, 2252, 1980.

131. **Helland, S. and Ueland, P. M.,** Inactivation of S-adenosylhomocysteine hydrolase by 9-β-D-arabinofuranosyladenine in intact cells, *Cancer Res.,* 42, 1130, 1982.

132. **Helland, S. and Ueland, P. M.,** Reactivation of S-adenosylhomocysteine hydrolase activity in cells exposed to 9-β-D-arabinofuranosyladenine, *Cancer Res.,* 42, 2861, 1982.

133. **Schanche, J.-S., Schanche, T., Ueland, P. M., and Montgomery, J. A.,** Inactivation and reactivation of intracellular S-adenosylhomocysteinase in the presence of nucleoside analogues in rat hepatocytes, *Cancer Res.,* 44, 4297, 1984.

134. **Hershfield, M. S., Small, W. C., Premakumar, R., Bagnara, A. S., and Fetter, J. E.,** Inactivation of S-adenosylhomocysteine hydrolase: mechanism and occurrence *in vivo* in disorders of purine nucleoside catabolism, in *The Biochemistry of S-Adenosylmethionine and Related Compounds,* Usdin, E., Borchardt, R. T., and Creveling, C. R., Eds., MacMillan Press, London, 1982, 657.

135. **Young, G. J., Hallam, L. J., Jack, I., and Van Der Weyden, M. B.,** S-Adenosylhomocysteine hydrolase inactivation and purine toxicity in cultured human T- and B-lymphoblasts, *J. Lab. Clin. Med.,* 104, 86, 1984.

136. **Juranka, P., Meffe, F., Guttman, S., Archer, S. M., and Chan, V.-L.,** An adenosine kinase mutation in baby hamster kidney cells causing increased sensitivity to adenosine, *Mutat. Res.,* 129, 397, 1984.

137. **Chan, V.-L. and Guttman, S.,** Codominant and recessive 9-β-D-arabinofuranosyladenine-resistant mutations of baby hamster cells, *Mut. Res.,* 149, 141, 1985.

138. **Shipman, C., Jr., Tong, S.-L., Smith, S. H., Katlama, N. B., and Drach, J. C.,** Establishment of a murine cell line resistant to arabinosyladenine and devoid of adenosine deaminase activity, *Antimicrob. Agents Chemother.,* 24, 947, 1983.

139. **Yeung, C.-Y., Ingolia, D. E., Bobonis, C., Dunbar, B. S., Riser, M. E., Siciliano, M. J., and Kellems, R. E.,** Selective overproduction of adenosine deaminase in cultured mouse cells, *J. Biol. Chem.,* 258, 8338, 1983.

140. **Hoffee, P. A., Hunt, S. W., III, and Chiang, J.,** Isolation of deoxycoformycin-resistant cells with increased levels of adenosine deaminase, *Somatic. Cell Genet.,* 8, 465, 1982.

141. **Hunt, S. W., III and Hoffee, P. A.,** Adenosine deaminase from deoxycoformycin-sensitive and -resistant rat hepatoma cells. Purification and characterization, *J. Biol. Chem.,* 257, 14239, 1982.

142. **Hunt, S. W., III and Hoffee, P. A.,** Increased adenosine deaminase synthesis and messenger RNA activity in deoxycoformycin-resistant cells, *J. Biol. Chem.,* 258, 41, 1983.

143. **Hunt, S. W., III and Hoffee, P. A.,** Amplification of adenosine deaminase gene sequences in deoxycoformycin-resistant rat hepatoma cells, *J. Biol. Chem.,* 258, 13185, 1983.

144. **Rowland, P., III, Pfeilsticker, J., and Hoffee, P. A.,** Adenosine deaminase gene amplification in deoxycoformycin-resistant mammalian cells, *Arch. Biochem. Biophys.,* 239, 396, 1985.

145. **Rowland, P., III, Chiang, J., Jargiello-Jarrett, P., and Hoffee, P. A.,** Chromosome anomalies associated with amplification of the adenosine deaminase gene (ADA) in rat hepatoma cells, *Cytogenet. Cell Genet.,* 41, 136, 1986.

146. **LePage, G. A.,** Resistance to 9-β-D-arabinofuranosyladenine in murine tumor cells, *Cancer Res.,* 38, 2314, 1978.

147. **Ayusawa, D., Iwata, K., and Seno, T.,** Alteration of ribonucleotide reductase in aphidicolin-resistant mutants of mouse FM3A cells with associated resistance to arabinosyladenine and arbinosylcytosine, *Somat. Cell Genet.,* 7, 27, 1981.

148. **Iwata, K., Ayusawa, D., and Seno, T.,** Increased level of ribonucleotide reductase and associated resistance to aphidicolin in mouse FM3A cell mutants selected for simultaneous resistance to 9-β-D-arabinofuranosyladenine and 1-β-D-arabinofuranosylcytosine, *Gann,* 73, 167, 1982.

149. **Ayusawa, D., Iwata, K., and Seno, T.,** Unusual sensitivity to bleomycin and joint resistance to 9-β-D-arabinofuranosyladenine and 1-β--D-arabinofuranosylcytosine of mouse FM3A cell mutants with altered ribonucleotide reductase and thymidylate synthase, *Cancer Res.,* 43, 814, 1983.

150. **Liu, P. K., Chang, C.-C., Trosko, J. E., Dube, D. K., Martin, G. M., and Loeb, L. A.,** Mammalian mutator mutant with an aphidicolin-resistant DNA polymerase *alpha, Proc. Natl. Acad. Sci.,* 80, 797, 1983.

151. **Fridland, A.,** Selection of 9-β-D-arabinofuranosyladenine-resistant human T-lymphoblasts with altered ribonucleotide reductase activity, *Cancer Res.,* 44, 4328, 1984.

152. **North, T. W.,** Effects of 9-β-D-arabinofuranosyladenine and 1-β-D-arabinofuranosylcytosine on levels of deoxyribonucleic acid precursors in uninfected and herpes simplex virus-infected cells, *Biochem. Pharmacol.,* 32, 3862, 1983.

153. **Vishwanatha, J. K., and Mishra, N. C.,** Chinese hamster ovary cell mutants resistant to DNA polymerase inhibitors. I. Isolation and biochemical genetic characterization, *Mol. Gen. Genet.,* 200, 393, 1985.

154. **Hay, J. and Subak-Sharpe, J.,** Mutants of herpes simplex virus 1 and 2 that are resistant to phosphonoacetic acid induce altered DNA polymerase activities in infected cells, *J. Gen. Virol.,* 31, 145, 1976.

155. **Kufe, D., Herric, D., Crumpacker, C., and Schnipper, L.,** Incorporation of 1-β-D-arabinofuranosylcytosine in DNA from herpes simplex virus resistant to 9-β-D-arabinofuranosyladenine, *Cancer Res.,* 44, 69, 1984.

156. **Coen, D. M., Aschman, D. P., Gelep, P. T., Retondo, M. J., Weller, S. K., and Schaffer, P. A.,** Fine mapping and molecular cloning of mutations in the herpes simplex virus DNA polymerase locus, *J. Virol.,* 49, 236, 1984.

157. **Coen, D. M., Fleming, H. E., Jr., Leslie, L. K., and Retondo, M. J.,** Sensitivity of arabinosyladenine-resistant mutants of herpes simplex virus to other antiviral drugs and mapping of drug hypersensitivity mutations to the DNA polymerase locus, *J. Virol.,* 53, 477, 1985.

Chapter 10

## GUANINE AND HYPOXANTHINE ANALOGS

**K. John Morrow, Jr. and David A. Rintoul**

## TABLE OF CONTENTS

I.      Introduction.................................................................146

II.     Mechanism of Cytotoxicity .....................................................146

III.    Biochemical Basis of Resistance................................................147

IV.     Molecular Mechanism of Genetic Variation......................................150

V.      Mutagenesis Studies ..........................................................152

VI.     HRPT Gene Therapy............................................................154

VII.    Conclusions..................................................................154

References......................................................................155

# I. INTRODUCTION

The question of why somatic cells show variability in their patterns of phenotypic expression is an old one, whose roots go back to the 19th century. An understanding of this complex issue has implications for questions of malignancy, cell differentiation, and aging. The development of bacterial genetics during the 1940s and 1950s produced an intellectual framework which could be adapted to eukaryotic somatic cells, provided that methods of selecting rare genetic events from large cellular populations could be perfected. Therefore, it is not surprising that considerable interest in the genetic control of drug resistance in cultured cells has existed since the early days of cell culture research. These studies began in the late 1950s, and grew out of an attempt to understand drug refractory states arising in the course of cancer treatment. Purine analog resistance was among the earliest systems exploited, and resistance to analogs of guanine and hypoxanthine was the subject of enthusiastic and spirited investigation. As new innovative technical developments allowed design of more and more sophisticated experiments, a body of knowledge was accumulated at an increasingly profound level. Current descriptions of resistance to guanine and hypoxanthine analogs include molecular studies of responsible DNA sequences, mutagenesis investigations, knowledge of the biochemical basis of cytotoxicity and cytogenetic investigations. In this review, we will consider each in turn, and conclude with some discussion of the role of these genetic units in gene therapy.

Three purine base analogs have been used for most of the work to be reviewed here: 8-azaguanine (AG), 6-thioguanine (TG), and 6-mercaptopurine (MP). In addition, scattered reports have appeared describing cell lines resistant to 8-azahypoxanthine (AH) and its corresponding nucleoside, azainosine (AI). Their structures, and those of the natural bases hypoxanthine and guanine, are shown in Figure 1.

When exogenous purines or their analogs are metabolized by mammalian cells, they are converted to the respective phosphoribosylated forms and then participate in the formation of nucleic acids (Figure 2). The *de novo* pathway of purine synthesis provides purines in the absence of external sources. Thus inhibition of purine synthesis by folic acid analogs such as aminopterin or amethopterin will not result in a cessation of cellular proliferation, unless the cell type under study has lost the salvage pathway through a mutational alteration. This observation forms the basis of the reverse selective HAT (hypoxanthine, aminopterin and thymidine) system by which (1) revertants and (2) cell hybrids can be selected.

# II. MECHANISM OF CYTOTOXICITY

Exposure of mammalian cell lines to increasing levels of purine analogs results in inhibition of cellular proliferation at lower concentrations and eventual killing at higher levels, as shown by kill curves measuring inhibition of colony formation (Figure 3). The $LD_{50}$ for mammalian cell lines varies over a vast range of concentrations, and is dependent on a number of different factors:

1. Cell lines; mouse P388 and L1210 cells are insensitive to AG (4)
2. Level of exogenous purines in the medium;[5] this has occasioned the recommendation that dialyzed serum be used during AG selection
3. Presence of guanase in the medium; this causes the detoxification of AG but not TG[5]

Purines or their analogs are converted into nucleoside and then nucleotide bases and thence incorporated into DNA and RNA (Figure 2). In addition guanine plays a role in numerous biochemical reactions as a cofactor. Thus there are a number of points at which these agents could exert a cytotoxic effect. The hypothesis has long been entertained that AG exerts its

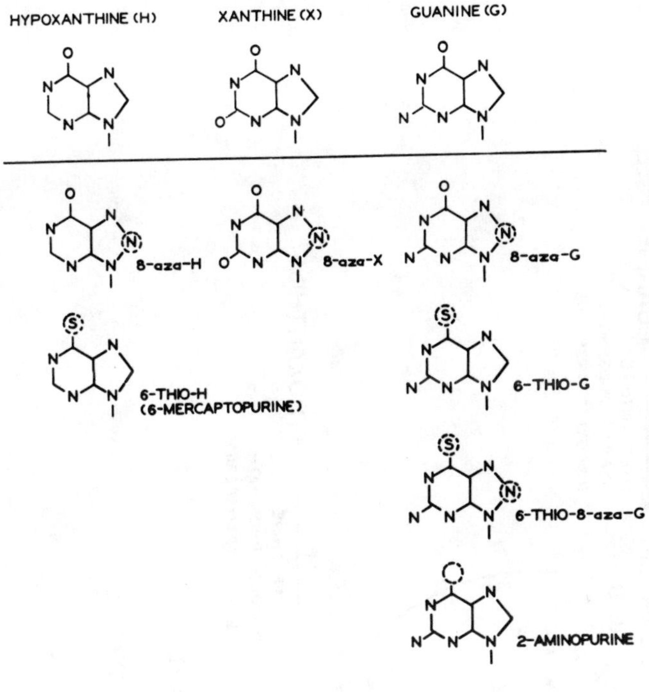

FIGURE 1. Analogs and naturally occurring purines bases. Adenine and its analogs are covered in the paper in this volume by Taylor.[28]

toxicity through incorporation into RNA, while thiopurines kill by incorporation into DNA. These beliefs are supported by the fact that inhibitors of DNA synthesis will protect cells from the cytotoxicity of thiopurines but not of AG.[6] It is likely that incorporation of TG into DNA results in an inability of the DNA to replicate.[7]

Chase experiments combining AG with actinomycin D indicate that up to 70% of the maturation of ribosomal RNA can be inhibited by AG, suggesting that this may be a major mechanism of toxicity of this substance.[8] Recent experiments[9] using L1210 mouse leukemia cells indicate that AG exerts its toxicity by inhibition of translation.

In the case of MP, there is ample evidence that the ribonucleotide and certain derivatives interfere with the further anabolism of IMP. Also, the synthesis of IMP can be inhibited through feedback inhibition by MP ribonucleotide; several of the enzymes involved in the biosynthesis of purines are inhibited by this mechanism.[10] It has not been established which (if any) of these effects has the major cytotoxicity,[7] nor have the mechanisms of cytotoxicity of AH and AI[11] been established.

## III. BIOCHEMICAL BASIS OF RESISTANCE

Initial studies demonstrated that mammalian cells resistant to guanine and hypoxanthine analogs could be isolated with relative ease.[12] Investigation of the biochemical basis of this resistance demonstrated that in most cases it could be attributed to a loss or decrease in the activity of the enzyme hypoxanthine guanine phosphoribosyltransferase (HPRT; IMP: pyrophosphate phosphoribosyltransferase; EC 2.4.2.8). This has proven to be the most common basis for resistance, and is now well understood at the gene level.

HPRT is usually measured by the conversion of radioactive hypoxanthine to IMP in the presence of PRPP and $Mg^{2+}$. The phosphorylated product has a decreased solubility and can be retained on filters under conditions which allow the removal of unreacted substrate.

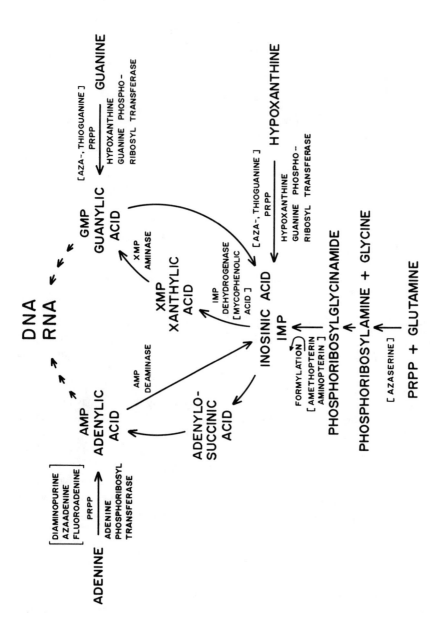

FIGURE 2.   Outline of purine metabolism in mammalian cells. Compounds indicated in parentheses are toxic analogs, resistance to which is obtained by loss of diminution of the corresponding enzyme.[35]

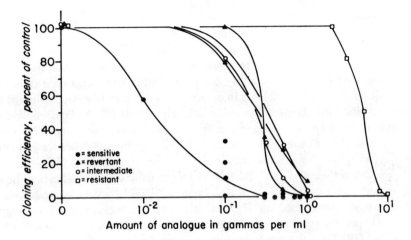

FIGURE 3.   Inhibition of cloning ability as a function of thioguanine concentration in transformed mouse fibroblast line.[3] An intermediate level of resistance can be selected with drug concentrations in the range of 0.1 μg/mℓ. Resistant lines selected in 1 μg/mℓ or higher have complete loss of HPRT and die in HAT medium. Note that revertants selected in HAT medium possess resistance profiles similar to the intermediate line.

In a variety of experimental systems, including human,[13] mouse,[3] hamster,[14] both diploid and transformed, loss or diminution of HPRT is associated with increased resistance. This is not, however, invariably the case, as double selection with AG followed by HAT resulted in the isolation of numerous clones with substantial HPRT levels.[14]

Other postulated resistance mechanisms include defects in transport,[15,16] increased levels of guanine deaminase,[10] 5′-nucleotidase (E.C. 2.4.2.1.)[17] or alkaline phosphatase (E.C. 3.1.3.1.).[18] The question of transport mutants for hypoxanthine and guanine has proven to be controversial. While their existence was suggested by the aforementioned studies, Plagemann and Wohlhuetter[19] have used rapid kinetic transport techniques to evaluate an AG resistant ts variant of Harris and Whitmore.[15] Although the biochemical basis of resistance of this mutant remains obscure, it does not reside in a transport defect. In fact, there are theoretical reasons for doubting the existence of transport mutants for AG; hypoxanthine is carried into cells by a saturable, carrier mediated transporter, but AG appears to enter the cell passively.[20]

Alkaline phosphatase elevation appears to be responsible, at least in part, for the resistance of a mouse sarcoma to the toxic effects of MP and TG.[21,22] Much of the enzyme is extracellularly located.[18] Moreover, isozymes with different antigenic properties are detectable in drug resistant sublines.[21,22] These observations bring to mind the findings of Santachiara-Benerecetti et al.[23] who determined that in human HeLa cell variants with widely disparate levels of alkaline phosphatase, different isozyme forms were preferentially increased. Henderson et al.[24] have also proposed that elevated levels of alkaline phosphatases are responsible for resistance to 6-methylmercaptopurine. Although this mechanism of resistance does not appear to be a common one in cultured cells, it may be of some significance in tumor cell populations.

There have been other scattered reports of 5′-nucleotidase and guanine deaminase figuring in purine analog resistance. For instance Berman et al.[25] attributed the greater sensitivity of rat liver epithelial cells to AG (but not TG) to decreased guanine deaminase and 5′-nucleotidase activities. Guanine deaminase converts AG to azaxanthine (which is not carcinostatic) but no correlation has been observed between resistance to AG and guanine deaminase levels.[26] More recently, guanine deaminase elevated variants have been examined by Meyers and Shin[27] with the finding that variation in AG resistance of cell lines is explained by variations in guanine deaminase levels. However, these were naturally occurring cell lines, and not drug resistant variants isolated following selection. The biochemical basis of resistance to AH[28] and azainosine[11] remains to be clarified.

The HPRT locus affected in drug resistant cell lines is the same as that responsible for the Lesch-Nyhan syndrome, as shown by complementation studies between cells from affected individuals and variants isolated in culture. This disorder is a rare, X-linked disease whose primary biochemical defect is a severe deficiency of HPRT. Afflicted individuals are characterized by mental retardation, spasticity, choreoatheosis, and compulsive self-mutilation.[29] The condition is incurable, untreatable, and is a prime candidate for gene therapy, although the pathophysiology of the disease has not been elucidated.

The differences between AG and TG with regard to their selective efficiency lie mainly in the decreased ability of AG to act as a substrate for HPRT, and in its greater instability when added to tissue culture medium. Hypoxanthine is an extremely effective noncompetitive inhibitor of AG phosphorylation, and that combined with the approximately tenfold differences in $K_m$ of HPRT for the two substrates accounts for the ineffectiveness of low concentrations of AG.[30] Thus it is possible to isolate AG resistant mutants which possess an increased $K_m$ for AG while still retaining wild type abilities to utilize hypoxanthine.[14] It should also be noted that mutant recovery is dependent on the density of cells plated for mutant selection, due to the effects of metabolic cooperation in confluent cells. This can be eliminated by the use of soft agar culture rather than the standard liquid medium culture.[31] These authors determined that greater than 95% of the TG resistant colonies isolated by this method were HAT sensitive.

A variety of other related compounds have been tested against HPRT⁻ and HPRT⁺ cell lines, with the result that most analogs related to hypoxanthine and guanine are less toxic to HPRT deficient cell lines (see Table 1).[72] Two exceptions are 6-methylthiopurine ribonucleoside and 6-ethylthiopurine ribonucleoside. These agents are apparently able to enter the cell intact, rather than degraded to their respective purine bases, which would make them substrates for HPRT. Another exception, 2-azaadenine, is doubtless a substrate for APRT rather than HPRT.

## IV. MOLECULAR MECHANISM OF GENETIC VARIATION

Over the years the genetic basis of hypoxanthine-guanine analog resistance has been the subject of great interest, and much of the research reported in this area has been concerned with indirect approaches to the resolution of this issue. These strategies include the measurement of mutation rates in cell lines of different ploidies[32] and analysis of partially resistant variants which often are unstable.[33,34] These and other studies[35] have produced interesting and suggestive findings, many of which are not easily reconcilable with simple molecular mechanisms such as base pair changes in the HPRT structural gene. This prompted the proposal of gene inactivation[36] as an explanation. Clearly, the resolution of these questions requires the cloning and molecular analysis of the responsible genetic elements. In those cases in which this has been carried out, the basis of hypoxanthine-guanine analog resistance is accountable without resort to epigenetic or other modulating mechanisms.

Prior to the availability of a cloned HPRT gene, characterization of mutants was aided through the use of polyclonal antibodies against HPRT which demonstrated the presence of immunologically cross reacting material in HPRT⁻ mutants.[37] Subsequent to this, a variety of biochemical techniques (SDS-PAGE, isoelectric focusing, high pressure liquid chromatography) provided strong evidence for structural gene mutations in cells resistant to AG and TG.[29,37-39]

Although other genetic elements involved in purine analog resistance have not been thoroughly analyzed, the HPRT gene has been the subject of much investigation. The mouse

**Table 1[a]**

## CYTOTOXICITY OF HYPOXANTHINE AND GUANINE ANALOGS TO H EP. NO. 2 CELLS AND A SUBLINE DEFICIENT IN HPRT[b]

| Compound | $ID_{50}$ ($\mu g/m\ell$)[c] | Ratio HPRT$^-$/HPRT$^{+}$ [d] |
|---|---|---|
| 6-Mercaptopurine | 0.2 | 2000 |
| 6-Mercaptopurine ribonucleoside | 0.4 | >250 |
| 6-Mercaptopurine ribonucleotide | 0.6 | >170 |
| 6-(Methylthio)purine ribonucleoside | 0.1 | 1 |
| 6-(Ethylthio)purine ribonucleoside | 0.3 | 1 |
| 6-(Benzylthio)purine ribonucleoside | 3.7 | 1.3 |
| 6-Thioguanine | 0.04 | 1300 |
| 6-Thioguanosine | 0.4 | >250 |
| 6-Thioguanylic acid | 0.3 | >330 |
| S-Methyl-6-thioguanine | 44 | 1.4 |
| Bis(thioinosine)-5′,5′′′-phosphate | 0.4 | 23 |
| 9-Butyl-6-mercaptopurine | 13 | 0.6 |
| 2-Azahypoxanthine | 0.4 | 600 |
| 2-Azainosine | 0.9 | 150 |
| 2′-Deoxy-2-azainosine | 0.6 | 200 |
| 2-Azaadenine | 11 | 1 |
| 2-Azaadenosine | 0.2 | 0.7 |
| 8-Azaadenine | 20 | 1—2 |
| 8-Azaadenosine | 0.8 | 70 |
| 8-Azahypoxanthine (8-AzaH) | 3· | >300 |
| 8-Azainosine (8-AzaHR) | 0.7 | 1—2 |
| 8-Azaguanine (8-AzaG) | 3 | 200 |
| 8-Azaguanosine (8-AzaGr) | 2 | 20—40 |
| 8-Aza-6-Thioinosine (8-AzaMPR) | (1) | 1 |

[a]   Modified from Montgomery.[72]
[b]   Resistant to MP; deficient in HPRT.
[c]   Dose required to inhibit treated to 50% of control cell growth.
[d]   Ratio of $ID_{50}$ for resistant cells to $ID_{50}$ for sensitive cells.

HPRT gene has been cloned and its structure determined.[40] It is a large gene, containing 9 exons spread over 33 kb of DNA. Its promotor has been sequenced, and it contains neither TATA or CAAT boxes, but rather the region immediately upstream from the cap site is rich in G/C sequences. It has been suggested[41] that the function of these clusters is to provide a cooperative means of minimizing chance *de novo* methylation in the regulatory regions. As these regions are a feature of housekeeping genes, control of their transcription may occur by a different mechanism from the differentiated gene functions so widely studied. Thus the G/C clusters could serve as irreversible switches to maintain continuous activity of housekeeping genes.

With the availability of the cloned gene[42] from mouse and human sources, it became possible to investigate not only the structure of the HPRT gene, but also the properties and mechanisms of forward and reverse mutation. Because of the unusual features of AG and TG resistant cell lines, it was not clear what the molecular basis of resistance could be. The hypothesis of either epigenetic mechanisms, or of mutation in regulatory or promotor elements was supported by various data. These included high mutation rates and activation of previously silenced HPRT genes as a result of cell hybridization.[43-45] On the other hand several studies, including the characterization of temperature sensitive mutants[46] established that at least some HPRT variants were the result of point mutation in the structural gene. Use of cloned HPRT probes has substantiated this belief. HPRT$^-$ mutations in cultured cells are thought to result from either deletions (often combined with rearrangements) or with point mutations.[40] In patients with the Lesch-Nyhan syndrome, a variety of different, independently occurring lesions have been demonstrated, including deletions and base pair substitutions.[40] Further details of these alterations are covered in the next section on mutagenesis.

Reverse mutation has been shown[47,48] to be due to gene amplification of the defective locus. Temperature sensitive variants with low but detectable levels of the enzyme will produce phenotypic revertants which overproduce the defective gene product at levels commensurate with growth in HAT medium. As shown by experiments using cDNA probes, such variants overproduce both the gene and the mRNA for HPRT, and tend to be unstable, losing their phenotype when cultivated in the absence of HAT medium. The fact that such variants produce only a few fold over the level of the parent mutant is probably due to the fact that a greater level of enzymatic activity is not required for growth in HAT.

Other revertants selected in HAT medium appear to result from second site mutations within the HPRT locus which restore partial activity.[49] The original mutation is one leading to a reduction in the molecular weight and a complete loss of enzymatic activity, and is most probably a missense mutation.

No information is available on the molecular nature of other resistance mechanisms, such as increases in levels of phosphatases.

## V. MUTAGENESIS STUDIES

Because the HPRT gene is well analyzed at the molecular level, because efficient selection in both the forward and reverse direction can be carried out, and because good evidence for a hemizygous condition exists, this locus lends itself particularly well to quantitative mutagenesis studies, and a substantial literature in this area has developed.[35] Studies on both spontaneous and induced mutations have added to our understanding of the structure of the mammalian genome, and to the HPRT locus in particular.

Notwithstanding these advantages, however, the system also carries some uncertainties and difficulties. One of the most significant of these is that resistant clones appearing during selection may have a heterogeneous nature; especially in the case of AG where several biochemical mechanisms may be responsible for resistance. Moreover, the genetic basis of a single biochemical defect (HPRT deficiency) may reside in multiple causes, including point mutation, deletion, gene inactivation, and modulation of expression. As mammalian cells are large and complex, and the mutagenic agent must undertake an epic voyage to reach the sensitive genetic element, the investigator could not expect that mutagens having known and direct mechanisms of action in bacterial or viral assay systems to have the same effects in mammalian cells. Lacking extensive molecular analysis of every variant arising in a large mutagenized sample, it would be premature to derive simple, unitary models of induced genetic change. Given these caveats, however, it has still been possible for investigators over the years to develop a coherent body of data describing many aspects of the mutational process involved in purine analog resistance.

Pioneering studies on spontaneous mutation rates in D98 heteroploid human cells (a HeLa variant) were carried out by Szybalski and Szybalska.[28] These landmark studies established the principle that mammalian cells could be subjected to quantitative mutational analysis, as had been so successfully performed in bacterial cell lines during the preceding decade. These studies took advantage of the fluctuation test[50] which measures mutation rates while at the same time establishing whether a particular variant is preexisting or induced by the selecting agent. In all cases of purine analog resistance it has been determined that AG and TG resistant cells are pre-existing in the population and are selected by the drug. This conclusion is now so widely accepted that it is no longer a debatable issue.[35]

Subsequently a variety of studies established that the spontaneous mutation rate varied widely among permanent cell lines, over more than three orders of magnitude.[51] This variation derives from a number of causes:

1.   Differences in selecting agents and presence of serum[52] and other interfering factors in the medium. This would allow the expression of partial HPRT loss or amplification of nucleotidase levels which would appear with greater frequency.
2.   Differences in ploidy level.[32,53] Whether of male or female origin, one would expect the original cell line to possess a single functional HPRT allele. However, many cell lines, including human lines may possess multiple copies of the X chromosome, either singly or as part of a duplication of the entire chromosome set.
3.   Differences in medium, trypsinization schedules, fluctuation in temperature, and other growth conditions. These could be mutagenic themselves, augmenting the spontaneous rate.
4.   Differences in seeding density, reflecting the influences of metabolic cooperation.

Induced mutagenesis was first considered by Szybalski and Szybalska,[28] with negative results. However, subsequent studies by Chu and Malling[54] using X-rays gave positive results. The failure to observe an increase in the incidence of mutant clones in the earlier studies could be due to an insufficiently long lag period between the application of the mutagen and addition of the selecting agent.[55] Experiments by Thilly et al.[56] substantiate this conclusion; these workers demonstrated an extremely long phenotypic lag in the case of TG resistance in human transformed lymphoblasts. In the case of ICR-191 induced mutations, full expression of all mutations required up to 20 days and 16 generations.

The analysis of reverse mutation at the HPRT locus began as early as did forward mutational studies; Szybalski and Szybalska[28] measured reversion rates using HAT medium. Later studies reported large variation in reversion rates, some of them higher than the forward rates.[57] Reversion could arise from repair of the original mutation, an intragenic suppressor mutation, or an intergenic suppressor mutation, such as a regulatory mutation. This latter possibility appears to be quite unlikely in this case, as no regulatory loci appear to govern the expression of the HPRT gene. Gene amplification, discussed above, could also result in a phenotypic revertant, capable of surviving in HAT medium. Another possibility would be a mutation in another gene, such as a gene governing resistance to aminopterin. With so many possibilities, it is not surprising that large variations in reversion rates have been recorded.

Expression time of reversion is much shorter than for forward mutation as would be expected; 2 days was sufficient to obtain optimal expression of reversion induced by chemical mutagens in the L5178Y line.[58] This observation suggests that the long lag required for expression of forward mutations is because of a need to dilute out pre-existing HPRT, rather than because of a need to fix induced changes into the DNA.

Careful cytogenetic analysis of X-ray induced TG resistance[59] indicates that at least 40% of the variants are due to deletions or gene rearrangements. X-rays are potent chromosome breakers, and it is not surprising that HPRT deficiency could be produced through this mechanism. Recently Stone-Wolff et al.[60] reported the characterization of two V79 cell lines, isolated after mutagenesis and growth in thioguanine, which can be used to distinguish between frame-shift and base-substitution mutagens. These lines, after further molecular characterization, could be used to assess the mutagenic capacity of previously uncharacterized carcinogens and mutagens.

The depth of genetic and biochemical characterization of this locus has enabled various investigators to use the HPRT system as an assay for mutagens, or in studies designed to assess the effects of other variables (anoxia, cell cycle parameters, etc.) on mutagen effectiveness. For example, forward mutation to TG resistance has been used as an assay for mutagen activation by rat liver microsome preparations.[61,62] The effects of heavy metals (cadmium) on mutation to TG resistance were studied by Ochi et al.[63] Finally, irradiation mutagensis of this locus has been studied in conjunction with cell cycle phase[64] in conjunction with hyperoxia and inhibition of cellular antioxidant systems,[65] and in lymphoma cell strains with differing UV sensitivities.[66] These and related studies, in addition to yielding more information about the HPRT locus, also provide data on mutagen mechanisms and synergism between various mutagen types.

## VI. HPRT GENE THERAPY

In recent years there has developed great interest and agitation among the general public, as well as within scientific circles, concerning prospects for treatment of genetic disorders using cloned segments of DNA. Ideally, such disorders would be recessive inborn errors of metabolism which would be correctable using bone marrow cells from the afflicted individual. The cells would be taken from the subject, treated with the appropriate genetic structural elements and promoters, and reinserted in the patient so as to achieve expression and palliation of the disorder. In order to merit such "desperate appliances"[67] a qualifying condition would have to be devastating, untreatable, and independent of spacial architecture of the tissue. To some extent the Lesch-Nyham syndrome appears to qualify for this dubious honor, however, the fact that the condition exerts its damage through the nervous system makes it less attractive as a candidate for genetic engineering.

Nonetheless, a number of studies have been published which have demonstrated the technical feasibility of various aspects of this protocol. Willis et al.[68] have designed a retrovirus vector carrying the human HPRT gene which will infect 100% of human lymphoblasts isolated from a patient with the Lesch-Nyhan syndrome. Gruber et al.[69] have shown that glial cells can cooperate metabolically with HPRT deficient fibroblasts to transfer labeled purines to these deficient cells. The use of glial cells in this study was motivated by the belief that metabolic defects in these cells might be important determinants of the neurological symptoms of the Lesch-Nyhan Syndrome. These data indicate that gene replacement therapy could be effective in this syndrome, since it should not be necessary to replace the defective gene in all cells of the patient. At present two laboratories are leading the way in these studies, that of Friedmann at the University of California at San Diego, and the group headed by Caskey at Baylor College of Medicine in Houston. The ethical, legal, and political ramifications of these studies are reviewed by Culliton.[70]

## VII. CONCLUSIONS

We have endeavored in this brief review to cover a wide range of studies, extending over three decades, during which time genetics and molecular biology have made such dramatic progress that certain subdisciplines (somatic cell genetics) are almost unrecognizable from their early origins. Despite these advances (or perhaps because of them) our understanding of hypoxanthine-guanine analog resistance has moved more rapidly at the molecular level than at the level of cellular physiology. Thus, the exact mechanism by which these analogs exert their toxicty is still unclear, and no prospect for its resolution appears forthcoming.

Research conducted over this period has repeatedly shown that resistant variants can be selected using mainly aza or thioguanine (AG or TG); while revertants can be isolated in medium containing HAT (hypoxanthine, aminopterin, and thymidine). The cellular toxicity of AG is thought to be the result of inhibition of ribosomal synthesis, due to the breakdown in feedback regulation of purine biosynthesis, while TG is believed to interfere with DNA replication. The mode of action of other analogs (mercaptopurine, azahypoxathine, azainosine) is in doubt.

The biochemical mechanisms by which cells circumvent this toxicity may be due to a loss of the enzyme hypoxanthine guanine phosphoribosyl transferase (HPRT), overproduction of alkaline phosphatases or overproduction of 5'-nucleotidases. Claims of resistance resulting from defects in purine transport have been made, but remain controversial.

The study of the molecular biology of the HPRT locus indicates that models of variation which propose regulatory mutations are unlikely. Gene inactivation as the result of transposition and the interruption of transcription cannot be entirely rule out. However, all the mutants that are thoroughly understood appear to be the result of gene deletion or missense and nonsense mutations. Reversion can occur by way of missense or nonsense repair, or by gene amplification of the defective (but still partially active) HPRT gene to levels sufficient to allow growth in HAT medium. Spontaneous and induced mutagenesis studies have demonstrated that the HPRT locus is stable, but yields drug-resistant variants with a low incidence; this can be increased by chemical mutagens and ionizing and UV radiation. The fluctuation test has repeatedly established that these variants are preexisting in the population rather than induced by the selecting agent.

Given the unlikeliness of controller elements in the HPRT locus, the search for mutations in regulatory genes governing drug resistance may require the analysis of such loci as the thymidine kinase gene, which shows wide ranging variation in activity levels as a function of growth state.

The HPRT gene has been cloned from a number of sources and employed in gene transfer protocols, and a great deal of information concerning its properties has been published. However, some mechanisms of resistance (increases in alkaline phosphatase levels) have not been studied at all on the molecular level, and the significance of others (guanine deaminase, and 5'-nucleotidase) is fragmentary, at best. There have been reports of resistant variants with partial and transient depression in HPRT levels.[30] Although these conditions bear some similarities to gene amplification variants, chromosomal characterization of phosphatase overproducing cell lines failed to reveal any cytogenetic evidence of gene amplification.[71]

Finally, the dearth of information concerning the mechanism of toxicity of hypoxanthine-guanine analogs is an issue of interest. It is not clear whether the main mechanism of killing is through the incorporation into nucleic acids, into cofactors, or by inhibiting feedback mechanisms. An understanding of the means of killing by these drugs would have important implications for the development of rational strategies in the design of chemotherapeutic agents. After three decades of investigation purine analog resistance still provides fertile areas of investigation.

# REFERENCES

1. **Hakala, M.,** Prevention of toxicity of amethopterin for sarcoma 180 cells in tissue culture, *Science,* 126, 255, 1957.
2. **Littlefield, J.,** Selection of hybrids from matings of fibroblasts in vitro and their presumed recombinants, *Science,* 145, 709, 1964.
3. **Morrow, J.,** Genetic analysis of azaguanine resistance in an established mouse cell line, *Genetics,* 65, 279, 1970.
4. **Anderson, D.,** Attempts to produce systems for isolating spontaneous and induced variants in various mouse lymphoma cells using a variety of selective agents, *Mutation Res.,* 33, 407, 1975.
5. **Van Zeeland, A. and Simons, J.,** The role of azaguanine in the selection from human diploid cells of mutants deficient in hypoxanthine guanine phosphoribosyl transferase, *Mutation Res.,* 24, 55, 1975.
6. **Nelson, J., Carpenter, J., Rose, L., and Adamson, D.,** Mechanism of action of 6-thioguanine, 6-mercaptopurine, and 8-azaguanine, *Cancer Res.,* 35, 2872, 1975.

7. **Brockman, R.,** Mechanisms of resistance to anticancer agents, *Adv. Cancer Res., 7*, 130, 1963.
8. **Weiss, J. and Pitot, H.,** Inhibition of ribosomal ribonucleic acid maturation by 5-azacytidine and 8-azaguanine in Novikoff hepatoma cells, *Arch. Biochem. Biophys., 160*, 119, 1974.
9. **Rivest, R., Irwin, D., and Mandel, H.,** Inhibition of initiation of translation in L1210 cells by 8-azaguanine, *Biochem. Pharm., 31*, 2505, 1982.
10. **Bennett, L. and Montgomery, J.,** Design of anticancer agents: Problems and approaches, *Methods Cancer Res., 3*, 549, 1967.
11. **Bennett, H., Vail, M., Allan, P., and Laster, W.,** Studies with 8-azainosine, a cytotoxic nucleoside with antitumor activity, *Cancer Res., 33*, 465, 1973.
12. **Thompson, L. and Baker, R.,** Isolation of mutants of cultured mammalian cells, in *Methods in Cell Physiology,* Vol 6, Prescott, D., Ed., Academic Press, New York, 1973, 209.
13. **DeMars, R. and Held, K.,** The spontaneous azaguanine resistant mutants of human diploid fibroblasts, *Humangenetik, 16*, 87, 1972.
14. **Morrow, J., Colofiore, J., and Rintoul, D.,** Chinese hamster cells resistant to azaguanine not deficient in hypoxanthine guanine phosphoribosyl transferase, *J. Cell. Physiol., 81*, 97, 1973.
15. **Harris, J. and Whitmore, G.,** Chinese hamster cells exhibiting a temperature sensitive dependent alteration in purine transport, *J. Cell Physiol., 83*, 43, 1974.
16. **Prasad, R., Shopsis, C., and Hochstadt, J.,** Distinct mechanisms of hypoxanthine transport in membrane vesicles isolated from CHO and 3T3 cells, *Biochem. Biophys. Acta, 643*, 306, 1981.
17. **Wolpert, M., Damle, S., Brown, J., Sznycer, E., Agrawal, K., and Sartorelli, A.,** The role of phosphohydrolases in the mechanism of resistance of neoplastic cells to 6-thiopurines, *Cancer Res., 31*, 1620, 1971.
18. **Lee, S., Shansky, C., and Sartorelli, A.,** Evidence for the external location of alkaline phosphatase activity on the surface of Sarcoma 180 cells resistant to 6-thioguanine, *Biochem. Pharm., 29*, 1859, 1980.
19. **Plagemann, P. and Wohlhuetter, R.,** Metabolic properties of an azaguanine-resistant variant of Chinese hamster ovary cells (aza'ts) with normal levels of hypoxanthine-guanine phosphoribosyltransferase activity, *J. Cell. Biochem., 27*, 109, 1985.
20. **Plagemann, P., Marz, R., Wohlhueter, R., Graff, J., and Zylka, J.,** Facilitated transport of 6 mercaptopurine and 6 thioguanine and non-mediated permeation of 8 azaguanine in Novikoff rat hepatoma cells and relationship to intracellular phosphorylation, *Biochem. Biophys. Acta, 647*, 49, 1981.
21. **Lee, M., Huang, Y., and Sartorelli, A.,** Immunological studies on alkaline phosphatases of 6-thiopurine sensitive and resistant sublines of sarcoma 180, *Cancer Res., 38*, 2419, 1978.
22. **Lee, M., Huang, Y., and Satorelli, A.,** Alkaline phosphatase activities of 6-thiopurine sensitive and resistant sublines of sarcoma 180, *Cancer Res., 38*, 2413, 1978.
23. **Santachiara-Benerecetti, S., Cesari, I., and DeCarli, L.,** Some properties of alkaline phosphatase from a human cell strain and from a clonal derivative with low activity, *J. Cell. Physiol., 69*, 169, 1967.
24. **Henderson, J., Caldwell, I., and Paterson, A.,** Decreased feedback inhibition in a 6(methylmercapto) purine resistant tumor, *Cancer Res., 27*, 1773, 1967.
25. **Berman, J., Tong, C., and Williams, G.,** Differences between rat liver epithelial cells and fibroblast cells in sensitivity to 8-azaguanine, *In Vitro, 16*, 661, 1980.
26. **Mandel, H.,** The physiological disposition of some anticancer agents, *Pharmacol. Rev., 11*, 743, 1959.
27. **Meyers, M. and Shin, S.,** Specific resistance to 8-azaguanine in cells with normal hypoxanthine-guanine phosphoribosyl transferase activity: the role of guanine deaminase, *Cytogenet. Cell Genet., 30*, 118, 1981.
28. **Szybalski, W. and Szybalska, E.,** Drug sensitivity as a genetic marker for human cell lines, *Univ. Mich. Med. Bull., 28*, 277, 1962.
29. **Caskey, C. and Kruh, G.,** The HPRT locus, *Cell, 16*, 1, 1979.
30. **Fox, M. and Hodgkiss, R.,** Mechanism of cytotoxic action of azaguanine and thioguanine in wild type V79 cell lines and their relative efficiency in selection of structural gene mutants, *Mutation Res., 80*, 165, 1981.
31. **Nishi, Y., Hasegawa, M., and Inui, N.,** Forward mutational assay of V79 cells to thioguanine resistance in a soft agar technique that eliminates the effects of metabolic cooperation, *Mutation Res., 125,*.105, 1984.
32. **Harris, M.,** Mutation rates in cells at different ploidy levels, *J. Cell. Physiol., 78*, 177, 1971.
33. **Carson, M., Vernick, D., and Morrow, J.,** Clones of Chinese hamster cells cultivated in vitro not permanently resistant to azaguanine, *Mutation Res., 24*, 47, 1974.
34. **Fox, M., and Radacic, M.,** Adaptational origin of some purine-analog resistant phenotypes in cultured mammalian cells, *Mutation Res., 49*, 275, 1978.
35. **Morrow, J.,** *Eukaryotic Cell Genetics,* Academic Press, 1983.
36. **Morrow, J.,** Gene inactivation as a mechanism for the generation of variability in somatic cell cultivated in vitro, *Mutation Res., 44*, 391, 1977.
37. **Beaudet, A., Roufa, D., and Caskey, C.,** Mutations affecting the structure of hypoxanthine-guanine phosphoribosyltransferase in cultured Chinese hamster cells. *Proc. Natl. Acad. Sci. U.S.A., 70*, 320, 1972.

38. **Capecchi, M., Haar, R., von der, Capecchi, N., and Sveda, M.,** Isolation of suppressible nonsense mutant in mammalian cells, *Cell,* 12, 371, 1977.
39. **Milman, G., Krauss, S., and Alson, A.,** Tryptic peptide analysis of normal and mutant forms of hypoxanthine phosphoribosyl transferase from HeLa cells, *Proc. Natl. Acad. Sci. U.S.A.,* 74, 926, 1977.
40. **Melton, D., Konecki, D., Brennand, J., and Caskey, C.,** Structure, expression and mutation of the hypoxanthine phosphoribosyltransferase gene, *Proc. Natl. Acad. Sci.,* 81, 2147, 1984.
41. **Wolf, S. and Migeon, B.,** Clusters of CpG dinucleotides implicated by nuclease hypersensitivity as control elements of housekeeping genes, *Nature,* 314, 467, 1985.
42. **Stout, J. and Caskey, C.,** HPRT: gene structure, expression and mutation, *Annu. Rev. Genetics,* 19, 127, 1985.
43. **Shin, S.,** Nature of mutations conferring resistance to 8-azaguanine in mouse cell lines, *J. Cell Sci.,* 14, 235, 1974.
44. **Croce, C., Bakay, B., Nyhan, W., and Koprowski, H.,** Reexpression of the rat hypoxanthine phosphoribosyl transferase gene in rat-human hybrids, *Proc. Natl. Acad. Sci.,* 70, 2590, 1973.
45. **Watson, B., Gormley, S., Gardiner, S., Evans, H., and Harris, H.,** Reappearance of murine hypoxanthine guanine phosphoribosyl transferase activity in mouse A9 cells after attempted hybridisation with human cell lines, *Exp. Cell Res.,* 75, 401, 1972.
46. **Fenwick, R. and Caskey, C.,** Mutant Chinese hamster cells with a thermosensitive hypoxanthine-guanine phosphoribosyl transferase, *Cell,* 5, 115, 1975.
47. **Fenwick, R., Fuscoe, J., and Caskey, C.,** Amplification versus mutation as a mechanism for reversion of an HGPRT mutation, *Som. Cell Mol. Genet.,* 10, 71, 1984.
48. **Zownir, O., Fuscoe, J., Fenwick, R., and Morrow, J.,** Gene amplification as a mechanism of reversion at the HPRT locus in V79 Chinese hamster cells, *J. Cell. Physiol.,* 119, 341, 1984.
49. **Fenwick, R.,** Reversion of a mutation affecting the molecular weight of HGPRT: intragenic suppression and localization of X-linked genes, *Som. Cell Genet.,* 6, 477, 1980.
50. **Luria, S. and Delbrück, M.,** Mutation of bacteria from virus sensitivity to virus resistance, *Genetics,* 28, 491, 1943.
51. **Morrow, J.,** On the relationship between spontaneous mutation rates in vivo and in vitro, *Mutation Res.,* 33, 367, 1975.
52. **Wild, D.,** Serum effects on the yield of chemically induced 8-azaguanine resistant mutant in Chinese hamster cell cultures, *Mutation Res.,* 25, 229, 1974.
53. **Morrow, J., Stocco, D., and Barron, E.,** Spontaneous mutation rate to thioguanine resistance is decreased in polyploid hamster cells, *J. Cell Physiol.,* 96, 81, 1978.
54. **Chu, E. and Malling, H.,** Mammalian cell genetics II. Chemical induction of specific locus mutations in Chinese hamster cells in vitro, *Proc. Natl. Acad. Sci. U.S.A.,* 61, 1306, 1968.
55. **Knaap, A. and Simons, J.,** A mutational assay system for L5178Y mouse lymphoma cells using hypoxanthine-guanine phosphoribosyl transferase (HGPRT) deficiency as marker. The occurrence of a long expression time for mutations induced by X-rays and EMS, *Mutation Res.,* 30, 97, 1975.
56. **Thilly, W., DeLuca, J., Furth, E., Hoppe, H., Kaden, D., et al.,** Gene-locus mutation assays in diploid human lymphoblast lines, in *Chemical Mutagens,* Vol. 6, De Seeres, F. and Hollander, A., Eds., Plenum, N.Y., 1979, 351.
57. **Chu, E.,** Mammalian cell genetics. III. Chemical induction of specific locus mutations in Chinese hamster cell cultures, *Mutation Res.,* 11, 23, 1971.
58. **Knapp, A., Khan, P., and Simons, J.,** Establishment of a dose response relationship for reverse mutation at the HPRT (hypoxanthine guanine phosphoribosyl transferase) locus in L5178Y mouse lymphoma cells, *Mutation Res.,* 96, 259, 1982.
59. **Cox, R. and Masson, W.,** Do radiation induced thioguanine resistant mutants of cultured mammalian cells arise by HGPRT mutation or X-chromosome rearrangement?, *Nature,* 276, 629, 1978.
60. **Stone-Wolff, D., Klein, C., and Rossman, T.,** HGPRT⁻ of V79 cells that revert specifically by base pair substitution and frame shift mutations, *Environ. Mutagens,* 7, 281, 1985.
61. **Chen, D., Okinaka, R., Strniste, G., and Barnhart, B.,** Induction of 6-thioguanine resistant mutations by rat liver homogenate (S9) activated promutagens in human embryonic skin fibroblasts, *Mutation Res.,* 101, 87, 1982.
62. **Huang, S. and Waters, M.,** Two methods to induce 6-thioguanine resistance in human fibroblasts in the presence of rat liver microsomes, *Mutation Res.,* 121, 71, 1983.
63. **Ochi, T. and Ohsawa, M.,** Induction of 6-thioguanaine resistant mutants and single stranded scission of DNA by cadmium chloride in cultured Chinese hamster cells, *Mutation Res.,* 111, 69, 1983.
64. **O'Neill, J. P. and Flint, K.,** X-ray induction of 6-thioguanine resistant mutants in division arrested, G0/G1 phase Chinese hamster ovary cells, *Mutation Res.,* 149, 119, 1985.
65. **Lesko, S., Trpis, L., and Yang, S.,** Induction of 6-thioguanine resistant mutants by hyperoxia and gamma-irradiation: effects of compromising cellular antioxidant systems, *Mutation Res.,* 149, 119, 1985.

66. **Jacobsen, E., Krell, K., Olemska-Beer, Z., and Beer, J.,** UV-induced mutagenesis at the hypoxanthine-guanine phosphoribosyl transferase locus in two L5178Y mouse lymphoma cells strains with different UV sensitivities, *Mutation Res.,* 129, 259, 1985.
67. **Robertson, M.,** Gene therapy: desperate appliances, *Nature,* 320, 213, 1986.
68. **Willis, R., Jolly, D., Miller, A., Plent, M., Esty, A., et al.,** Partial phenotypic correction of human Lesch Nyhan syndrome (hypoxanthine guanine phosphoribosyl transferase deficient) lymphoblasts with a transmissible retrovirus vector, *J. Biol. Chem.,* 259, 7842, 1984.
69. **Gruber, H., Koenher, R., Luchtman, L., Willis, R., and Seegmiller, J.,** Glial cells metabolically cooperate: a potential requirement for gene replacement therapy, *Proc. Natl. Acad. Sci.,* 82, 6662, 1985.
70. **Culliton, B.,** Gene therapy: research in public, *Science,* 227, 493, 1985.
71. **Fox, M. and Ockey, C.,** Modulation of enzyme activity in azaguanine resistant V79 cells selected by chronic drug exposure, *Exp. Cell Res.,* 153, 413, 1984.
72. **Montgomery, J.,** Studies on the biological activity of purine and pyrimidine analogs, *Medicinal Res. Rev.,* 2, 271, 1982.

Chapter 11

# HALOGENATED AND OTHER 5-POSITION SUBSTITUTED PYRIMIDINES

**Elliot R. Kaufman**

## TABLE OF CONTENTS

I.      Introduction ................................................................. 160

II.     5-Bromo-2'-Deoxyuridine ..................................................... 160

III.    5-Iodo-2'-Deoxyuridine ...................................................... 162

IV.     5-Fluorouracil .............................................................. 163

V.      5-Hydroxymethyl-2'-Deoxyuridine ............................................. 164

VI.     Conclusions ................................................................. 168

References ........................................................................ 169

# I. INTRODUCTION

Initial interest in the halogenated pyrimidine analogs derived from their potential use as antiviral agents and chemotherapeutic agents. However, the identification of drug-resistant variants in cell populations treated with these agents resulted in these compounds becoming powerful tools for somatic cell geneticists.[1] In the late 1950s and early 1960s a number of cell lines resistant to pyrimidine analogs were isolated. In many cases, they were found to maintain their phenotype in the absence of selection, and were shown to result from the loss of a nucleoside kinase activity. In this review, we will briefly discuss some of the 5-position substituted pyrimidine analogs in the light of other more novel mechanisms of resistance.

# II. 5-BROMO-2′-DEOXYURIDINE

The thymidine analog, 5-bromo-2′-deoxyuridine (BrdUrd) (Figure 1) produces a variety of biological effects in mammalian cells. In addition to being toxic at high concentrations, BrdUrd has been shown to induce latent viruses,[2] inhibit or induce differentiated functions,[3] and inhibit ribonucleotide reductase (EC 1.17.4.1) activity.[4] The close structural and chemical similarities between thymidine and BrdUrd allows the utilization of BrdUrd and its phosphorylated derivatives as substrates for the various enzymes involved in the biosynthesis of DNA. Thus, wild-type cells exposed to BrdUrd readily incorporate 5-bromouracil (BrUra) into their DNA in place of thymine residues. Numerous studies have demonstrated a correlation between the incorporation of BrdUrd into DNA and the occurrence of its biological effects. As a result, it was generally assumed that all or most of the biological effects of BrdUrd resulted from the presence of BrUra in DNA. The subsequent demonstration[4] of the ability of BrdUTP to act as an inhibitor of the ribonucleotide reductase-catalyzed reduction of CDP to dCDP, resulting in a deoxycytidineless state and inhibition of DNA synthesis, provided another mechanism by which BrdUrd could affect cells.

A number of cell lines resistant to high concentrations of BrdUrd have been isolated, and, in general, the ability of the cells to survive has been associated with either the loss of thymidine kinase (EC 2.7.1.21) activity[5] or a deficiency in thymidine transport.[6] However, more recently, a number of clones of the Syrian hamster melanoma cell line RPMI 3460 were selected by their resistance to high concentrations of BrdUrd and were found to have novel phenotypes.[7] The BrdUrd-resistant lines obtained were characterized as to the percentage of thymine residues in DNA replaced by BrUra when grown in high concentrations of BrdUrd, the level of assayable thymidine kinase activity, and the ability to utilize exogenous thymidine for growth, as determined by growth in HAT medium,[8] which requires functional thymidine kinase activity for growth. In contrast to the BrdUrd-resistant cells generally reported in the literature, most of the cell lines isolated had high levels of BrUra incorporated in their DNA when grown in the presence of high concentrations of BrdUrd, and/or had significant levels of assayable thymidine kinase activity. The ability of the cells to utilize exogenous thymidine, as measured by growth in HAT medium, was shown to correlate well with the level of substitution of BrUra for thymine in DNA. These findings clearly demonstrated that exclusion of BrUra from DNA is not a necessary condition for survival in the presence of high concentrations of BrdUrd and that the generally accepted assumption that most of the disruptive effects of BrdUrd were due to its incorporation into DNA may not be entirely correct. As BrdUrd toxicity has been linked to deoxycytidine starvation,[4] these BrdUrd-resistant mutants may have alterations involving ribonucleotide reductase activity.

The relationship between ribonucleotide reductase activity and BrdUrd resistance suggested above was examined by the study of mutants with alterations in ribonucleotide reductase activity. A series of mutants resistant to hydroxyurea, an inhibitor of ribonucleotide

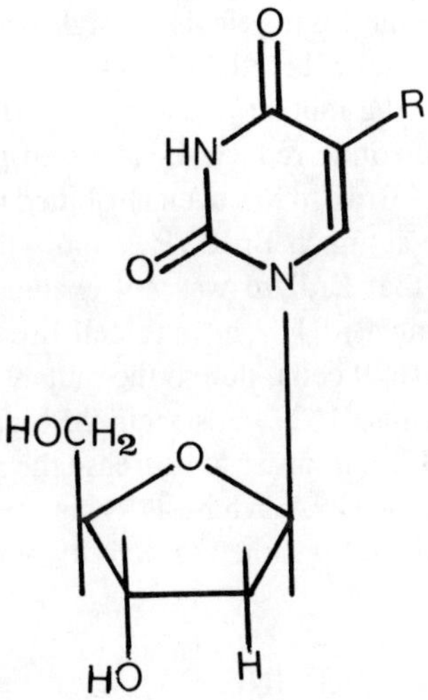

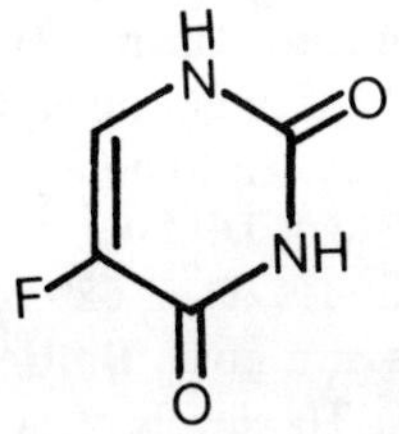

5−Fluorouracil

5−Iodo-2′-deoxyuridine : R= I

5−Bromo-2′-deoxyuridine: R= Br

5−Hydroxymethyl-2′-deoxyuridine : R=CH₂OH

FIGURE 1.

reductase activity, was selected from the Syrian hamster melanoma cell line RPMI 3460. A number of mutants resistant to 0.3 m$M$ hydroxyurea were isolated, and, from some of these, second-step mutants resistant to 1.0 m$M$ hydroxyurea were isolated.[9] The resistant cells were tested for their responses to BrdUrd in terms of toxicity, mutagenesis, and incorporation of BrdUrd into DNA. All of the hydroxyurea-resistant lines showed increased resistance to the toxic effects of BrdUrd. In addition, the hydroxyurea-resistant cells were all found to be resistant to BrdUrd mutagenesis. Overall, there was a good correlation among the levels of resistance to hydroxyurea toxicity, BrdUrd toxicity, and BrdUrd mutagenesis in the hydroxyurea-resistant cells. These tests were carried out under conditions which insured that the parental and hydroxyurea-resistant cells incorporated equal amounts of BrdUrd into their DNA, so that the resistance to BrdUrd cannot be attributable to decreased incorporation of BrdUrd into DNA in the resistant cells.

The ribonucleotide reductase activities of the hydroxyurea-resistant mutants were also studied using an in vitro assay of CDP reductase activity.[10] Seven of nine mutants were found to have increased specific activities of CDP reductase, ranging from 1.5 to 4 times that of the parental cells. All of the second-step mutants had activities greater than the single-step mutants from which they were derived. Enzyme assays were performed to test for qualitative, as well as quantitative, changes in the CDP reductase activity in some of the mutants. In no case was the activity from a mutant cell extract more resistant to an inhibitor, such as BrdUTP or hydroxyurea, than was the wild-type enzyme. Therefore, the resistance to hydroxyurea and BrdUrd in these cells appears to be associated with increased levels of the wild-type ribonucleotide reductase activity.

In more recent studies, a mutant V79 Chinese hamster fibroblast cell line, called 1629, with an altered CTP synthetase activity was isolated by selection for resistance to 5-fluorouracil.[11] (These cells will be discussed in detail below in the section on 5-fluorouracil.)

The 1629 cells were found to be cross resistant to the toxic effects of high concentrations of BrdUrd. The resistance of 1629 cells to BrdUrd can be directly attributed to the increased levels of intracellular dCTP that were generated by the mutant phenotype. As BrdUTP has been shown to be a potent inhibitor of the ribonucleotide reductase-catalyzed reduction of CDP to dCDP,[4] the toxicity of high concentrations of BrdUrd has been attributed to starvation for dCTP. The 1629 cells were shown to generate as much BrdUTP as did wild-type V79 cells at a given BrdUrd concentration, indicating that BrdUrd was not excluded from the cells. The levels of dCTP decreased with increasing BrdUTP in both cell lines, however, the absolute levels of dCTP were always higher in 1629 cells, due to the mutant phenotype, which involves increased CTP and dCTP pools. Thus, 1629 cells required higher concentrations of BrdUrd to generate higher levels of BrdUTP in order to decrease the intracellular levels of dCTP to a level inhibitory to or limiting for DNA synthesis. This report was the first to describe the association between an altered CTP synthetase activity and resistance to high concentrations of BrdUrd.

## III. 5-IODO-2'-DEOXYURIDINE

The relatively close chemical and structural similarities between thymidine and its analog 5-iodo-2'-deoxyuridine (IdUrd) (Figure 1) allows for the utilization of this compound and its phosphorylated derivatives as substrates for the biosynthetic pathway leading to DNA. IdUrd has been shown to be incorporated into mammalian DNA in place of thymine residues,[12] however, comparison of the relative uptake of thymidine and IdUrd into mammalian DNA showed a significant preference for thymidine.[13-16]

Early work with thymidine kinase deficient cells indicated that they were resistant to IdUrd and were shown to exclude IdUrd from incorporation into DNA.[5] Mutants specifically selected for resistance to IdUrd were also found to lack thymidine kinase activity.[17-19] In more recent studies, cells resistant to IdUrd were isolated that did not lack thymidine kinase activity.[20] Briefly, a clone of Syrian hamster melanoma cells was selected for resistance to high concentrations of IdUrd. Unlike the IdUrd-resistant cell lines previously isolated these cells were found to express normal levels of thymidine kinase activity. They were also shown to have the ability to grow in HAT medium and to incorporate exogenous thymidine and other thymidine analogs into their DNA. These findings indicated that these cells did not have a general block to the incorporation of all 5-position substituted deoxypyrimidines. However, these IdUrd-resistant cells were found to preferentially exclude IdUrd from their DNA. Analyses of the acid-soluble nucleotide pools of wild-type and IdUrd-resistant cells showed that the resistant cells were able to take up and phosphorylate exogenous thymidine as well as did the wild-type cells, and that both the resistant and wild-type cells accumulated dTTP as the major phosphorylated metabolite. In contrast, while the wild-type cells accumulated significant levels of both IdUMP and IdUTP when exposed to exogenous IdUrd, the IdUrd-resistant cells were found to only accumulate IdUMP. Thus, the resistant cells appeared to have a markedly decreased ability to phosphorylate IdUrd beyond the monophosphate level. Assays of thymidylate kinase (EC 2.7.4.9) activity in extracts of wild-type cells indicated a slight preference for dTMP as a substrate over IdUMP. When the IdUrd-resistant cells were assayed for thymidylate kinase activity, it was found that their thymidylate kinase activity had a much reduced affinity for IdUMP as a substrate, while retaining the ability to efficiently phosphorylate dTMP and the monophosphates of other thymidine analogs, such as BrdUMP. The van der Waals radius of the 5-methyl group of thymidine is 2.0 angstroms, the 5-Br group of BrdUrd is 1.95 Å, and the 5-I group of IdUrd is 2.15 Å. Thus, the larger size of the I-atom may be the basis by which the thymidylate kinase discriminates between the analogs. It is also possible that differences in the electronegativity of these 5-position groups may be involved. These IdUrd-resistant cells appear to be the first example of resistance to a halogenated pyrimidine analog based on enzymatic changes subtle enough to discriminate between different analogs.

## IV.5-FLUOROURACIL

The pyrimidine analog 5-fluorouracil (FUra) (Figure 1) and its derivative nucleosides, 5-fluorouridine (FUrd) and 5-fluoro-2'-deoxyuridine (FdUrd), were first investigated in 1957.[21] Since their inception, the primary mechanism of cytotoxicity of these drugs has been considered to be thymidylate starvation and inhibition of DNA synthesis caused by anabolism of these compounds to their active form, FdUMP, an irreversible inhibitor of thymidylate synthetase.[22] However, much importance has also been attributed to the incorporation of FUra into RNA.[23,24]

The fluorinated pyrimidines, FUra, FUrd, and FdUrd, have been shown to be active against many animal tumors,[25] and are used clinically in the treatment of breast and gastrointestinal cancers.[26] The effectiveness of these drugs as clinical palliatives has often been limited by the development of resistance in the tumor cell populations. Recent reports of cellular resistance to the fluoropyrimidines include (1) resistance to FUra as a result of decreased orotate phosphoribosyltransferase activity,[27-29] (2) resistance to FUrd as a result of decreased uridine kinase activity,[27,28] and (3) resistance to FdUrd due to decreased thymidine kinase activity.[27,28] All of these resistant cell lines block the anabolism of these analogs to their active nucleotide forms by the loss of an enzymatic activity.

Resistance to FUra has also been associated with increased CTP levels in mutant V79 Chinese hamster fibroblast cells.[11] A clone, called 1629, stably resistant to the toxic effects of FUra was isolated from mutagenized V79 cells by a single-step selection procedure in high concentrations of FUra. The 1629 cells were found to (1) be resistant to high concentrations of FUra, (2) also be resistant to FUra, but not to FdUrd, (3) be cross resistant to the toxic effects of cytosine arabinoside and to high concentrations of thymidine, (4) incorporate less FUra into RNA than do the wild-type cells, (5) have increased intracellular levels of CTP and dCTP, and decreased levels of UTP, and (6) have an auxotrophic requirement, when grown in medium lacking all pyrimidines, that was satisfied by the addition of thymidine to the medium. The primary lesion in these FUra-resistant cells was an altered CTP synthetase (EC 6.3.4.2) activity which was no longer sensitive to negative feedback regulation by CTP. The resulting increased CTP levels appeared to be responsible for the varied phenotypic characteristics of the 1629 cells, including the resistance to FUra.

The FUra-resistant 1629 cells were phenotypically distinct from the majority of FUra-resistant cell lines described in the literature, with the exception of cells isolated as resistant to cytosine arabinoside and subsequently shown to be cross resistant to FUra and have increased CTP levels.[30,31] The pleiotropic nature of the altered CTP synthetase activity causes changes in nucleotide metabolism that resulted in the varied phenotypic characteristics briefly described above. The loss of negative feedback regulation of CTP synthetase by CTP caused increased levels of CTP to accumulate in the cells. The increased CTP levels caused higher levels of dCTP by providing more CDP as substrate for reduction by ribonucleotide reductase. This effect served to protect the cells against inhibition by high concentrations of thymidine, which is known to inhibit the ribonucleotide reductase-catalyzed reduction of CDP to dCDP[32] and thereby starve the cells for dCTP. In addition, the high dCTP levels protected the cells against the toxic effects of cytosine arabinoside by completing with araCTP for incorporation into DNA. The auxotrophic requirement for thymidine was probably caused by competitive inhibition of the ribonucleotide reductase-catalyzed reduction of UDP by the high levels of CDP.[30] In addition, the high levels of CTP, which is known to exert negative feedback inhibition on the pyrimidine biosynthetic pathway,[33] resulted in reduced levels of UTP and possibly UDP in the cells. Thus, an insufficient supply of dUMP, necessary for thymidylate synthesis, was the probable cause of the thymidine auxotrophy. It should be noted that V79 cells lack dCMP deaminase activity and, therefore, cannot obtain dUMP via the deamination of dCMP.

It was found that in the wild-type V79 cells the addition of thymidine did not protect against the toxicity of FUra, strongly suggesting that the toxicity involved RNA and not any effects due to the formation of FdUMP and inhibition of thymidylate synthetase. This was supported by the finding that the FUra-resistant 1629 cells were also resistant to FUrd, but not to FdUrd. The resistance of the 1629 cells to FUra was due to decreased anabolism resulting in lower levels of FUTP formed and less incorporation into RNA. The terminal product of pyrimidine ribonucleotide biosynthesis, CTP, regulates pyrimidine biosynthesis by acting as a specific inhibitor of the first step of the *de novo* pyrimidine pathway[33] as well as the salvage pathway.[34] Thus, the decreased anabolism of FUra in the resistant cells was probably due to feedback inhibition of the pyrimidine biosynthetic and salvage pathways caused by the increased levels of CTP.

This mutation describes a new mechanism by which cells in culture have become resistant to FUra. This work also suggests that populations of cells with high intracellular levels of CTP may be resistant to FUra. It is possible that this mechanism is the cause of a significant portion of the FUra resistance observed clinically in tumor cell populations. Increased CTP levels have been associated with the rapid growth of hepatomas and kidney tumor cells.[35,36] It may be possible to screen tumor cell populations for CTP levels in an effort to predict whether a tumor will respond to FUra therapy. It may also be profitable to devise protocols that lower the levels of intracellular CTP, thus increasing the anabolism of FUra and thereby increasing the sensitivity of the cells to FUra killing. Such a protocol might prove useful in treating tumors which were resistant to FUra therapy due to a mechanism similar to that described above.

## V. 5-HYDROXYMETHYL-2′-DEOXYURIDINE

The analog 5-hydroxymethyl-2′-deoxyuridine (hmdUrd) (Figure 1), although not an halogenated pyrimidine, will be included for discussion due to its being a 5-position substituted thymidine analog and because of the unique mode of resistance expressed in mammalian cells. HmdUrd is a naturally occurring component of the DNA of certain bacteriophage of *B. subtilis*[37] and of members of the Pyrrophyta (dinoflagellates).[38,39] In the bacteriophage 5-hydroxymethyuracil (hmUra) replaces all of the thymine residues in the phage DNA, while in the Pyrrophyta as much as 70% of the thymine residues are replaced by hmUra. Although hmUra has been found to be a normal component of the DNA of these organisms, hmdUrd has been shown to have cytotoxic effects on some mammalian cells in culture.[40-45] It has been suggested that the toxic effects of hmdUrd are due to its incorporation into DNA.[41-45]

Although hmUra and hmdUrd had been identified only as minor products of irradiated solutions of thymine and thymidine at neutral pH,[46,47] recent analysis of DNA from γ-irradiated Hela cells showed the major thymine derivative to be hmUra.[48,49] These findings together with the identification and purification of an hmUra-DNA glycosylase activity from mouse plasmacytoma cells[50] suggested that the formation of hmUra in DNA by exposure to ionizing radiation may contribute to the cytotoxic effects of the radiation.

In recent studies[44] involving cellular and biochemical analyses of the toxic effects of hmdUrd using V79 Chinese hamster cells, it was found that the toxic effects of hmdUrd could be totally suppressed by the addition of thymidine at 1/10th the concentration of hmdUrd. When other pyrimidines were tested, deoxyuridine was found to also suppress toxicity, although not as well as thymidine, while orotate, uridine, cytidine, and deoxycytidine did not have significant effect. Biochemical analyses of the metabolic fate of hmdUrd demonstrated low but significant levels of hmdUTP and the incorporation of hmUra residues into DNA. Surprisingly, in addition to these metabolites, relatively high levels of free hmUra were also detected in the acid-soluble cell extracts. Further analysis demonstrated that when V79 cells were exposed to hmdUrd, significant amounts of hmUra were released into the culture medium. In vitro assays provided evidence that hmdUrd was first phosphorylated to its monophosphate and then degraded to hmUra, possibly via the action of a new enzymatic activity, hydroxymethyldeoxyuridylate phosphorylase. Exposure of cells to hmUra alone, at concentrations as high as 3 m$M$, had no effect on viability. However, when V79 cells were simultaneously exposed to low, nontoxic concentrations of hmdUrd and high, nontoxic concentrations of hmUra, a synergistic reduction in viability was observed. This synergistic effect was found to correlate with increased incorporation of hmUra into DNA, possibly via end-product inhibition of an hmUra-DNA glycosylase.

These findings suggested that hmdUrd was metabolized by the thymidine salvage pathway and that competitors for uptake and phosphorylation by this pathway could provide protection against hmdUrd toxicity. In support of this suggestion was the previous observation[43] that thymidine kinase deficient cells were resistant to hmdUrd toxicity. The results presented also demonstrated a correlation between incorporation of hmdUrd into DNA and toxicity. It is unlikely that hmdUrd toxicity was due to the inhibition of thymidylate synthetase by hmdUMP and subsequent starvation for thymidine nucleotides. Although many 5-substituted analogs of dUMP have been shown to be potent inhibitors of this enzyme, when tested, hmdUMP was not found to be among this group.[51] It was also shown that the ability of 1 $\mu M$ thymidine, an adequate source of thymidine nucleotides, to protect V79 cells from hmdUrd toxicity could be overcome by concentrations of hmdUrd that raised the hmdUrd/thymidine concentration ratio to values >10. This would not be the case if hmdUrd toxicity was caused by the inhibition of *de novo* thymidylate biosynthesis by hmdUMP.

When the metabolic fate of hmdUrd in V79 cells was investigated, results both expected and unexpected were obtained. As was expected, hmdUrd was anabolized to its triphosphate and ultimately incorporated into cellular DNA. The ability of V79 cells to anabolize hmdUrd was low when compared to their ability to anabolize thymidine. The levels of hmdUTP that were generated were approximately 30-fold lower than those of dTTP generated from equimolar concentrations of exogenous hmdUrd and thymidine, respectively. Likewise, the amount of hmdUrd incorporated into DNA was low relative to the thymidine residues incorporated during the same time period. These results indicated a significant degree of discrimination between thymidine and hmdUrd by the anabolic pathway. The results also indicated that hmdUrd nucleotides accumulated primarily as hmdUMP, while thymidine nucleotides were found primarily in the dTTP pool. These findings were similar to those obtained with another thymidine analog, IdUrd.[20] In these studies, the accumulation of IdUMP was apparently due to its being a poor substrate for thymidylate kinase, the enzyme that phosphorylates dTMP to dTDP. A similar situation may exist with hmdUMP, thus providing at least part of the mechanism by which the cells discriminate between the incorporation of hmdUrd and thymidine into DNA. Unexpectedly, hmdUrd was also found to be catabolized to hmUra at a relatively high rate. This catabolic pathway did not utilize thymidine as a substrate, as thymine was never detected either in acid-soluble cell extracts or in the culture medium. When cell-free extracts of V79 cells were tested for their ability to metabolize hmdUrd in vitro, the results clearly indicated that it was first necessary to phosphorylate hmdUrd to hmdUMP before it could be degraded to hmUra, and this degradation was dependent upon the presence of $Mg^{2+}$ and ATP. Therefore, it is unlikely that a thymidine phosphorylase activity was involved. It is also unlikely that thymidylate synthetase was involved in the degradation of hmdUrd to hmUra, as preincubation of the cells in the presence of FdUrd, which results in irreversible inhibition of this enzyme,[52] had no effect on the ability of the cells to produce hmUra. Another possible source of hmUra could be due to the action of an enzyme, such as a pyrimidine phosphoribosyltransferase, which was capable of cleaving the *N*-glycosidic bond of a pyrimidine nucleotide. However, one might have also expected such an activity to be reversible and, therefore, also be capable of converting the free pyrimidine base to its nucleotide. That this was not the case was suggested by the lack of toxicity of high concentrations of hmUra in the absence of hmdUrd. Therefore, it seemed unlikely that a pyrimidine phosphoribosyltransferase-like activity was responsible for the observed generation of hmUra from hmdUrd. The results suggested the possibility of a new enzymatic activity that could be termed a pyrimidine nucleotide phosphorylase, or more specifically an hydroxymethyldeoxyuridylate phosphorylase, which acted irreversibly.

Another mechanism by which hmUra could have been generated was cleavage from DNA by the action of an hmUra-DNA glycosylase activity. Such a DNA glycosylase has been described in mammalian cells,[50] and presumably functions to eliminate hmUra, a major thymine-derived DNA lesion produced by ionizing radiation and oxidative damage.[49] It is unlikely that a DNA glycosylase could account for the large amounts of hmUra generated by the cells and excreted into the culture medium, and could certainly not account for the generation of hmUra in the in vitro reactions, because the in vitro reactions do not support DNA synthesis and DNA glycosylases do not utilize nucleoside monophosphates as substrates.[53] However, an hmUra-DNA glycosylase activity could be acting upon any hmUra residues incorporated into DNA, and thereby, have significant effects on hmdUrd toxicity. This suggestion is supported by the observations that (1) high concentrations of exogenous hmUra, while itself not toxic, produced a synergistic effect with hmdUrd, which increased toxicity by many orders of magnitude; (2) this synergistic effect on toxicity was specific for hmUra, as other pyrimidines, such as uracil and thymine, had no effect; (3) high concentrations of unlabelled hmUra increased the level of incorporation of [³H] hmdUrd detected in DNA without having any significant effects on hmdUTP levels; and (4) the uracil-DNA glycosylase has been shown to be sensitive to end-product inhibition by uracil.[53]

Resistance to the toxic effects of hmdUrd has been observed in Hela cells,[40] in thymidine kinase-deficient mouse cells,[43] and in a Syrian hamster melanoma cell line, HM-3, selected in a multistep procedure by continuous exposure to 1, 10, and 100 μ*M* hmdUrd, respectively.[43] In more recent studies,[45] a spontaneously arising clone, stably resistant to the toxic effects of hmdUrd, was isolated from V79 Chinese hamster fibroblast cells by a single-step selection procedure. The hmdUrd-resistant cells were selected in the continuous presence of 30 μ*M* hmdUrd, a concentration which reduces the plating efficiency of wild-type cells to <1% after a 24-hr exposure. A line of human Hela cells were also found to be intrinsically resistant to concentrations of hmdUrd as high as 100 μ*M*. All of the hmdUrd-resistant cells were found to (1) grow normally in HAT medium, which requires the expression of thymidine kinase activity; (2) be sensitive to the toxic effects of high concentrations of BrdUrd, another thymidine analog; (3) have unaltered hmdUrd nucleotide metabolism, as measured by HPLC analysis of acid-soluble cell extracts; and (4) have decreased levels of hmdUrd incorporation into DNA. Although high concentrations of hmUra were found to be nontoxic for both wild-type and hmdUrd-resistant cells, the resistant phenotype could be suppressed by exposing the cells to hmdUrd and high concentrations of hmUra simultaneously.

Neither the hmdUrd-resistant V79 cells nor the Hela cells were found to be resistant to hmdUrd due to decreased uptake and metabolism of the analog, as was the case in thymidine kinase deficient cells.[43] Evidence to support this finding included the ability of hmdUrd-resistant V79 cells to grow in HAT medium, which requires thymidine kinase activity for growth, and their sensitivity to BrdUrd, another thymidine analog which is toxic to cells expressing thymidine kinase activity. Hela cells were also found to be resistant to HAT medium and sensitive to BrdUrd. In addition to these cellular tests, the ability of hmdUrd-resistant V79 and Hela cells to metabolize hmdUrd was directly determined by HPLC analysis of the acid-soluble nucleotide pools of cells exposed to [³H] hmdUrd. It was found that the wild-type V79 cells, the hmdUrd-resistant V79 cells and the Hela cells all generated approximately the same levels of hmdUTP when exposed to hmdUrd. Thus, resistance to hmdUrd was not found to be associated with decreased uptake and anabolism of the analog.

The catabolic conversion of hmdUrd to hmUra by V79 cells was discussed above.[44] As hmUra was shown to be nontoxic to the cells even at very high concentrations, it was suggested that this catabolic conversion might serve to detoxify the hmdUrd for the cells. Therefore, the hmdUrd-resistant cells were tested to determine whether increased catabolism of hmdUrd was involved in their mechanism of resistance. It was found that wild-type V79 cells, hmdUrd-resistant V79 cells and Hela cells all generated hmUra at approximately the same rate when exposed to hmdUrd. Thus, it appeared unlikely that the catabolism of hmdUrd to hmUra is involved in the mechanism of resistance to the analog. This finding was in agreement with those described above in which the levels of hmdUTP accumulating in all three cell lines were found to be similar. If the hmdUrd-resistant cells catabolized hmdUrd at a much greater rate, one might expect this to be reflected in lower levels of hmdUTP, and this was not the case. It should also be noted that the presence of high concentrations of unlabeled hmUra in the culture medium did not appear to have a very significant effect on the rates of hmdUrd catabolism. As high concentrations of hmUra in the medium was shown to have a very significant effect on hmdUrd toxicity in all of the cell lines tested, it seems unlikely that the anabolic conversion of hmdUrd to hmUra is involved in the mechanism of resistance to hmdUrd toxicity.

The wild-type and hmdUrd-resistant cells were also tested for their ability to incorporate hmdUrd into cellular DNA. It was found that hmdUrd-resistant V79 cells incorporated 3-fold less hmdUrd into cellular DNA than did the wild-type V79 cells, and that Hela cells incorporated 25-fold less hmdUrd than V79 cells when exposed to a given concentration of hmdUrd. These differences in incorporation were observed even though the three cell lines had been shown to accumulate the same levels of hmdUTP, the direct precursor of DNA. Thus, the result demonstrated a strong correlation between relative resistance to hmdUrd and incorporation of hmdUrd into DNA. The results also suggested that the differences observed in incorporation of hmdUrd into DNA were not due to differences in the ability to generate the DNA precursor hmdUTP.

Another strong correlation was observed between the ability of high concentrations of hmUra to increase hmdUrd toxicity and incorporation into DNA. High, but nontoxic, concentrations of hmUra were found to (1) increase the toxicity of hmdUrd in wild-type V79 cells, (2) suppress the resistant phenotype in hmdUrd-resistant V79 and Hela cells, and (3) cause a fivefold increase in the level of incorporation of hmdUrd into DNA in all three cell lines. It had been shown that these concentrations of hmUra had no significant effect on the hmdUTP levels in V79 cells.[44] The results suggested that hmdUrd toxicity was due to its incorporation into DNA and that the hmdUrd-resistant V79 cells and the Hela cells were resistant to hmdUrd because they do not incorporate as much hmdUrd into their DNA.

One possible mechanism by which the hmdUrd-resistant cells could have been preventing hmdUrd incorporation was a decreased ability to utilize hmdUTP as a precursor for DNA synthesis, e.g., a DNA polymerase with a higher $K_m$ for hmdUTP. It is unlikely that this mechanism was involved in the hmdUrd-resistant V79 or the Hela cells as it is unclear how high concentrations of hmUra could cause increased incorporation and suppress the hmdUrd-resistant phenotype. As hmUra was itself shown not to be incorporated in to DNA,[44] there is no simple mechanism by which hmUra could be acting to increase the affinity of a DNA polymerase for hmdUTP as a substrate for DNA synthesis. Another mechanism by which hmdUrd-resistant cells could have been excluding hmdUrd from their DNA was to incorporate hmdUrd into DNA at a rate equal to that of wild-type cells and then remove it more efficiently. This could have been accomplished by the cleavage of hmUra residues from DNA by the action of an hmUra-DNA glycosylase activity. Such DNA glycosylase has been described in mammalian cells,[50] and presumably functions to eliminate hmUra, a major thymine-derived DNA lesion produced by ionizing radiation and oxidative damage.[49] An hmUra-DNA glycosylase activity could have been acting upon hmUra residues incorporated into DNA, and thereby, have had significant effects on hmdUrd toxicity. This suggestion was supported by the observations that (1) high concentrations of exogenous hmUra, while itself not toxic, produced a synergistic effect with hmdUrd, which increased toxicity by many orders of magnitude and suppressed the hmdUrd-resistant phenotype; (2) this synergistic effect on toxicity was specific for hmUra, as other pyrimidines, such as uracil and thymine, had no effect;[44] (3) high concentrations of unlabeled hmUra increased the level of incorporation of [³H] hmdUrd detected in DNA without having any significant effects on hmdUTP levels; and (4) the uracil-DNA glycosylase has been shown to be sensitive to end-product inhibition by uracil[53] and, therefore, the hmUra-DNA glycosylase may be sensitive to inhibition by hmUra. The hmdUrd-resistant V79 cells and the Hela cells might, therefore, be thought to be resistant because they were expressing higher levels of this hmUra-DNA glycosylase activity than were the wild-type cells. This would allow the more efficient removal of hmUra from their DNA, resulting in a lower steady-state level of hmUra residues, thereby avoiding the toxic effects. This hypothesis can be tested directly by assaying for hmUra-DNA glycosylase activity in both hmdUrd-sensitive and resistant cells. These assays are necessary before hmUra-DNA glycosylase can be implicated in the mechanism of resistance to hmdUrd.

## VI. CONCLUSIONS

Pyrimidine analogs have provided the somatic cell geneticist with a fertile field of investigation, as well as providing powerful tools for the selection of cell lines with useful genetic markers. The commonly observed mechanism by which a mammalian cell line can become resistant to the toxic effects of these analogs has been the loss of a kinase activity resulting in exclusion of the analog from the anabolic pathway necessary to convert it to its active form, usually a nucleoside triphosphate. In this review, we have briefly described some novel mechanisms by which mammalian cells have become resistant to pyrimidine analogs. Resistance to BrdUrd appeared to involve mechanisms which avoided the decreased dCTP levels resulting from the inhibition of the ribonucleotide reductase-catalyzed reduction of CDP to dCDP by BrdUTP. Two such mechanisms were discussed (1) increased expression of ribonucleotide reductase resulting in less inhibition by BrdUTP, and (2) high intracellular levels of dCTP, resulting from an altered CTP synthetase activity, that required higher levels of BrdUTP to generate enough inhibition to cause the dCTP levels to become limiting. Resistance to IdUrd was shown to involve the exclusion of IdUrd from DNA. This, however, was due to an altered thymidylate kinase activity that still functioned to phosphorylate dTMP, a function necessary for viability, but no longer utilized IdUMP as a substrate. Resistance to FUra resulted from decreased incorporation into RNA. This was due to an altered CTP synthetase activity, no longer sensitive to negative feedback control by CTP, which generated increased levels of intracellular CTP. The high CTP levels resulted in an inhibition of the pyrimidine salvage pathway necessary to anabolize FUra to its triphosphate and, thus, inhibited the incorporation of FUra into RNA. Resistance to hmdUrd did not appear to result from decreased anabolism and inhibition of incorporation into DNA, however, the resistant cells were found to accumulate less hmUra in their DNA. This could have been due to increased hmUra-DNA glycosylase activity in the resistant cells, which served to remove hmUra residues from DNA at a greater rate than in the wild-type cells. Clearly, the potential genetic response of mammalian cells to selection by pyrimidine analogs is still worthy of active investigation.

# REFERENCES

1. **Harris, M.,** *Cell Culture and Somatic Variation,* Holt, Rinehart and Winston, New York, 1964.
2. **Hampar, B., Derge, J. G., Martos, L. M., and Walker, J. L.,** Persistence of a repressed Epstein-Barr virus genome in Burkitt lymphoma cells made resistant to 5-bromodeoxyuridine, *Proc. Natl. Acad. Sci., U.S.A.,* 68, 3185, 1971.
3. **Rutter, W. J., Pictet, R. L., and Morris, P. W.,** Toward molecular mechanisms of developmental processes, *Annu. Rev. Biochem.,* 26, 601, 1973.
4. **Meuth, M. and Green, H.,** Induction of a deoxycytidineless state in cultured mammalian cells by bromodeoxyuridine, *Cell,* 2, 109, 1974.
5. **Dubbs, D. R. and Kit, S.,** Effect of halogenated pyrimidines and thymidine on growth of L-cells and a subline lacking thymidine kinase, *Exp. Cell Res.,* 33, 19, 1964.
6. **Breslow, R. E. and Goldsby, R. A.,** Isolation and characterization of thymidine transport mutants of Chinese hamster cells, *Exp. Cell Res.,* 55, 339, 1969.
7. **Kaufman, E. R. and Davidson, R. L.,** Novel phenotypes arising from selection of hamster melanoma cells for resistance to BUdR, *Exp. Cell Res.,* 107, 15, 1977.
8. **Littlefield, J.,** Selection of hybrids from matings of fibroblasts in vitro and their presumed recombinants, *Science,* 145, 709, 1964.
9. **Davidson, R. L. and Kaufman, E. R.,** Resistance to bromodeoxyuridine mutagenesis and toxicity in mammalian cells selected for resistance to hydroxyurea, *Somat. Cell Genet.,* 5, 873, 1979.
10. **Ashman, C. R., Reddy, G. P. V., and Davidson, R. L.,** Bromodeoxyuridine mutagenesis, ribonucleotide reductase activity, and deoxyribonucleotide pools in hydroxyurea-resistant mutants, *Somat. Cell Genet.,* 7, 751, 1981.
11. **Kaufman, E. R.,** Resistance to 5-fluorouracil associated with increased cytidine triphosphate levels in V79 Chinese hamster cells, *Cancer Res.,* 44, 3371, 1984.
12. **Matthias, A. P., Fischer, G. A., and Prusoff, W. H.,** Inhibition of growth of mouse leukemia cells in culture by 5-iodo-deoxyuridine, *Biochim. Biophys. Acta,* 36, 560, 1959.
13. **Prusoff, W. H.,** Incorporation of iododeoxyuridine into the deoxyribonucleic acid of mouse Ehrlish-ascites-tumor cells in vivo, *Biochim. Biophys. Acta,* 39, 327, 1960.
14. **Hughes, W. L., Commerford, S. L., Gitlin, D., Krueger, R. C., Schultze, B., Shah, V., and Reilly, P.,** Deoxyribonucleic acid metabolism in vivo. I. Cell proliferation and death as measured by incorporation and elimination of iododeoxyuridine, *Fed. Proc.,* 23, 640, 1964.
15. **Fox, B. W. and Prusoff, W. H.,** The comparative uptake of $^{125}$I labeled 5-iodo-2'-deoxyuridine and thymidine-$^3$H into tissues of mice bearing hepatome-129, *Cancer Res.,* 25, 234, 1965.
16. **Baugnet-Manieu, L. and Goutier, R.,** Mechanisms responsible for the low incorporation into DNA of the thymidine analogue, 5-iodo-2'-deoxyuridine, *Biochem. Pharmacol.,* 17, 1017, 1968.
17. **Fox, M.,** Spontaneous and X-ray induced genotypic and phenotypic resistance to 5-iodo-2'-deoxyuridine in lymphoma cells in vitro, *Mutation Res.,* 13, 403, 1971.
18. **Fox, M. and Anderson, D.,** Characteristics of spontaneous and induced thymidine and 5-iodo-2'-deoxyuridine resistant clones of mouse lymphoma cells, *Mutation Res.,* 25, 89, 1974.
19. **Anderson, D. and Fox, M.,** The induction of thymidine and IUdR-resistant variants in P388 mouse lymphoma cells by X-rays, UV, and mono- and bi-functional alkylating agents, *Mutation Res.,* 25, 107, 1974.
20. **Kaufman, E. R. and Davidson, R. L.,** Altered thymidylate kinase substrate specificity in mammalian cells selected for resistance to iododeoxyuridine, *Exp. Cell Res.,* 123, 355, 1979.
21. **Heidelberger, C., Chaudhuri, N. K., Dannenberg, P., Mooren, D., Griesbach, L., Duschinsky, R., Schnitzer, R. J., Plevin, E., and Scheiner, T.,** Fluorinated pyrimidines, a new class of tumor-inhibitory compounds, *Nature,* 179, 663, 1957.
22. **Cohen, S. S., Flaks, J. G., Barner, H. D., Loeb, M. R., and Lichtenstein, J.,** The mode of action of 5-fluorouracil and its derivatives, *Proc. Natl. Acad. Sci. U.S.A.,* 44, 1004, 1958.
23. **Ardalan, B., and Glazer, R.,** An update on the biochemistry of 5-fluorouracil, *Cancer Treat. Rev.,* 8, 157, 1981.
24. **Myers, C. E.,** The pharmacology of the fluoropyrimidines, *Pharmacol. Rev.,* 33, 1, 1981.
25. **Heidelberger, C., Griesbach, L., Montag, B. J., Mooren, D., Cruz, O., Schnitzer, R. J., and Grunberg, E.,** Studies on fluorinated pyrimidines. II. Effects on transplanted tumors, *Cancer Res.,* 18, 305, 1958.
26. **Heidelberger, C.,** Fluorinated pyrimidines and their nucleosides, in *Handbook of Experimental Pharmacology,* Vol. 38, part 2, Sartorelli, A. C. and Johns, D. G., Eds., Springer Verlag, Berlin, 1975, 193.
27. **Mulkins, M. A. and Heidelberger, C.,** Isolation of fluoropyrimidine-resistant murine leukemic cell lines by one-step mutation and selection, *Cancer Res.,* 42, 956, 1982.
28. **Mulkins, M. A. and Heidelberger, C.,** Biochemical characterization of fluoropyrimidine-resistant murine leukemic cell lines, *Cancer Res.,* 42, 965, 1982.

29. **Patterson, D.,** Isolation and characterization of 5-fluorouracil resistant mutants of Chinese hamster ovary cells deficient in the activities of orotate phosphoribosyltransferase and orotidine 5'-monophosphate decarboxylase, *Somat. Cell Genet.,* 6, 101, 1980.

30. **de Saint Vincent, R., Dechamps, M., and Buttin, G.,** The modulation of the thymidine triphosphate pool of Chinese hamster cells by dCMP deaminase and UDP reductase, *J. Biol. Chem.,* 255, 162, 1980.

31. **Meuth, M., Goncalves, O., and Thom, P.,** A selection system specific for Thy mutator phenotype, *Somat. Cell Genet.,* 8, 423, 1982.

32. **Bjursell, G., and Reichard, P.,** Effects of thymidine on deoxyribonucleoside triphosphate pools and deoxyribonucleic acid synthesis in Chinese hamster ovary cells, *J. Biol. Chem.,* 248, 3904, 1973.

33. **Gerhart, J. C. and Pardee, A. B.,** The enzymology of control by feedback inhibition, *J. Biol. Chem.,* 237, 891, 1962.

34. **Orengo, A.,** Feedback regulation in the ribopyrimidine "salvage" pathway, *Exp. Cell Res.,* 41, 338, 1966.

35. **Weber, G., Olah, E., Jui, M. S., and Tzeng, D.,** Biochemical programs and enzyme-pattern-targeted chemotherapy in cancer cells, *Adv. Enzyme Regul.,* 17, 1, 1978.

36. **Williams, J. C., Kizaki, H., Weber, G., and Morris, H., P.,** Increased CTP synthetase activity in cancer cells, *Nature,* 271, 71, 1978.

37. **Kallen, R. G., Simon, M., and Marmur, J.,** Occurrence of a new pyrimidine base replacing thymine in bacteriophage DNA: 5-hydroxymethyluracil, *J. Mol. Biol.,* 5, 248, 1962.

38. **Rae, P. M. M.,** 5-Hydroxymethyluracil in the DNA of a dinoflagellate, *Proc. Natl. Acad. Sci. U.S.A.,* 70, 1141, 1973.

39. **Rae, P. M. M.,** Hydroxymethyluracil in eukaryote DNA: A natural feature of the Pyrrophyta (dinoflagellates), *Science,* 194, 1062, 1976.

40. **Waschke, S., Reefschlager, J., Barwolff, D., and Langen, P.,** 5-Hydroxymethyl-2'-deoxyuridine, a normal DNA component in certain *Bacillus subtilis* phages is cytostatic for mammalian cells, *Nature,* 255, 629, 1975.

41. **Matthes, E., Barwolff, D., Preussel, B., and Langen, P.,** The incorporation of hydroxymethyldeoxyuridine into DNA of Ehrlich ascites carcinoma cells and some of its consequences, in *Antimetabolites in Biochemistry, Biology and Medicine,* Skoda J. and Langen, P., Eds., Pergamon Press, Oxford, 1979, 115.

42. **Kahilainen, L. I., Bergstrom, D. E., and Vilpo, J. A.,** 5-Hydroxymethyl-2'-deoxyuridine. Cytotoxicity and DNA incorporation studied by using a novel [2-$^{14}$C]-derivative with normal and leukemic hematopoietic cells, *Acta Chem. Scand.,* B 39, 477, 1985.

43. **Kaufman, E. R. and Davidson R. L.,** Effects of thymidine analogs on Syrian hamster melanoma cells: phenotypes arising from selection for analog resistance, *Somat. Cell Genet.,* 3, 649, 1977.

44. **Kaufman, E. R.,** Biochemical analysis of toxic effects of 5-hydroxymethyl-2'-deoxyuridine in mammalian cells, *Somat. Cell Molec. Genet.,* 12, 501, 1986.

45. **Kaufman, E. R.,** Resistance to toxic effects of 5-hydroxymethyl-2'-deoxyuridine in mammalian cells, *Somat. Cell Molec. Genet.,* 13, 101, 1987.

46. **Cadet, J. and Teoule, R.,** Radiolyse gamma de la thymidine en solution aqueuse aeree, III. Aspects quantitatifs et mecanisme, *Bull. Soc. Chim. Fr.,* 3-4, 891, 1975.

47. **Myers, L. S., Jr., Ward, J. F., Tsukamoto, W. T., Holmes, D. E., and Julca, J. R.,** Radiolysis of thymine in aqueous solutions: Change in site of attack with change in pH, *Science,* 148, 1234, 1965.

48. **Teebor, G. W., Frenkel, K., and Goldstein, M. S.,** Identification of radiation-induced thymine derivatives in DNA, *Adv. Enzyme Regul.,* 20, 39, 1982.

49. **Teebor, G. W., Frenkel, K., and Goldstein, M. S.,** Ionizing radiation and tritium transmutation both cause formation of 5-hydroxymethyl-2'-deoxyuridine in cellular DNA, *Proc. Natl. Acad. Sci. U.S.A.,* 81, 318, 1984.

50. **Hollstein, M. C., Brooks, P., Linn, S., and Ames, B. N.,** Hydroxymethyluracil DNA glycosylase in mammalian cells, *Proc. Natl. Acad. Sci. U.S.A.,* 81, 4003, 1984.

51. **Wataya, Y., Santi, D. V., and Hansch, C.,** Inhibition of *Lactobacillus casei* thymidylate synthetase by 5-substituted 2'-deoxyuridylates. Preliminary quantitative structure-activity relationship, *J. Med. Chem.,* 20, 1469, 1977.

52. **Danenberg, P. V.,** Thymidylate synthetase — a target enzyme in cancer chemotherapy, *Biochim. Biophys. Acta,* 473, 73, 1977.

53. **Lindahl, T.,** DNA repair enzymes, *Annu. Rev. Biochem.,* 51, 61, 1982.

Chapter 12

# CYTOSINE ARABINOSIDE, DEOXYCOFORMYCIN, AND COFORMYCIN

**Gérard Buttin, Michelle Debatisse, and Bruno Robert De Saint Vincent**

## TABLE OF CONTENTS

I.    Cellular Resistance to Cytosine Arabinoside ...................................172
    A.    Cytosine Arabinoside Resistance of Deoxycytidine Kinase
        Deficient Rodent Cells .....................................................172
    B.    Cytosine Arabinoside Resistance of Rodent Cells with an
        Expanded dCTP Pool: Cross Resistance to Thymidine ..................172
    C.    Cytosine-Arabinoside Resistance of Rodent Cells Selected for
        Aphidicolin-Resistance: Multiple Cross-Resistance to
        Nucleosides ................................................................175
    D.    Cytosine-Arabinoside Resistance of Rodent Cells with
        Unidentified Biochemical Defects .......................................176
    E.    Cytosine Arabinoside Resistance in Human Tumor Cells...............176
    F.    Conclusions ...............................................................177

II.   Cellular Resistance to Deoxycoformycin and Coformycin .....................177
    A.    Amplification of the ADA Gene in Deoxycoformycin-Resistant
        Cells.......................................................................178
        1.    Detoxification to Excess Ado ....................................178
        2.    Utilization of dAdo as the Sole Purine Source ..................179
        3.    Utilization of Ado as the Purine Source by an
                Adenosine-Kinase Deficient Line .............................179
    B.    Amplification of Adenylate-Deaminase Gene or Altered
        Regulation of Purine Biosynthesis in Cells Resistant to High
        Coformycin Concentrations..............................................180
    C.    Conclusions ...............................................................180

Acknowledgments .................................................................180

References.........................................................................181

# I. CELLULAR RESISTANCE TO CYTOSINE ARABINOSIDE

Cytosine-arabinoside (1-β-D-arabinofuranosylcytosine; cytarabine) is a potent inhibitor of DNA synthesis in mammalian cells; its ability to block viral growth and tumor cell proliferation is well documented.[1] The nucleoside is presently a major drug in the treatment of human acute lymphoblastic leukemia.[2] The molecular mechanism by which cytosine-arabinoside (AraCyt) interferes with DNA synthesis is complex and still controversial but there is growing agreement that the analog exerts a dual action.[1,7] Competition of Ara-CTP with dCTP restricts dCTP incorporation by DNA polymerases, especially α-DNA polymerase; incorporation of Ara-CTP by DNA polymerases distorts the primer-template and blocks further synthesis by chain termination.

AraCyt is a substrate for cytidine (Cyd)-deaminase, an enzyme widely distributed in mammalian cells and sera;[3,4] the product of the deamination reaction is not cytotoxic.

## A. Cytosine Arabinoside Resistance of Deoxycytidine Kinase Deficient Rodent Cells

The first biochemical mechanism of AraCyt resistance characterized in mammalian cells was the impaired capacity of mutant of the mouse leukemia cell line L 5178Y to phosphorylate AraCyt and deoxycytidine (dCyd).[5] Decreased conversion of AraCyt to phosphorylated nucleotides has been observed in other resistant lines, and shown by Drahowsky and Kreis to be due to almost complete absence of AraCyt kinase activity.[6] Subsequent work again identified dCYD-kinase as the phosphorylating activity deficient in these murine neoplasms.[8,9] The same biochemical defect has been demonstrated in resistant clones selected from a variety of mammalian cell lines;[10-13] genetic and biochemical[14] analysis agree to indicate that AraCyt behaves as a metabolic analog of dCyd. Cells unable to phosphorylate AraCyt are very efficiently protected against the cytotoxicity of the drug. Thus, subclones of the CCL39 Chinese hamster lung cell lines selected for their ability to grow in medium containing 5 μg/mℓ of AraCyt (20 × 10⁻ $M$) were all found both deficient in AraCyt kinase activity and able to form colonies at AraCyt concentrations as high as 50 μg/mℓ.[15] The observation that an important level of dCyd-kinase is preserved in these cells disclosed the presence of a mitochondrial isozyme of dCyd-kinase, which does not utilize AraCyt as a substrate.[10,16]

Although AraCTP appears to be the active derivative, no resistant mutant line has been characterized so far with a defect in AraCyt phosphorylation at a step beyond monophosphate formation. A complete loss of activity of the nucleoside diphosphate kinase is expected to be lethal, and dCyd-monophosphate kinase is also likely to be a nondispensable enzyme. Moreover, monophosphate formation is the rate-limiting step in AraCyt and dCyd metabolism.[17] Therefore, partial defects in the activity of the enzymes governing further steps of drug phosphorylation may escape detection.

## B. Cytosine Arabinoside Resistance of Rodent Cells with an Expanded dCTP Pool: Cross Resistance to Thymidine

Because AraCyt is an analog of dCyd, it can be predicted that changes in the intracellular pool of dCyd derivatives will interfere with AraCyt metabolism and with its efficiency as a toxic drug. dCTP and AraCTP are competitors at the level of DNA polymerases;[1] moreover, dCTP is a potent feed back inhibitor of the dCyd-AraCyt kinase.[8,14] Therefore, an increase in the dCTP pool level may also drastically reduce the conversion of AraCyt to AraCMP.

A mutant with a 4-fold increased pool of phosphorylated dCyd derivatives was first isolated by Momparler et al. from L 5178Y mouse cells exposed to 2.4 × 10⁻⁶ $M$ AraCyt for 12 days.[18] We selected such mutants from the Chinese hamster line CCL 39.[15] This line is devoid of Cyd-deaminase activity, a phenotypic trait that limits changes in the actual drug concentration supplied to the cells during selective growth, but does not permit to determine

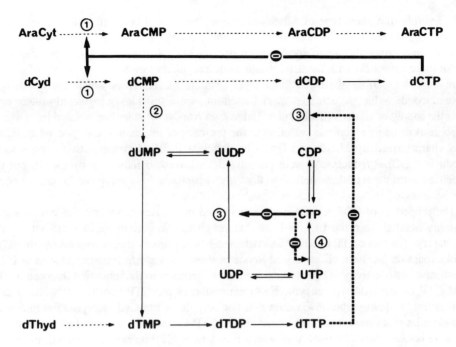

FIGURE 1.    Identified pathways of pyrimidine and AraCyt metabolism in CCL39.—►: endogenous metabolism; ·······►: metabolism of exogenously supplied nucelosides; ⊶►: feed-back inhibitions in wild-type cells; ⊶►: feed-back inhibitions characterized in mutant cells. ① : dCyd-AraCyt-kinase; ② : dCMP-deaminase; ③ : ribonucleotide-reductase; ④ : CTP-synthetase.

to what extent alterations in the activity of this detoxifying enzyme can modulate resistance. Special care was taken to analyze single step mutants and to screen for mutants with low resistance to the drug. Selections from the mutagenized wild-type line were carried out in the presence of 0.5 μg/mℓ of AraCyt, a drug concentration only five times above that required to kill all wild-type cells under the chosen plating conditions. This selection yielded mutants able to survive in medium supplemented with 50 μg/mℓ of AraCyt ("high resistance" phenotype); these clones were devoid of dCyd-AraCyt kinase activity. But a more frequent class of mutants was recovered, which did not resist AraCyt concentrations higher than 1 μg/mℓ ("low resistance" phenotype). Several of these clones were further analyzed. All exhibited a pattern of common traits showing that they were not leaky kinase mutants: (1) they possessed normal dCyd-AraCyt kinase activity, yet they incorporated about 20 times less dCyd into DNA than the wild-type line; (2) in contrast to wild-type cells, their growth was not inhibited by 1 m*M* thymidine (dThd); (3) the dCTP pool of these cells was 4 to 5 times larger than in wild-type cells. An AraCyt resistant mutant selected after several passages in $1 \times 10^{-7}$ *M* AraCyt had been previously reported by Bach to be 4-fold more resistant to fluorodeoxyuridine and 30-fold more resistant to thymidine (dThd) than its parent but its dCTP pool level was not determined.[19] The expansion of the dCTP pool simply accounts for the joint resistance to AraCyt and dThd (Figure 1). As pointed out above, this change is sufficient to determine AraCyt resistance; moreover, the toxic effect of dThd in excess is to deplete the dCTP pool, because it generates excess dTTP that inhibits the production of dCDP by the ribonucleotide-reductase.[20] Cells overproducing dCTP may withstand such a regulation better than wild-type cells. In support to this interpretation, mutants with the same cross-resistance phenotype were isolated as cells resistant to a selective medium containing 1 m*M* dThd. With a second selection step, it was possible to isolate mutants which cumulate the biochemical defects of "high resistance" and "low resistance" mutants. These double mutants were obtained either as clones with increased AraCyt resistance from a "low resistance" line or as dThd-resistant derivatives of a dCyd-AraCyt kinase deficient line.

In hybrids, the phenotype of "high resistance" to AraCyt behaved as a recessive trait, in good agreement with the identification of the primary defect as the loss of an enzyme activity. In contrast, the phenotype of joint resistance to AraCyt and dThd was semidominant, a trait more consistent with the manifestations of a regulatory mutation. A variety of genetic changes can modulate the dCTP pool level. Among the enzymes which can be altered, ribonucleotide reductase deserves special attention, since this highly regulated protein controls the supply of all deoxynucleotides. Indeed, an AraCyt resistant line isolated from mouse fibroblasts through a stepwise selection in the presence of increasing AraCyt concentrations was characterized by Meuth and Green as deficient in dCyd-kinase activity and also as producing a CDP reductase protein partially desensitized to inhibition by dATP, but the specific contribution of these defects to the "high resistance" phenotype of the mutant could not be assessed.[21]

The properties of CDP-reductase were examined in extracts of several "low resistance" mutants isolated from the CCL39 lines, but no change in activity or in sensitivity to the regulatory effectors dATP or dTTP was detected.[15] The primary defect responsible for dCTP pool expansion has been characterized in one of these lines as an altered regulation of CTP-synthetase. This activity is half-desensitized in cell extracts to the inhibition imposed by 0.2 mM CTP on the wild-type enzyme.[22] An expansion of the CTP pool was first discovered in this line, following the observation that not only dCyd but Cyd incorporation into macromolecules is severely decreased in these cells. CTP-synthetase was identified as the altered enzyme because the UTP pool from which it generates CTP remained unaltered; the nature of the defect was characterized by direct "in vitro" assays.

Definitive evidence that this defect is responsible for the resistant phenotype was supplied by the isolation of revertants which simultaneously regained wild-type sensitivity of the enzyme to CTP and wild-type sensitivity of cell proliferation to AraCyt and dThd. They were obtained by exploiting the discovery that, when associated to a defect in dCMP-deaminase activity, CTP overproduction imposes dThd auxotrophy.[23] As shown in Figure 1, excess CTP inhibits UDP reduction, making cells entirely dependent on the activity of dCMP deaminase for endogenous production of dTTP. We isolated by chance a dThd dependent clone from the CTP overproducing line and characterized it as dCMP-deaminase deficient. Survivors from a culture of this subline in dThd-less medium had regained a CTP-sensitive CTP-synthetase, wild-type pools of CTP and dCTP and wild-type sensitivity to both AraCyt and dThd.[22]

In the CCL39 line, dCTP pool expansion seems to be frequently caused by CTP pool expansion, as judged from the important fraction of mutants selected for "low resistance" to AraCyt or for dThd resistance, which are deficient in exogenous Cyd incorporation. Other biochemical alterations increasing the dCTP pool level remain indeed to be identified in mutants which do not manifest this particular phenotypic trait. It is of interest that dThd auxotrophs of the Chinese hamster ovary (CHO) cell line isolated through selection for AraCyt resistance[26] have also been characterized more recently as mutants with a deregulated CTP-synthetase.[24] Because they are cross-resistant to 5-fluorouracil, these mutants (designated: "thy⁻") can be specifically recovered from the CHO line through selection in growth medium supplemented with both AraCyt and 5-fluorouracil.[25] The thy⁻ mutants require dThd for their growth, have a five- to tenfold expanded dCTP pool and frequently revert to the wild-type state.[27] The high frequency of pleiotropic reversion prompted the authors to examine the rate of mutation at different independent gene loci; this study disclosed the remarkable property of the thy⁻ mutation to behave as a mutator with marked specificity of action. Although it was first considered that the thy⁻ phenotype was the manifestation of ribonucleotide reductase alterations,[27] further work showed that the CHO line is dCMP-deaminase deficient and established that thy⁻ mutants bear an additional defect similar to that altering CTP synthetase in the mutants described above.[24] In both cases, 50% of CTP synthetase activity remains CTP sensitive; an extensive study carried out on revertants of a thy⁻ mutant strongly supports the interpretation that the mutant cells express one wild-type and one mutant allele of the CTP-synthetase gene. Secondary thy⁻ mutants with an enzyme fully resistant to CTP were isolated; sensitivity to AraCyt and mutational rates at several loci are essentially identical in these mutants and in the primary thy⁻ mutants. The "mutator" phenotype of the mutants selected from CCL39 for low resistance to AraCyt has not been examined, but they have presumably an increased mutation rate since there is evidence that this is a rather general property of cells with unbalanced triphosphate pools.[28]

## C. Cytosine-Arabinoside Resistance of Rodent Cells Selected for Aphidicolin-Resistance: Multiple Cross Resistance to Nucleosides

Much effort has been devoted to characterize mutants resistant to aphidicolin, an inhibitor of DNA replication in vivo and of α-DNA polymerase activity in vitro. Such mutants isolated from the mutagenized mouse mammary carcinoma line FM3A and from a dThd-auxotroph derivative (thymidylate-synthetase deficient) showed cross resistance to AraCyt, dThd, adenine-arabinoside (AraAde) and deoxyadenosine (dAdo).[29]

Following a second cycle of selection for increased aphidicolin resistance, spontaneous secondary mutants were derived; they exhibited increased resistance to the same inhibitors, suggesting that the pattern of pleiotropic resistance was the manifestation of a single genetic alteration. This interpretation was strengthened by the observation that direct selection of AraCyt resistant clones from the same lines yielded not only clones jointly resistant to AraCyt and dThd and dCyd-AraCyt kinase deficient clones, but also a third class of mutants resistant to AraCyt, dThd, AraAde, dAdo, and aphidicolin. The aphidicolin-sensitive mutants resistant to AraCyt and dThd preserved normal sensitivity to AraAde and, like the Chinese hamster "low resistance" mutants, had an expanded dCTP pool. The phenotype of the AraCyt resistant mutants cross resistant to aphidicolin was undistinguishable from that of mutants selected for aphidicolin resistance. In hybrids, all resistances behaved as semidominant traits. Biochemical analysis revealed that, whatever the selection procedure, all aphidicolin-resistant mutants examined had a markedly expanded dATP pool, a slightly increased dCTP pool and unchanged dTTP and dGTP pools. In two mutants of this class, the level and regulation of ADP and CDP reductase activities were analyzed in vitro; reductase activity was found normal in these cells, but the enzyme was desensitized to dATP. This result accounts for resistance to adenylic nucleosides and aphidicolin. Resistance to dThd and Ara-Cyt was not directly explained by this analysis, because in vitro sensitivity of CDP-redutase to dTTP was unaltered. Despite reduced ability to incorporate exogenous dCyd into macromolecules, the CTP pool was little increased (at most twofold) as compared to its expansion (eightfold) in mutants from the same line which are resistant only to dThd and to comparable AraCyt concentrations. Further biochemical characterization of these mutants remains indeed desirable but the paradoxical situation may just illustrate incomplete knowledge of the influence of a reductase regulatory defect on deoxyribonucleotide supply. In vivo dThd resistance, contrasting with dTTP sensitivity of CDP-reductase in cell extracts has been also reported by Ullman et al. for a mouse tumor cell mutant. Using permeabilized cells, these authors showed that, in contrast to wild-type reductase, the mutated enzyme was dTTP resistant, if supplied with physiological low concentrations of ATP.[30]

The key role of ribonucleotide-reductase in the control of multiple nucleoside resistances is also illustrated by the properties of mutants with the same pattern of cross resistances, isolated from the CHO line.[31] Aphidicolin-resistant cells recovered from stepwise selection in the presence of increasing concentrations of the drug expressed at each step growing resistance to AraCyt, dThd, and Ara Ade. All four pools of dCTP, dTTP, dGTP, and dATP increased stepwise, in contrast to the situation observed in mutants recovered from FM3A which maintained normal dGTP and dTTP pools. Ribonucleotide reductase studied in one

CHO mutant was normally sensitive to dATP but eight- to ninefold more active than in the parental line, a property accounted for by overproduction of the protein. Thus both accumulation of the reductase or its desensitization to dATP appear to govern resistance to multiple nucleosides toxic to wild-type cells, including AraCyt.

## D. Cytosine-Arabinoside Resistance of Rodent Cells with Unidentified Biochemical Defects

Mutants which appear to disclose a new mechanism of AraCyt resistance were recovered as spontaneous mutants or after mutagenesis from the cytidine-deaminase deficient CHO-K$_1$ hamster line, following single step selection in 1 $\mu$g/m$\ell$ of AraCyt.[32] They show reduced growth rate (or survival) in the presence of 5 $\mu$g/m$\ell$ of AraCyt and remain sensitive to Ara Ade and aphidicolin. They preserve normal AraCyt-kinase activity and appear to take up normally AraCyt; AraCyt resistance behaves as a dominant trait. Concentration dependent inhibition by AraCTP of all four deoxyribonucleoside-triphosphates was observed when dialyzed mutant extract were utilized for a $\alpha$-DNA polymerase assay. In contrast, AraCTP inhibited only dCTP incorporation when the enzyme source was a wild-type extract. These results are consistent with the interpretation that $\alpha$-DNA polymerase is altered in these cells, but further investigations remain necessary for definitive characterization.

Spontaneous mutants jointly resistant to AraCyt and Ara Ade were also isolated by the same group from CHO-K$_1$ cells growing in 1 $\mu$g/m$\ell$ of AraCyt and 20 $\mu$g/m$\ell$ of Ara Ade; one mutant was utilized for the selection of aphidicolin-resistant derivatives.[33] It is claimed to have wild-type AraCyt kinase, AraCyt deaminase and ribonucleotide reductase activities, and a normal dCTP pool; unfortunately, no data are supplied and some of these properties are established on the basis of very indirect evidence.

## E. Cytosine Arabinoside Resistance in Human Tumor Cells

The development of clinical AraCyt resistance may be an important source of failures in the treatment of human acute myelogenous leukemia; yet, analysis of AraCyt resistance in human cells is still at an early stage. Attempts have been made to discover correlations between the failure of patients to respond to an AraCyt containing regimen and some biochemical properties of their tumor cells; attention was mostly paid to the efficiency of AraCyt transport, phosphorylation, retention, and deamination by these cells. Reduced dCyd-kinase activity was found to correlate best with AraCyt refractoriness, but resistance was also found for patients with tumor cells exhibiting full activity of this enzyme.[34] The isolation of AraCyt resistant mutants from established human cells has been recently reported by two groups. Bhalla et al. recovered a stable resistant line from cultures of the HL60 promyelocytic leukemic line grown for several weeks in the presence of AraCyt concentrations stepwise increasing from $5 \times 10^{-8} M$ to $10^{-6} M$.[12] The HL60/AraC subline is dCyd-AraCyt-kinase deficient. As expected, it cannot be protected against dThd inhibition of proliferation by exogenous supply of dCyd, suggesting the possibility to exploit this property for in vivo cradication of dCyd-AraCyt kinase deficient cells by dThd perfusion. Eradication of dCyd-AraCyt kinase deficient hamster cells by dThd has been previously demonstrated and exploited to devise a selective system for hybrids between these cells and thymidine-kinase or HGPRT deficient cells.[35]

Human epidermoid carcinoma KB cells resistant to AraCyt (KB/araC) have also been established by continuous exposure of a cell culture to concentrations of AraCyt increasing from $5 \times 10^{-8}$ to $9 \times 10^{-6} M$.[13] AraCyt-kinase activity was reduced in sublines cloned from the heterogenous surviving population and was below 1% of the wild-type level in some clones. No marked increase in cytidine-deaminase activity was detected in the resistant clones and no clone cross-resistant to amethopterin or cis-platinum was identified. KB cells doubly resistant to AraCyt and vincristine were established by continuous exposure of the heterogeneous KB/AraC cell population to increasing doses of vincristine.[36] The surviving population was unstably cross resistant to a variety of drugs, and gained increased resistance to AraCyt; survivors from KB cells treated according to the same protocol exhibited low AraCyt resistance. These observations are best accounted for by the emergence of ''multidrug resistant'' mutants (please see Biedler et al., in Volume 2) implying that the intracellular concentration of AraCyt is controlled by the level of $mdr_1$ gene expression, but clarification of this phenotype must await the analysis of clonal populations.

## F. Conclusions

Three enzyme defects leading to AraCyt resistance have been so far unambiguously identified. Complete deficiency of dCyd-AraCyt kinase is sufficient to cause ''high resistance'' to the drug in both rodent and human cells. Deregulation of CTP-synthetase activity, and alterations in the level of activity or in the regulation of ribonucleotide-reductase determine lower resistance to AraCyt. Because these mutations are dominant, and can be easily expressed in diploid or aneuploid cells, their importance in the emergence of AraCyt resistant clones during prolonged chemotherapy deserves precise evaluation. Studies on rodent cells also showed that mutants with hyperactive CTP-synthetase entirely rely on the activity of dCMP-deaminase for their survival in dThd deprived media. Because increased CTP-synthetase activity has been demonstrated in some rapidly growing tumor cells,[37] strategies exploiting dCMP-deaminase inhibitors may prove useful for the eradication of these tumors. Whatever its enzymatic origin, low resistance to AraCyt is frequently the manifestation of altered control in dCTP synthesis; one should expect that other still unidentified biochemical defects can lead to the manifestation of the same phenotypic trait. Their occurrence, as well as that of other mechanisms for AraCyt resistance, may be cell type dependent. Isolation of resistant mutants from established human cancer lines, and establishment of cells taken from patient tumors may represent in the future two complementary approaches for the identification of defects with clinical significance. They should allow a more complete screening of biochemical alterations responsible for specific or nonspecific AraCyt resistance and an estimate of the contribution of genetically determined AraCyt resistance vs. that of reduced cell proliferation rates to the survival of malignant cells.

## II. CELLULAR RESISTANCE TO DEOXYCOFORMYCIN AND COFORMYCIN

Adenosine-deaminase (adenosine aminohydrolase) is an important interconversion enzyme in mammalian cells. Children with a deficiency in ADA activity undergo a severe combined immunodeficiency disease characterized by the loss of B and T cell functions.[38] Another genetic disorder, hereditary hemolytic anemia, has also been associated with abnormally high levels of ADA activity.[39] The availability of ADA inhibitors is of considerable importance to develop model systems for the study of these clinical defects and for potentiating the action of adenosine (Ado) analogs with antiviral or with cytotoxic activity, which are substrates of ADA. Two classes of very potent ADA inhibitors are available: the antibiotics coformycin (Cof) and 2'-deoxycoformycin (covidarabin; dCof). These antibiotics have the properties of transition state analogs[40] and 9-(hydroxyalkyl)adenines, such as *erythro*-9(2-hydroxy-3-nonyl) adenine (EHNA), which presumably bind to a region adjacent to the catalytic site of ADA.[41] Cof and dCof are tight-binding inhibitors of ADA with $K_i$ values in the range of 2.5 to $15 \times 10^{-12}\ M$; EHNA is a semitight binding inhibitor with $K_i$ values on the order of 2 to $4 \times 10^{-9}\ M$.[42,43] Commercially available EHNA is a mixture of two chiral isomers with markedly different inhibitory properties.[45] So far dCof (and Cof) have been preferred for genetical and clinical studies because inhibition of ADA by EHNA is more readily reversible and EHNA affects several aspects of purine metabolism which are not accounted for by ADA inhibition.[44]

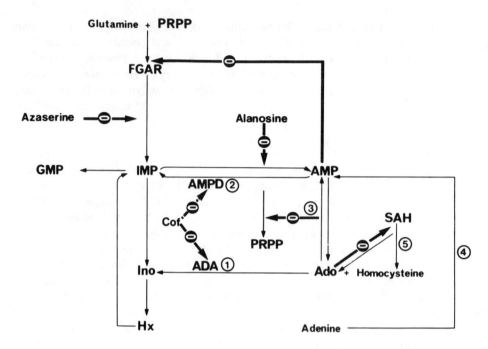

FIGURE 2.    dAdo metabolism in CCL39.—⊖—▶: action of natural or drug inhibitors.

## A. Amplification of the ADA Gene in Deoxycoformycin-Resistant Cells

ADA activity is not required for the proliferation of mammalian cells in the usual culture media; addition of ADA inhibitors does not alter their growth rate.[46,47] But several media supporting only growth of cells expressing ADA have been developed. Such selections rely on two physiological functions of ADA: (1) ADA activity governs the production of inosinic and guanylic derivatives from adenylic nucleosides; and (2) ADA detoxifies potentially cytotoxic adenylic purines by converting them to inosinic purines. Natural adenylic purines have been shown to interfere with the activity of several important biochemical pathways (Figures 2 and 3). In cells with an active adenosine kinase, exogenous Ado blocks PRPP synthesis and thereby endogenous pyrimidine biosynthesis through some incompletely reconstructed mechanism, thereby imposing uridine (Urd) auxotrophy.[46,48,49] dAdo phosphorylation generates as a final product dATP, a powerful inhibitor of ribonucleotide-reductase; dAdo and Ado in excess have also been shown to respectively inactivate or inhibit the activity of S-adenosyl-homocysteine hydrolase (SAH) an enzyme controlling methylation reactions.[50,51,52] Three main strategies have been exploited with success to isolate mutants overproducing ADA.

### 1. Detoxification to Excess Ado[53]

This protocol relies on a modification of the "AAU medium" which selects for adenosine kinase expression.[54] In AAU medium, generation of AMP by endogenous purine biosynthesis is blocked by alanosine; AMP is derived from 0.1 m*M* exogenous Ado, Urd is added to compensate for inhibition of pyrimidine biosynthesis. Raising Ado concentration creates an absolute requirement for ADA activity; addition of 10 n*M* dCof becomes lethal and survivors are recovered which overproduce ADA. From mouse cell cultures growing in the presence of stepwise increasing dCof concentrations (up to 12 μ*M*), clones with up to 11,000-fold the wild-type activity of ADA were recovered. Further work identified these cells as mutants with a comparable amplification of the ADA gene, producing 75% of their whole protein as ADA.[55,56] In this selection, ADA activity is assumed to avoid accumulation of cytotoxic Ado concentrations.

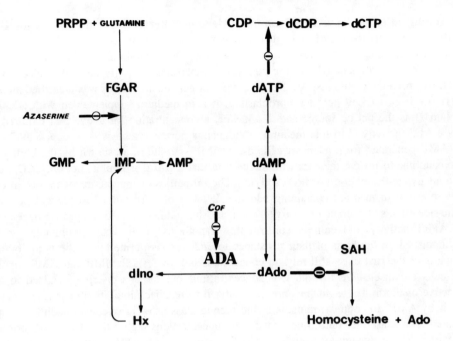

FIGURE 3.   Ado metabolism in CCL39.—⊝→: action of natural or drug inhibitors.   ① :
adenosine-deaminase;   ② : adenylate-deaminase;   ③ : adenosine-kinase;   ④ : APRT;
⑤ : SAH hydrolase.

## 2. Utilization of dAdo as the Sole Purine Source

In CCL39 Chinese hamster fibroblasts, with endogenous purine biosynthesis deliberately
blocked by azaserine, dAdo can be used as a guanylic and riboadenylic purine source only
through a pathway (Figure 2) initiated by ADA.[46,49] Cells grow in medium supplemented
with azaserine, dAdo and dCyd — added to compensate for inhibition of CDP-reductase —
but die if Cof (20 n$M$) is further added. Following transfer of surviving clones to medium
with 1 µ$M$ Cof, second step spontaneous mutants expressing 100-fold higher than wild-type
ADA activity were recovered.[57] These mutants are more resistant than the wild-type line to
low Ado concentrations, even when ADA activity is fully turned off by Cof, indicating that
they bear an additional unidentified defect. Cof resistance is unstable in these lines; they
overproduce an ADA protein with unaltered kinetic properties, suggesting that ADA hy-
peractivity is the manifestation of gene amplification. ADA gene amplification was indeed
demonstrated in mutants isolated from the P815 mouse mammary tumor line using a very
similar selection protocol.[58] The selective medium contained azaserine, dAdo, DCyd, and
Urd; dCof was used as the ADA inhibitor. Mutants with 100-fold amplification of the ADA
gene were recovered upon three selection steps. They may also bear an additional defect —
possibly correcting for SAH inactivation by dAdo — because P815 cells divided at a normal
rate in the medium containing azaserine and the nucleoside mixture only after a period of
adaptation.

## 3. Utilization of Ado as the Purine Source by an Adenosine Kinase Deficient Line

Stable overproduction of ADA (up to 2000-fold) was observed by Hoffee et al. in adenosine-kinase deficient Novikoff rat hepatoma cells surviving growth in medium supplemented
with Ado and increasing dCof concentrations.[47] The choice of this line was made to insure
that Ado would be metabolized by ADA and to avoid the inhibitory effect of Ado on cell
growth (Figure 3). In all but one examined resistant mutants, ADA gene copy number was
increased to a degree similar to the increase in enzyme activity.[59]

## B. Amplification of Adenylate-Deaminase Gene or Altered Regulation of Purine Biosynthesis in Cells Resistant to High Coformycin Concentrations

As just illustrated above, restrictions imposed by ADA inhibitors to the channeling of nucleosides from the adenylic to the guanylic compartment strongly favor the selection of ADA overproducing mutants. A different pattern of genetic alterations was identified among survivors from CCL39 hamster fibroblasts grown in medium supplemented with adenine (0.1 m$M$) as the purine source and 2 $\mu M$ Cof, a concentration far above that required to block ADA activity.[60] In this medium, endogenous purine synthesis is feedback inhibited by AMP generated from adenine; cells die of IMP starvation, as shown by the ability of hypoxanthine to restore their growth, suggesting that 2 $\mu M$ Cof inhibits not only ADA but also adenylate-deaminase (AMPD) activity. The properties of mutants recovered from one step selection in medium containing adenine, 2 $\mu M$ Cof, Urd (added to prevent possible toxic side effects of adenine derivatives) and alanosine (added to make cell growth dependent on APRT activity) did entirely confirm this hypothesis. Two types of mutants can be distinguished on the basis of their resistance to endogenous purine biosynthesis inhibitors. Mutants of the first class still rely on endogenous biosynthesis for IMP and GMP supply; the cells are insensitive to high Cof concentrations but die if azaserine is added to the selective medium. These mutants are desensitized to feedback inhibition of purine biosynthesis by AMP. In contrast, mutants of the second class grow in selective medium supplemented with azaserine, but do not resist Cof concentrations higher than that used for their selection. These mutants overproduce AMPD. Mutants with AMPD activity increased up to 150-fold were recovered by stepwise selection for increasing Cof resistance.[61] Several proteins physiologically unrelated to the purine salvage pathway frequently coaccumulate with AMPD. Isolation of c-DNA probes was possible for four genes coding for these unidentified proteins; the probes allowed to demonstrate amplification of these genes in the overproducing lines[62] and to propose a putative map of the amplifiable chromosomal sequence.[63] This map has been confirmed and amplification of the AMPD gene established by "walking" along the chromosomal amplifiable region.[65]

## C. Conclusions

Partial inhibition of ADA and AMPD by the tight-binding inhibitors dCof and Cof is clearly a very efficient approach for the selection of cells which amplified the genes coding for these target enzymes. This strategy allowed cloning of the ADA gene c-DNA, which can be used as a dominant selectable marker for foreign DNA transfer and amplification in mammalian cells.[64] Release of ADA from overproducing cells also permitted to devise an improved assay for cytotoxicity mediated by T lymphocytes.[58] Overproduction of AMPD in lung fibroblasts has been observed under conditions which can presumably be exploited to select for amplification of the genes coding for the different AMPD isozymes. This study also identified changes in natural purine concentrations which are sufficient to convert Cof or dCof to toxic analogs. This information may prove useful in understanding the clinical properties of these drugs. Less tightly binding inhibitors, such as EHNA, with a possibly different pattern of secondary effects, may allow the selection of a markedly different collection of mutants with interesting physiological properties.

## ACKNOWLEDGMENTS

Work performed by the authors was supported in part by the CNRS, the DGRST, the Université P. et M. Curie, the INSERM, the Ligue Nationale Francaise contre le Cancer, and the Fondation pour la Recherche Médicale. The expert secretarial assistance of Mrs. M. Mahérou is gratefully acknowledged.

# REFERENCES

1. **Cozzarelli, N. R.,** The mechanism of action of inhibitors of DNA synthesis, *Ann. Rev. Biochem.,* 46, 641, 1977.
2. **Bodey, G. P., Freireich, E. J., Monto, R. W., and Hewlett, J. S.,** Cytosline arabinoside therapy for acute leukemia in adults. *Cancer Chemother. Rep.,* 53, 59, 1969.
3. **Camiener, G. W. and Smith, C. G.,** Studies on the enzymatic deamination of cytosine-arabinoside. I. Enzyme distribution and species specificity, *Biochem. Pharmacol.,* 14, 1405, 1965.
4. **Ho, D. H. W.,** Distribution of kinase and deaminase of 1-β-D-arabinofuranosylcytosine in tissues of man and mouse, *Cancer Res.,* 33, 2816, 1973.
5. **Chu, M. Y. and Fischer, G. A.,** Comparative studies of leukemic cells sensitive and resistant to cytosine arabinoside, *Biochem. Pharmacol.,* 14, 333, 1965.
6. **Drahowsky, D. and Kreis, W.,** Studies on drug resistance. II. Kinase patterns in P815 neoplasma sensitive and resistant to 1-β-D-arabinofuranosylcytosine, *Biochem. Pharmacol.,* 19, 940, 1970.
7. **Major, P. P., Egan, E. M., Beardsley, G. P., Minden, M., and Kufe, D. W.,** Lethality of human myeloblasts correlates with the incorporation of araC into DNA, *Proc. Natl. Acad. Sci. U.S.A.,* 78, 3235, 1981.
8. **Schrecker, A. W.,** Metabolism of 1-β-D-arabinofuranosylcytosine in leukemia L1210: nucleoside and nucleotide kinases in cell-free extracts, *Cancer Res.,* 30, 632, 1970.
9. **Schrecker, A. W. and Urshel, M. J.,** Metabolism of 1-β-D-arabinofuranosylcytosine in leukemia L1210: studies with intact cells, *Cancer Res.,* 28, 793, 1968.
10. **Robert de Saint Vincent, B. and Buttin, G.,** Studies on 1-β-D-arabinofuranosylcytosine resistant mutants of Chinese hamster fibroblasts. A mitochondrial deoxycytidine kinase devoid of activity on arabinocytosine, *Eur. J. Biochem.,* 37, 481, 1973.
11. **Rogers, A. M., Hill, R., Lehmann, A. R., Arlett, C. F., and Burns, V. W.,** The induction and characterisation of mouse lymphoma L5178Y cell lines resistant to 1-β-D-arabinofuranosylcytosine, *Mutation Res.,* 69, 139, 1980.
12. **Bhalla, K., Nayak, R., and Grant, S.,** Isolation and characterization of a deoxycytidine-kinase deficient human promyelocytic leukemic cell line highly resistant to 1-β-D-arabinofuranosylcytosine, *Cancer Res.,* 44, 5029, 1984.
13. **Tsuruo, T., Naganuma, K., Iida, H., Sone, S., Ishii, K., Tsubura, E., Tsukagoshi, S., and Sakurai, Y.,** Establishment of human KB cells resistant to 1-β-D-arabinofuranosylcytosine and mechanisms of cellular resistance in isolated clones, Gann, 75, 690, 1984.
14. **Momparler, E. L. and Fischer, G. A.,** Mammalian deoxycytidine-kinase I. Deoxycytidine kinase purification, properties and kinetic studies with cytosine arabinoside, *J. Biol. Chem.,* P. 4298, 1968.
15. **Robert de Saint Vincent, B. and Buttin, G.,** Studies on 1-β-D-arabinofuranosylcytosine resistant mutants of Chinese hamster fibroblasts. III. Joint resistance to arabinofuranosylcytosine and to excess thymidine, a semidominant manifestation of deoxycytidine tripyphosphate pool expansion, *Somat. Cell Genet.,* 5, 67, 1979.
16. **Cheng, Y. C., Domin, B., and Lee, L. S.,** Human deoxycytidine kinase. Purification and characterization of the cytoplasmic and mitochondrial isozymes from blast cells of acute myelocytic leukemia patients, *Biochem. Biophys. Acta,* p. 481, 1977.
17. **Plageman, P. G. W., Marz, R., and Wohlheuter, R. M.,** Transport and metabolism of deoxycytidine and 1-β-D-arabinofuranosylcytosine into cultured Novikoff rat hepatoma cells, relationship to phosphorylation, and regulation of triphosphate synthesis, *Cancer Res.,* 38, 978, 1981.
18. **Momparler, R. L., Chu, M. Y., and Fischer, G. A.,** Studies on a new mechanism of resistance of L5178Y murine leukemia cells to cytosine arabinoside, *Biochem. Biophys. Acta,* 161, 481, 1968.
19. **Bach, M. K.,** Biochemical and genetic studies of a mutant strain of mouse leukemia L1210 resistant to 1-β-D-arabinofuranosylcytosine (cytarabine), *Cancer Res.,* 29, 1036, 1969.
20. **Bjursell, G. and Reichard, P.,** Effects of thymidine on deoxyribonucleoside triphosphate pools and deoxyribonucleic acid synthesis in Chinese hamster ovary cells, *J. Biol. Chem.,* 248, 3904, 1973.
21. **Meuth, M. and Green, H.,** Alterations leading to increased ribonucleotide resistance in cells selected for resistance to deoxynucleosides, *Cell,* 3, 367, 1974.
22. **Robert de Saint Vincent, B., and Buttin, G.,** Studies on 1-β-D-arabinofuranosyllcytosine resistant mutants of Chinese hamster fibroblasts. IV. Altered regulation of CTP synthetase generates arabinosylcytosine and thymidine resistance, *Biochem. Biophys. Acta,* 610, 352, 1980.
23. **Robert de Saint Vincent, B., Dechamps, M., and Buttin, G.,** The modulation of the thymidine triphosphate pool of Chinese hamster cells by cCMP deaminase-deficient lines, *J. Biol. Chem.,* 255, 162, 1980.
24. **Trudel, M., Van Genechten, T., and Meuth, M.,** Biochemical characterization of the hamster thy mutator gene and its revertants, *J. Biol. Chem.,* 259, 2355, 1984.

25. **Meuth, M., Gonçalves, O., and Thom, P.,** A selection system specific for the thy mutator phenotype, *Somat. Cell Genet.,* 8, 423, 1982.

26. **Meuth, M., Trudel, M., and Siminovitch, L.,** Selection of Chinese hamster cells auxotrophic for thymidine by 1-β-D-arabinofuranosylcytosine, *Somat. Cell Genet.,* 5, 303, 1979.

27. **Meuth, M., L'Heureux-Huard, N., and Trudel, M.,** Characterization of a mutator gene in Chinese hamster ovary cells, *Proc. Natl. Acad. Sci. U.S.A.,* 76, 6505, 1979.

28. **Weinberg, G., Ullman, B., and Martin, D. W., Jr.,** Mutator phenotypes in mammalian cell mutants with distinct biochemical defects and abnormal dNTP pools, *Proc. Natl. Acad. Sci., U.S.A.,* 78, 2447, 1981.

29. **Ayusawa, D., Iwata, K., and Seño, T.,** Alteration of ribonucleotide reductase in aphidicolin resistant mutants of mouse FM3A cells with associated resistance to arabinosyladenine and arabvinosylcytosine, *Somat. Cell Genet.,* 7, 27, 1981.

30. **Ullman, B., Clift, S. M., Gudas, L. T., Levison, B. B., Wormsted, M. A., and Martin, D. W.,** Alteration in deoxyribonucleotide metabolism in cultured cells with ribonucleotide reductase activities refractory to feedback inhibition by 2'-deoxyadenosine triphosphate, *J. Biol. Chem.,* 255, 8308, 1980.

31. **Sabourin, C. L. K., Bates, P. F., Glatzer, L., Chang, C. C., Trosko, J. E., and Boezi, J. A.,** Selection of aphidicolin resistant CHO cells with altered levels of ribonucleotide-reductase, *Somat. Cell Genet.,* 7, 255, 1981.

32. **Mishra, N. C., Hinnant, K., and Cason, E.,** New AraC resistant mutants of Chinese hamster ovary cells, *Genet. Res.,* 95, 1, 1985.

33. **Smith, D. B. and Mishra, N. C.,** A Chinese hamster ovary cell mutant resistant to aphidicolin, *Cell. Biol.,* 9, 331, 1985.

34. **Tattersale, M. N. H., Ganeshaguru, K., and Hoffbrand, A. V.,** Mechanisms of resistance of human acute leukemia cells to cytosine arabinoside, *Br. J. Haematol.,* 27, 39, 1977.

35. **Dechamps, M., Robert de Saint Vincent, B., Evrard, C., Sassi, M., and Buttin, G.,** Studies on 1-β-D-arabinofuranosylcytosine resistant mutants of Chinese hamster fibroblasts. II. High resistance to AraC as a genetic marker for cellular hybridization, *Expt. Cell Res.,* 86, 269, 1974.

36. **Sone, S., Ishii, K., and Tsuruo, T.,** Augmentation of 1-β-D-arabinofuranosylcytosine resistance in human KB epidermoid carcinoma cells upon induction of a second resistance to vincristine, *Cancer Res.,* 46, 3099, 1986.

37. **Williams, J. C., Kizaki, H., Weber, G., and Morris, H. P.,** Increased CTP synthetase activity in cancer cells, *Nature,* 271, 71, 1978.

38. **Kellems, R. E., Yeung, C. Y., and Ingolia, D. E.,** Adenosine-deaminase deficiency and severe combined immunodeficiencies. *Trends Genet.,* 1, 278, 1985.

39. **Valentine, W. N., Paglia, D. E., Tartaglia, A. P., and Gilsany, F.,** Hereditary hemolytic anemia with increased red cell adenosine deaminase (45 to 70 fold) and decreased adenosine triphosphate, *Science,* 195, 783, 1977.

40. **Cha, S., Agarwal, R. P., and Parks, R. E., Jr.,** Tight-binding inhibitors. II. Non steady state nature of inhibition of milk xanthine oxidase by allopurinol and alloxanthine and of human erythrocyte adenosine deaminase by coformycin, *Biochem. Pharmacol.,* 24, 2187, 1975.

41. **Schaeffer, H. J. and Vince, R.,** Enzyme inhibitors, XVIII. Studies on the stereoselectivity of inhibition of adenosine deaminase by DL-D- and L-9-(2-hydroxypropyl)adenine., *J. Med. Chem.,* 10, 689, 1965.

42. **Agarwal, R. P., Spector, T., and Parks, R. E., Jr.,** Tight-binding inhibitors. IV. Inhibition of adenosine deaminase by various inhibitors, *Biochem. Pharmacol.,* 26, 359, 1977.

43. **Agarwal, R. P., Cha., S., Crabtree, G. W., and Parks, R. E., Jr.,** in *Chemistry and Biology of Nucleosides and Nucleotides,* Harmon, R. E., Robins, R. K., and Townsend, L. B., Eds., Academic Press, New York, 1978, 159.

44. **Henderson, F., Brox, L., Zombor, G., Hunting, D., and Lomax, C.,** Specificity of adenosine deaminase inhibitors, *Biochem. Pharmacol.,* 26, 1967, 1977.

45. **Bessodes, M., Bastian, G., Abushanab, E., Panzica, R. P., Berman, S. F., Marcaccio, E. J., Jr., Chen, S. F., Stoeckler, J. D., and Parks, R. E., Jr.,** Effect of chirality of EHNA on adenosine deaminase inhibition, *Biochem. Pharmacol.,* 31, 879, 1982.

46. **Debatisse, M. and Buttin, G.,** The control of cell proliferation by preformed purines: a genetic study. II. Pleiotropic manifestations and mechanism of a control exerted by adenylic purines on PRPP synthesis, *Somat. Cell Genet.,* 3, 513, 1977.

47. **Hoffee, P. A., Hunt, S. W., III, and Chiang, J.,** Isolation of deoxycoformycin-resistant cells with increased levels of adenosine-deaminase, *Somat. Cell Genet.,* 8, 465, 1982.

48. **Ishii, K. and Green, H.,** Lethality of adenosine for cultured mammalian cells by interference with pyrimidine biosynthesis, *J. Cell Sci.,* 13, 429, 1973.

49. **Debatisse, M. and Buttin, G.,** The control of cell proliferation by preformed purines: a genetic study. I. Isolation and preliminary characterization of Chinese hamster lines with single or multiple defects in purine salvage pathways, *Somat. Cell Genet.,* 3, 497, 1977.

50. **Kredich, N. M. and Martin, D. W., Jr.,** Role of S-adenosylhomocysteine in adenosine mediated toxicity in cultured mouse T lymphoma cells, *Cell,* 12, 931, 1977.
51. **Hershfield, M. S.,** Apparent suicide inactivation of human lymphoblasts S-adenosylhomocysteine hydrolase by 2'-deoxyadenosine and adenine arabinoside, *J. Biol. Chem.,* 254, 22, 1979.
52. **Kajander, E. O., Kubota, M., Carrera, C. J., Montgomery, J. A. and Carson, D. A.,** Resistance to multiple adenine nucleoside and methionine analogues in mutant murine lymphoma cells with enlarged S-adenosylmethionine pools, *Cancer Res.,* 46, 2866, 1986.
53. **Yeung, C. Y., Ingolia, D. E., Bobonis, C., Dunbar, B. S., Riser, M. E., Siciliano, M. J., and Kellems, R. E.,** Selective overproduction of adenosine-deaminase in cultured mouse cells, *J. Biol. Chem.,* 258, 8338, 1983.
54. **Chan, T. S., Cregan, R. P., and Reardon, P.,** Adenosine-kinase as a new selective marker in somatic cell genetics: isolation of adenosine-kinase deficient mouse cell lines and human-mouse hybrids cell lines containing adenosine kinase, *Somat. Cell Genet.,* 4, 1, 1978.
55. **Yeung, C. Y., Frayne, E. G., Al-Ubaidi, M. R., Hook, A. G., Ingolia, D. E., Wright, D. A., and Kellems, R. E.,** Amplification and molecular cloning of murine adenosine deaminase gene sequences, *J. Biol. Chem.,* 258, 15179, 1983.
56. **Ingolia, D. E., Yeung, C. Y., Orengo, I. F., Harrison, M. L., Frayne, E. G., Rudolph, F. B., and Kellems, R. E.,** Purification and characterization of adenosine deaminase from a genetically enriched mouse cell line, *J. Biol. Chem.,* 260, 13261, 1985.
57. **Fernandez-Mejia, C., Debatisse, M., and Buttin, G.,** Adenosine-resistant Chinese hamster fibroblast variants with hyperactive adenosine-deaminase: an analysis of the protection against exogenous adenosine afforded by increased activity of the deamination pathway, *J. Cell. Physiol.,* 120, 321, 1984.
58. **Vielh, P. and Castellazzi, M.,** Use of a P815-derived line with an amplified adenosine deaminase gene: an improved target for cellular cytotoxicity, *Eur. J. Immunol.,* 15, 981, 1985.
59. **Hunt, S. W. III, and Hoffee, P. A.,** Amplification of adenosine-deaminase gene sequences in deoxy-coformycin-resistant rat hepatoma cells, *J. Biol. Chem.,* 258, 13185, 1983.
60. **Debatisse, M., Berry, M., and Buttin, G.,** The potentiation of adenine toxicity to Chinese hamster cells by coformycin: suppression in mutants with altered regulation of purine biosynthesis or increased adenylate-deaminase activity, *J. Cell. Physiol.,* 106, 1, 1981.
61. **Debatisse, M., Berry, M., and Buttin, G.,** Stepwise isolation and properties of unstable Chinese hamster cell variants overproducing adenylate deaminase, *Mol. Cell. Biol.,* 2, 1346, 1982.
62. **Debatisse, M., Robert de Saint Vincent, B., and Buttin, G.,** Expression of several amplified genes in an adenylate-deaminase overproducing variant of Chinese hamster fibroblasts, *EMBO J.,* 3, 3123, 1984.
63. **Debatisse, M., Hyrien, O., Petit-Koskas, E., Robert de Saint Vincent, B., and Buttin, G.,** Segregation and rearrangement of coamplified genes in different lineages of mutant cells that overproduce adenylate-deaminase, *Mol. Cell. Biol.,* 6, 1776, 1986.
64. **Kaufman, R. J., Murtha, P., Ingolia, D. E., Yeung, C. Y., and Kellems, R. E.,** Selection and amplification of heterologous genes encoding adenosine-deaminase in mammalian cells, *Proc. Natl. Acad. Sci. U.S.A.,* 83, 3136, 1986.
65. **Debatisse, M.,** in preparation.

Chapter 13

# CYCLIC AMP AND OTHER EFFECTORS OF CYCLIC AMP-DEPENDENT PATHWAYS

**Bernard P. Schimmer**

## TABLE OF CONTENTS

I.  Introduction ................................................................. 186
    A.  The Role of Cyclic AMP as a Second Messenger ...................... 186
    B.  Metabolism and Action of Cyclic AMP ............................... 187

II.  Mutants of the Mouse Adrenocortical Tumor Cell Line, Yl ............... 189
    A.  General Properties of Yl Cells ..................................... 189
    B.  Adenylate Cyclase Mutants .......................................... 190
    C.  Protein Kinase Mutants ............................................. 192

III.  Mutants of the Mouse Lymphoma Cell Line, S49 ........................ 194
    A.  General Properties of S49 Cells .................................... 194
    B.  Protein Kinase Mutants ............................................. 194
    C.  Adenylate Cyclase Mutants .......................................... 196
    D.  Other S49 Mutants ................................................. 197

IV.  Mutants of the Chinese Hamster Ovary Cell Line (CHO) ................. 198
    A.  General Properties of CHO Cells .................................... 198
    B.  Cyclic AMP-Resistant Mutants ...................................... 198

V.  Other Mutant Cell Lines ............................................... 200
    A.  Variants of the Macrophage Cell Line, J774.2 ...................... 200
    B.  Variants of the Canine Kidney Cell Line, MDCK ..................... 201

VI.  Summary and Prospects ................................................ 201

Acknowledgments .......................................................... 201

References ............................................................... 202

# I. INTRODUCTION

The enzymes involved in the metabolism and action of cyclic AMP (adenosine 3′,5′-monophosphate; cAMP) provide one of the important interfaces through which cells recognize and respond to many hormones and drugs. These enzymes, which are described in more detail below, have been studied extensively and many of the cells' responses to cAMP have been well characterized. Mutants with defects in the enzymes of the cAMP-dependent pathway have been isolated from a variety of mammalian cell lines, and the consequences of these mutations on cAMP metabolism and action have been evaluated. The first mutants of this type were spontaneous, stable variants isolated from the Y1 mouse adrenocortical tumor cell line.[1] Later, Tomkins and his co-workers developed a strategy for the systematic selection of cAMP-resistant mutants from the S49 mouse lymphoma cell line.[2] These early studies led to the isolation and characterization of cAMP-defective mutants from other cell types, including neuroblastoma cells,[3] macrophage cells,[4] Chinese hamster ovary (CHO) cells,[5] rat pituitary cells,[6] dog and porcine kidney cells,[7,8] and pheochromocytoma cells.[9] Because of the pleiotropic effects of cAMP in mammalian cells, these mutations predictably influenced a large set of cellular end responses to many effector molecules.

The study of mutations affecting the cAMP-dependent pathways of animal cells has provided us with a number of important insights into the mechanisms of hormone and drug actions. These studies have led to the isolation and identification of the guanyl nucleotide-binding regulatory proteins important in signal transduction, and they have provided genetic evidence for the obligatory roles of adenylate cyclase, cAMP, and cAMP-dependent protein kinase in hormonal control of a number of regulated end responses. This review will discuss the isolation of mutants resistant to a variety of compounds which affect cAMP formation or action (viz., ACTH, isoproterenol, prostaglandin $E_1$, forskolin, cholera toxin, and cAMP analogs), and the various consequences of these mutations.

## A. The Role of Cyclic AMP as a Second Messenger

Sutherland and his colleagues[10,11] postulated that cAMP mediated the actions of a hormone or drug on its target tissue, providing that several criteria were met. These criteria are embodied in what is now known as Sutherland's Second Messenger Hypothesis, and can be summarized as follows:

> A hormone (or drug) thought to act via cyclic AMP should elevate the intracellular levels of the cyclic nucleotide at all concentrations of agonist that produce a biological effect.

> Cyclic AMP (or other agents which raise the intracellular level of cyclic AMP), when added to the target tissue, should mimic all the effects of the hormone or drug.

Using these criteria, Sutherland established cAMP as an important intracellular mediator of the actions of a variety of peptide hormones and amines on target cells. A partial list of end-effects ascribed to cAMP in various target cells has been compiled.[11] Kuo and Greengard[12] extended Sutherland's hypothesis by postulating that all of the actions of cAMP in animal cells resulted from activation of cAMP-dependent protein kinase and consequent enhancement of protein phosphorylation. Kuo and Greengard's hypothesis was prompted by the observations that a broad spectrum of mammalian cells contained this enzyme, and that the activation of this enzyme was the only well-documented action of cAMP in animal cells.

As we have noted previously,[13] however, Sutherland's hypothesis is incomplete since it only identifies *potential* second messengers in hormone and drug action. The hypothesis, as stated, does not exclude the existence of other mediators, acting either concomitantly with or independently of cAMP and the cAMP-dependent protein kinase, nor does it evaluate the importance of cAMP relative to other mediators in regulating specific metabolic pathways.

As other intracellular mediators of hormone and drug action have emerged, e.g., cyclic GMP, calcium and calmodulin, diacylglycerol, and protein kinase C, it has been difficult to decide which pathways are most important, or obligatory for the regulation of cell functions. For example, both epinephrine and glucagon, whose actions in the liver classically have been ascribed to cAMP-dependent mechanisms,[11] in fact may act via a pathway involving calcium, diacylglycerol, and protein kinase C.[14,15] Therefore, we have suggested that another criterion must be applied to establish the relative importance of cAMP as a second messenger:

> Pharmacological reagents or genetic mutations which *specifically* interfere with the formation or action of cAMP should inhibit all the effects of the agonist on its target cell.

Reagents that specifically inhibit the formation or action of cAMP in target cells, however, generally are not available. Therefore, the development of mammalian cell lines with specific mutations in the pathways of cAMP metabolism has provided the means to specifically disrupt the cAMP-dependent pathway and to clearly define the relative importance of cAMP in hormone and drug action.

## B. Metabolism and Action of Cyclic AMP

The intracellular levels of cAMP in mammalian cells are determined by the rates of synthesis, degradation, and secretion of the cyclic nucleotide. cAMP is synthesized from ATP by the cyclizing action of the plasma membrane enzyme, adenylate cyclase. The activity of this enzyme is regulated (both positively and negatively) by polypeptide hormones, biogenic amines, prostaglandins, nucleosides and nucleotides, bacterial toxins, and diterpenes. With the possible exception of the diterpene forskolin,[16] these agents impinge on the adenylate cyclase system through discrete receptors, coupled to the enzyme through the heterotrimeric guanyl nucleotide-binding regulatory proteins, Gs and Gi.[17] Gs mediates the activation of adenylate cyclase, and is composed of an $\alpha$ subunit, a $\beta$ subunit, and a $\gamma$ subunit. The $\alpha$ subunit binds guanyl nucleotides, exists in at least two forms (45 kDa and 52 kDalton polypeptides), and appears to be the subunit directly responsible for activation of adenylate cyclase. The $\beta$ and $\gamma$ subunits of Gs are 35 and 8 kDa polypeptides, respectively, and exert a direct, negative regulatory influence on the $\alpha$ subunit of Gs.[17] Gi is a negative regulator of adenylate cyclase activity. The $\alpha$ subunit of Gi (a 41 kDa polypeptide) is distinct from the $\alpha$ subunit of Gs, while the $\beta$ and $\gamma$ subunits of Gs and Gi are functionally identical. The guanyl nucleotide-binding regulatory proteins and the receptors for the toxins and diterpenes have broad tissue distribution, whereas the hormone receptors are distributed in a tissue-specific manner.

cAMP is degraded to 5'-AMP by a family of cAMP-phosphodiesterases. At least three forms of cAMP-phosphodiesterase have been identified on the basis of physical properties, subcellular distribution, substrate specificity, and regulatory properties.[18] One form of the enzyme appears in the soluble fraction of cell homogenates, has a low affinity for cAMP, a higher affinity for cGMP and is dependent upon calcium and calmodulin for activity. A second form of the enzyme has a high affinity for cAMP, is a particulate enzyme which also appears to varying extents in the soluble fraction of cell homogenates, is activated by insulin and is induced by cAMP generating hormones. The third form of the enzyme is a soluble, cGMP-dependent cAMP phosphodiesterase. The cAMP phosphodiesterase activity of this enzyme is stimulated by low doses of cGMP. A partial list of inhibitors of the cAMP-phosphodiesterases have been assembled by Weiss and Levin[19] and by Miller et al.[20] These include competitive inhibitors of the methylxanthine family such as theophylline and 3-isobutyl-1-methylxanthine, noncompetitive inhibitors such as papaverine, and phenothiazine derivatives such as trifluoperazine. The phenothiazines interfere with the actions of calcium and calmodulin on the low Km enzyme, and also competitively inhibit the activity of the high Km phosphodiesterase.[21] cAMP is extruded from mammalian cells by an active process which has not been well characterized. A variety of drugs including probenecid and the phophodiesterase inhibitors theophylline and papaverine interfere with the egress of cAMP, but the egress of cAMP from cells appears to contribute only modestly to the overall turnover of the cyclic nucleotide.[22]

As noted above, cAMP exerts its diverse actions in animal cells primarily by activating a family of cAMP-dependent protein kinases. The activated protein kinases, in turn, regulate cellular activity by catalyzing the phosphorylation of various cellular proteins. The reversible, covalent modification of proteins by phosphorylation-dephosphorylation is regarded as an important mechanism by which mammalian cells regulate many of their complex biochemical processes.[23] The patterns of proteins phosphorylated within each cell determine, in part, the specificity of response of various target tissues to cAMP. In bacteria, cAMP directly regulates gene transcription by forming a complex with a specific protein which binds to DNA.[24] The recent findings that one of the regulatory subunits of the mammalian cAMP-dependent protein kinase is homologous to the bacterial cAMP binding protein in its cAMP binding domains[25] and may have topoisomerase activity[26,26a] has prompted the suggestion that cAMP may influence transcription in animal cells by a similar mechanism.[27]

Although the cAMP-dependent protein kinases have been most studied, they represent only a fraction of the protein phosphotransferases which influence phosphorylation reactions in vivo. Other important phosphotransferases include protein kinase C, cGMP-dependent protein kinase, calcium/calmodulin-dependent protein kinase, double-stranded, RNA-dependent protein kinase, and a number of messenger-independent protein kinases.[28,29]

Two major classes of cAMP-dependent protein kinases have been described in mammalian tissues, and are designated type-1 and type-2 on the basis of distinguishing physical and chemical properties.[30-34] These enzymes have different cellular distributions. In some tissues, such as rabbit skeletal muscle, the type-1 enzyme predominates;[35] in other tissues, such as bovine cardiac muscle, the type-2 enzyme predominates;[36] in yet other tissues, such as porcine skeletal muscle and bovine brain, the two classes of enzyme are present in equal amounts.[37,38] Recently, subclasses of the type-2 enzyme have been described in bovine brain,[39] rat adipose tissue,[40] and in rat ovarian granulosa cells.[41] The major isozyme forms of cAMP-dependent protein kinase also are distributed intracellularly between soluble and membrane-associated fractions, the exact distribution depending upon the cell type and animal species under investigation.[42,43] Both cAMP-dependent protein kinase isozymes are asymmetric tetramers composed of one dimeric regulatory subunit and two catalytic subunits. The different properties of the two protein kinase isozymes—molecular size, requirements for association and dissociation of subunits, binding of MgATP, and autophosphorylation—reflect differences in the regulatory subunits of each enzyme.[30,32-34] The two cAMP-dependent protein kinase isozymes seem to utilize the same catalytic subunit. Although much is known about the structures of the cAMP-dependent protein kinase isozymes, it is not known if the different isozymes each have unique functions within cells.

Both the type-1 regulatory subunit ($R^I$) and the type-2 regulatory subunit ($R^{II}$) have distinct domains which bind cAMP, participate in dimer formation, and bind the catalytic subunit.[29,44-46] $R^I$ and $R^{II}$ each contain two cAMP-binding sites per monomer; these binding sites can be distinguished by their different specificities for cAMP analogs and different cAMP binding properties.[47] $R^I$ and $R^{II}$ are immunologically distinct[45] and are products of separate genes.[46] $R^I$ has an apparent molecular weight of 47,000 to 49,000; $R^{II}$ has an apparent molecular weight of 52,000 to 55,000.[50] Both $R^I$ and $R^{II}$ are phosphoproteins; however, an effect of phosphorylation on function has been demonstrated only for $R^{II}$.[51] In addition, amino acid sequences have been determined for $R^I$, $R^{II}$, and catalytic subunit[52-54] and cDNA clones of each subunit have been isolated.[55-57] In the absence of cAMP, the dimeric regulatory subunits of the enzyme are associated with two catalytic subunits, generating an inactive holoenzyme complex. Activation of the enzyme with cAMP involves the binding of cAMP to the regulatory subunits and the liberation of active catalytic subunits. Reassociation of the subunits leads to the inactivation of the enzyme and the dissociation of bound cAMP. Factors which determine the activity of cAMP-dependent protein kinase include the concentration of free cAMP, the activity of cAMP-phosphodiesterase, and the presence of inhibitors of cAMP-dependent protein kinase.[58-60] ATP and Mg together promote the reassociation of $R^I$ with catalytic subunit;[61] dephosphorylation favors the reassociation of $R^{II}$ with catalytic subunit.[51] The biosynthesis of individual subunits of cAMP-dependent protein kinase, as well as their subcellular distribution also can be regulated through increases in intracellular levels of cAMP.[62,63]

The cAMP-dependent protein kinase utilizes ATP and Mg to catalyze the phosphorylation of serine (and sometimes threonine) residues in appropriate acceptor proteins. Although the cAMP-dependent protein kinases phosphorylate a large number of proteins in vitro and in vivo, the enzymes show a distinct substrate specificity. As a general rule, the sites within a protein that are phosphorylated by the cAMP-dependent protein kinases have two basic amino acids (e.g., arginine) in the amino-terminal vicinity of the target serine residue.[64] In a variety of cell types including S49 lymphoma cells, rat adrenal cells, and rat hepatocytes, over 20 different proteins have been shown to serve as physiological substrates for cAMP-dependent phosphorylation based on an electrophoretic screening procedure.[65,66] The identities of only a few of these proteins, however, have been determined,[65,66] and for most actions of cAMP, the metabolic pathways leading to the measured end-response are poorly understood.

## II. MUTANTS OF THE MOUSE ADRENOCORTICAL TUMOR CELL LINE, Y1

### A. General Properties of Y1 Cells

The Y1 cell line is a well-characterized endocrine line derived from a minimally deviated mouse adrenocortical tumor.[67] The properties of this cell line have been detailed previously.[68] The cell line is nearly diploid, responsive to corticotropin (ACTH), and behaves in many respects like cells from a normal adrenal cortex. Early events in the action of ACTH on Y1 cells include binding to specific membrane receptors at the cell surface,[69,70] activation of adenylate cyclase[71] through the agency of a guanyl nucleotide regulatory protein,[72] and accumulation of cAMP.[73] The cAMP, in turn, activates cAMP dependent protein kinases[74] increasing the phosphorylation of cellular proteins. End-effects of ACTH on Y1 cells include enhanced synthesis and secretion of $C_{21}$ steroids,[75,76] inhibition of cell replication,[77] and striking changes in cell shape.[67] Y1 cells grow as flat epithelial cells well-attached to the culture vessel under basal conditions. When stimulated with ACTH, these cells retract, assume a rounded morphology, and slowly detach from the culture dish. ACTH-mediated growth arrest occurs early in the $G_1$ phase of the cell cycle (<6 hr) and is specific for DNA synthesis; total RNA and protein synthesis are not affected.[78,79] ACTH also brings about a number of other intracellular changes, some of which are supportive for one or more of the characteristic end-effects of the hormone. When stimulated with ACTH, the cell line utilizes glucose,[80] mobilizes cholesterol,[81] phosphorylates ribosomes,[82] and becomes depleted of ascorbic acid[83] at an increased rate. Stimulation of Y1 cells with ACTH also causes the rapid induction of ornithine decarboxylase and the induction of some of the enzymes of the steroidogenic pathway, including the 11β-hydroxylase and adrenodoxin.[84]

Because the Y1 cell line is representative of normal isolated adrenal cells, this system has been used to address some of the major questions regarding the regulation of adrenocortical functions.[68] One of these questions pertains to the relative importance of adenylate cyclase, cAMP, and cAMP-dependent protein kinase in the actions of ACTH on the adrenal cortex. It is well established that cAMP and its analogs, when added to isolated adrenal cells, mimic many of the hormone's effects.[13] Several observations, however, contribute to the uncertainties regarding the role of cAMP as a second messenger in ACTH's action. First, the concentrations of ACTH which are required to increase cAMP levels are greater than those required to stimulate the various end responses, suggesting separate actions of ACTH on cAMP accumulation and on the various end responses. Second, certain ACTH analogs can regulate adrenocortical functions while changing cAMP levels only marginally, suggesting that changes in cAMP levels are not very important in ACTH's actions. Third, a direct role for the cAMP-dependent protein kinase in ACTH's actions has not been demonstrated. Fourth, the specific phosphorylated proteins which serve as the targets of cAMP's actions in the hormonal response have not been defined.[13] Accordingly some investigators have suggested that other second messengers, i.e., calcium, diacyl glycerol and protein kinase C, or cGMP, may be more important than cAMP in regulating adrenocortical functions.[85,86] The ability to derive mutants from the Y1 adrenocortical cell line with specific lesions in the pathways of cAMP metabolism and action has permitted an assessment of the obligatory roles of adenylate cyclase, cAMP, and the cAMP-dependent protein kinase in various actions of ACTH.

## B. Adenylate Cyclase Mutants

Three groups of mutants, phenotypically similar and harboring defects in the ACTH-sensitive adenylate cyclase system have been isolated from Y1 cells. The first mutants of this type were clones Y6 and OS3.[1] Clone Y6 was isolated by randomly cloning cells from the transplantable mouse adrenocortical tumor; OS3 was cloned after it selectively overgrew the Y1 population in culture. These clones did not respond to ACTH with increased rates of steroidogenesis, and thus appeared to lose the capacity for organ-specific, differentiated functions. At the time, "dedifferentiation" of cells in culture was thought to be caused by the selective overgrowth of fibroblastic elements contaminating the population or by nutritional deficiencies in the culture environment.[87,88] Several lines of evidence, however, indicated that the loss of ACTH-regulated steroidogenic activity in these clones was related to a specific defect in cAMP synthesis. ACTH was unable to stimulate adenylate cyclase and increase cAMP levels in the mutants,[89] whereas general activators such as sodium fluoride and magnesium ions,[89] cholera toxin and guanyl nucleotides,[72,90,91] and forskolin[92] effectively stimulated the enzyme. The rest of the hormonally regulated steroidogenic pathway appeared to be intact in these mutants since cholera toxin or cAMP were able to stimulate steroidogenesis normally.[1,91,93,94] When ACTH-sensitive adenylate cyclase activity was restored in the mutant clones following passage of the mutants as tumors,[96] these mutants concomitantly recovered ACTH-stimulated steroidogenic activity.[1,96] Sato and his co-workers[97] previously had passaged cells in culture through a cycle of growth as tumors in animals to enhance the expression of differentiated functions. They presumed that animal passage either selected the few functional tumor cells left in a population overgrown with nonfunctional fibroblastic elements[97] or provided a nutritional requirement for glutamine and serum albumin.[67,88] The mechanism of recovery of ACTH-sensitivity in Y6 and OS3 cells after animal passage remains unexplained, but seemed not to involve selection from a population overgrown with fibroblasts or fulfillment of specific nutritional requirements missing from the culture medium.[1,96]

The observations obtained with the spontaneously derived mutants, Y6 and OS3, were subsequently confirmed with a second set of adenylate cyclase mutants isolated using a modification[98] of the selection protocol developed by Tomkins and his coworkers for S49 lymphoma cells.[2] Y1 cells, when treated with 8BrcAMP, normally stop growing, become rounded and eventually detach from the culture dish. The combined effects of 8BrcAMP on growth and morphology effectively reduce the plating efficiency of Y1 cells so that fewer than 1 in $10^6$ cells normally survive this treatment.[99] Following mutagenesis of the ACTH-responsive Y1 cell line with *N*-methyl-*N'*-nitro-*N*-nitrosoguanidine and growth of the cells in 1 m*M* 8BrcAMP (8-bromoadenosine 3',5'-monophosphate), a few cells in the Y1 population ($<$1 in $10^5$) grew into colonies of rounded cells. These colonies were partially resistant to the growth-inhibiting effects of 8BrcAMP, but were fully responsive to the steroidogenic effects of the cyclic nucleotide. Like the spontaneously derived mutants Y6 and OS3, however, these clones had specific defects in the ACTH-sensitive adenylate cyclase system, rendering them resistant to the steroidogenic effects of the hormone.[98] The emergence of adenylate cyclase-defective mutants from a selection with 8BrcAMP also has been observed in rat pituitary tumor cells.[6] The basis for these selections is not understood. Possibly, the defect in the adenylate cyclase system renders cells partially resistant to 8BrcAMP by lowering the endogenous level of cyclic nucleotide. These adenylate cyclase-defective clones also did not respond to ACTH with changes in cell shape[98] or with increases in ornithine decarboxylase activity,[100] though they responded normally to cAMP and to 8BrcAMP.

Analysis of the mutations in the adenylate cyclase-defective clones by somatic cell fusion indicated that they were recessive and noncomplementary.[92] When fused with the Y1 parent, each mutant clone formed a hybrid which retained ACTH-sensitive adenylate cyclase activity. When an 8BrcAMP-resistant mutant was fused with either Y6 or with OS3, the hybrids remained insensitive to ACTH. Virtually all of the hybrids formed by fusing Y6 with OS3 also remained insensitive to ACTH.[92,95] These observations suggested that each of the adenylate cyclase-defective clones harbored a defect affecting the same regulatory element of the adenylate cyclase system. One hybrid clone isolated from the fusions between Y6 and OS3 did recover ACTH-sensitive adenylate cyclase activity and ACTH-regulated steroidogenic activity.[92,95] The recovery of ACTH sensitivity in this one hybrid was a rare event and was not likely the result of complementation.[95]

Biochemical analyses of these clones have correlated the mutation affecting adenylate cyclase activity with the deficiency of a specific protein designated p68.[95,101] This protein had a relative molecular weight of 68,000, an isoelectric point of 7.2 and an avidity for plasma membrane fractions; the protein was found in the cytosol, however, when cells were disrupted under hypoosmotic conditions.[95,102] The adenylate cyclase-defective clones, including clones Y6 and OS3, contained considerably less p68 than did ACTH-responsive clones whether measured in purified plasma membranes or in total cell homogenates.[95] The one hybrid formed between the mutant clones Y6 and OS3 which recovered ACTH-regulated adenylate cyclase activity also recovered the capacity to synthesize p68.[95] Among a large number of independent clonal isolates from Y1, the amount of p68 correlated with the maintenance of an ACTH-responsive adenylate cyclase system.[95,101] While the precise role of p68 has yet to be determined, the available data suggest that this protein maintains hormone-sensitive adenylate cyclase activity by recycling the hormone receptor from an inactive, desensitized mode to an active mode.[101]

A third set of Y1 mutants harboring defects in the adenylate cyclase system have been isolated recently using the diterpene forskolin as a selective agent.[103] Forskolin activates adenylate cyclase activity and raises the intracellular levels of cAMP in Y1 adrenal cells[103,104] and in many other cell types.[105] Accordingly, forskolin has been used as a probe to study the mechanisms involved in the regulation of the enzyme[106-109] and also to evaluate the role of cAMP in the regulation of cell function.[105,110] Forskolin is thought to stimulate adenylate cyclase activity via a direct action on the catalytic subunit of the enzyme;[105,109] however, other components of the adenylate cyclase system, including the guanyl nucleotide binding regulatory proteins Gs and Gi, also have been implicated in forskolin's actions.[111] In Y1 cells, forskolin inhibited growth, changed cell shape, and stimulated steroidogenesis in a cAMP-dependent manner.[104] As a consequence of forskolin's actions on cell growth and morphology, the diterpene reduced the plating efficiency of Y1 cells over six orders of magnitude.[104] Forskolin-resistant mutants were isolated from Y1 cells by virtue of their resistance to the morphological and growth-inhibitory effects of forskolin.[103,104] These mutants also were resistant to the morphological and growth inhibiting effects of ACTH[92] but remained responsive to 8BrcAMP, indicating that the resistance to forskolin resulted from a defect in cAMP synthesis, rather than cAMP action.[103] The forskolin-resistant phenotype arose spontaneously within the Y1 population with a frequency of 2 mutants per million cells per generation, indicative of a mutational event at a single genetic locus, and appeared to be explained by a defect in the Y1 adenylate cyclase system.[103,104] The adenylate cyclase from mutant cells was partially resistant to forskolin—the diterpene increased adenylate cyclase activity in the mutants to 40% of the level achieved in parent Y1 cells—was totally resistant to ACTH and was stimulated normally by sodium fluoride. This behavior suggested that the defect affected the activity of a regulatory subunit of adenylate cyclase rather than the enzyme's catalytic subunit, and recent observations[104a] implicated the α subunit of Gs in this mutation. Clearly, an understanding of the mechanism of action of forskolin on the adenylate cyclase system and the basis for the mutation to forskolin resistance will be pertinent to understanding the mechanism of hormone action.

## C. Protein Kinase Mutants

Following mutagenesis with ethyl methanesulfonate or *N*-methyl-*N'*-nitro-*N*-nitrosoguanidine and selective growth in 1m*M* 8BrcAMP, a second family of mutants, distinct from the adenylate cyclase mutants, was recovered from Y1 cells. These mutants had cAMP-dependent protein kinases which were resistant to activation by cAMP, and which required 5- to 600-fold more cAMP for activation than required by the normal enzyme.[74,98,99] Adenylate cyclase activity in these mutants was regulated normally by ACTH. Designated Y1(Kin), these mutants were recovered as clones which not only were resistant to the growth inhibiting effects of 8BrcAMP, but which also continued to grow as adherent, well-stretched cells in the presence of the cyclic nucleotide. They arose with a frequency of approximately 1 to 2 mutants per 10⁶ cells following mutagenesis suggestive of a mutational event at a single genetic locus, but they occurred less frequently than did the adenylate cyclase mutants (*vide supra*). Mutations in a structural gene encoding R[I] appeared to account for the altered protein kinase activity and hence the cAMP-resistant phenotype in at least some of the Kin clones. In the mutant clones examined, only the activity of the type-1 enzyme (the major isozyme found in the cytosolic fraction of Y1 cells) was affected; the type-2 enzyme behaved normally.[49,74] On the basis of reconstitution studies using dissociated regulatory and catalytic subunits of the mutant enzymes, the mutation affecting protein kinase activity was further localized to the regulatory subunit of the type-1 enzyme; the catalytic subunit behaved normally.[50] The mutation was associated with structural changes in R[I], as evidenced by its altered electrophoretic mobility in isoelectric focusing gels. Kin mutant cells harbored both parental and charge-modified forms of R[I].[50,112] The mRNA from mutant cells, in a heterologous cell-free translation system, programmed the synthesis of the charge-modified forms of R[I] and wild-type RI in equal amounts. These latter observations ruled out the possibility that posttranslational events contributed to the charge-modification of R[I] in mutant cells, and indicated that the cAMP-resistant clones arose from a single mutational event affecting only one of two R[I] alleles.[112] The manifestation of a cAMP-resistant phenotype in cells that contained both wild-type and charge-modified forms of R[I] suggested that the Kin mutation was codominant. Nevertheless, the Kin mutation appeared to behave recessively when analyzed in cell fusion and gene transfer experiments.[113-115] When fused to a rat glioma cell line, hybrids recovered normal cAMP-dependent protein kinase activity, even though the mutant R[I] subunit was still present.[113] When transfected with genomic DNA from cAMP-responsive Y1 cells, transformants with normal cAMP-dependent protein kinase activity were recovered with an estimated frequency of 0.2 to 0.5 per 10³ transformation-competent cells.[114] These frequencies were comparable to those obtained when transferring single genes from total genomic DNA into fibroblasts.[116,117] The dominant or recessive expression of the Y1(Kin) mutation may depend upon phenomena of gene dosage. The mutant $R^I$ allele behave codominantly when present with one wild-type $R^I$ gene; in the presence of additional copies of the wild-type $R^I$ gene provided during cell fusion or transfection, the mutant allele may be excluded from holoenzyme complexes and behave recessively.

As a consequence of this mutation in the $R^I$ gene, the Kin mutants all were resistant to the steroidogenic effects of ACTH, cAMP, and its analogs.[98,99] The degree of resistance of the steroidogenic pathway to activation by hormone and cyclic nucleotide correlated closely with the degree of impairment of the cAMP-dependent protein kinase.[98,118] Furthermore, Kin mutants which recovered cAMP-dependent protein kinase activity after cell fusion or after DNA-mediated gene transfer with Y1 genomic DNA also recovered the capacity to respond to ACTH and to cAMP with increased steroidogenesis.[113-115] cAMP-responsive transformants of the Kin mutants obtained by transfection with total Y1 genomic DNA were not stable and gradually lost their cAMP-responsive protein kinase activity. In these transformants the capacity to respond to ACTH and cAMP with increased steroidogenesis segregated with the cAMP-dependent protein kinase.[115]

The Kin mutants also have been used to study the roles of cAMP and cAMP-dependent protein kinase in the regulation of growth and cell shape, and in the synthesis of ornithine decarboxylase and tetrahydrobiopterin. The Kin mutants were resistant to the growth-inhibitory and morphological effects of ACTH and cAMP,[98,110] and were resistant to the stimulatory effects of the hormone and cyclic nucleotide on ornithine decarboxylase and tetradihydrobiopterin synthesis.[100,119] Interestingly, in some of the Kin mutants regulation of ornithine decarboxylase activity was impaired to a greater extent than predicted on the basis of the impaired protein kinase and steroidogenic activities.[98,100] These latter observations led to a suggestion that regulation of ornithine decarboxylase activity may have resulted from an activity of $R^I$ distinct from its role in protein phosphorylation.[100]

The adenylate cyclase and protein kinase mutants of Y1 also have been used to evaluate the mechanisms by which other agonists, such as NPS [9-tryptophan (*o*-nitrophenylsulfenyl)-substituted]-ACTH, phorbol esters and vinblastin regulate various adrenocortical activities. NPS-ACTH is an ACTH derivative which stimulates steroidogenesis with 1/100th the potency of the native hormone, and to the same maximum level, but which stimulates cAMP accumulation only slightly.[120,121] Because of its marginal effects on cAMP accumulation, the NPS derivative of ACTH was thought to stimulate steroidogenesis via a cAMP-independent mechanism.[121] NPS-ACTH stimulated steroidogenesis in the Y1 adrenal tumor cell line as it did in normal adrenal cells, and was a weak partial agonist with respect to cAMP accumulation.[122] To test the role of cAMP and cAMP-dependent protein kinase in the steroidogenic actions of NPS-ACTH, the effects of this derivative were examined in two adenylate cyclase mutants and in two protein kinase mutants derived from Y1 cells.[122] In the adenylate cyclase and protein kinase mutants, the steroidogenic responses to NPS-ACTH were impaired in a manner which paralleled the steroidogenic responses to the native hormone and which reflected the degree of defect in the cAMP-regulated pathway. These observations indicated that NPS-ACTH, like ACTH, regulated adrenal steroidogenesis through a cAMP-dependent mechanism.

In Y1 cells, the phorbol ester TPA (12-O-tetradecanoylphorbol-13-acetate) stimulates steroidogenesis and the production of plasminogen activator, inhibits cell replication and causes cell rounding without producing measurable changes in cAMP levels.[123] TPA is thought to exert its effects in most target cells by replacing diacylglycerol, and stimulating protein kinase C;[124] however, the phorbol ester also can increase cAMP levels by inhibiting Gi activity.[125] In order to determine if cAMP participated in the various end-effects of TPA in Y1 cells, the effects of TPA in two Y1(Kin) mutants were evaluated.[123] In the Kin mutants, the effects of TPA on steroidogenesis and plasminogen activator production were impaired, whereas the morphological and growth inhibiting effects were not affected. On the basis of these studies, Estensen et al.[123] suggested that some of TPAs actions on Y1 cells may be mediated by cAMP whereas other effects of TPA occur via cAMP-independent mechanisms.

The microtubule poisons, colchicine and vinblastine, stimulate steroidogenesis in Y1 cells to levels approaching that achieved with ACTH, without producing measurable changes in the levels of cAMP.[126] These microtubule inhibitors, however, are known to increase the intracellular levels of cAMP in other cell types, particularly lymphoid elements.[127,128] Therefore, colchicine and vinblastine may have increased adrenal steroidogenesis by a cAMP-dependent mechanism involving changes in cAMP levels too small to be detected accurately. Accordingly, the steroidogenic actions of colchicine and vinblastine were evaluated in a Y1(Kin) mutant harboring a severely impaired protein kinase.[129] Colchicine and vinblastine stimulated steroidogenesis over basal levels in the Kin mutant to the same extent in the Y1 parent, though the absolute levels of steroid output were lower than the level achieved with the parent line.[129] As a consequence of these studies, Wolff[129] has suggested that colchicine and vinblastine stimulate steroidogenesis by a cAMP-independent mechanism, possibly involving the intramitochondrial translocation of substrate cholesterol to the cholesterol side-chain cleavage enzyme.

Taken together, the results obtained with the different adenylate cyclase-defective and protein kinase-defective mutants indicated that adenylate cyclase, cAMP, and the cAMP-dependent protein kinase were obligatory components in the actions of ACTH on adrenal steroidogenesis, replication, cell shape, ornithine decarboxylase synthesis, and tetrahydro-biopterin synthesis.[89,98,100,110,119] Inasmuch as ACTH's actions were mimicked by exogenously added cAMP,[13] we have suggested that the generation of cAMP and the subsequent activation of the cAMP-dependent protein kinase are both essential and sufficient for the regulation of these adrenocortical functions. Furthermore, these mutants have provided the tools to distinguish cAMP-dependent from cAMP-independent regulatory processes in the adrenal cortex.

## III. MUTANTS OF THE MOUSE LYMPHOMA CELL LINE, S49

### A. General Properties of S49 Cells

S49 is a pseudodiploid cell line originating from an oil-induced mouse lymphoma.[130] Agents which increase the intracellular levels of cAMP in these cells change the levels or the phosphorylation state of approximately 1% of total cellular proteins;[66] however, changes in only a few end-responses have been documented. Increasing the intracellular cAMP levels in these cells inhibits their growth in the G1 phase of the cell cycle,[131] inhibits their ornithine decarboxylase and S-adenosylmethionine decarboxylase activities,[132] increases their cAMP phosphodiesterase levels,[133] and eventually causes their cytolysis.[2] These changes occur whether cAMP levels are increased directly with dibutyryl cAMP, or secondarily by activation of adenylate cyclase with isoproterenol, or with cholera toxin.[134] Cytolysis also is triggered by glucocorticoids,[130] but by a mechanism that is distinct from cyclic nucleotide-induced lysis.[135]

Horibata and Harris[130] demonstrated the the cytolytic action of the glucocorticoids could be used to selectively isolate and grow steroid-resistant mutants from S49 cells. The properties and molecular bases of steroid-resistant mutants have been reviewed elsewhere.[136] This selection scheme provided the basis for the subsequent isolation of mutants defective in the cAMP-dependent, cytolytic pathway of S49 cells.[2]

### B. Protein Kinase Mutants

Three different classes of mutants defective in cAMP-dependent protein kinase were isolated from the S49 line by virtue of their resistance to growth inhibitory and cytolytic actions of dibutyryl cAMP.[2,137,138] These mutants have been the subject of earlier reviews by Bourne et al.[139] and Steinberg.[140] The cAMP-resistant, protein kinase-defective mutants could be isolated in a single-step selection procedure with a frequency of approximately 2 per $10^7$ cells per generation, consistent with a mutational event at a single genetic locus.[137]

One class of mutants, $V_{max}$ mutants, had reduced levels of a protein kinase activity which showed normal activation kinetics with cAMP. These variants comprised 25 to 100% of the cAMP-resistant isolates from S49 cells without mutagenesis.[138,140] They were largely unstable when maintained under nonselective conditions and readily reverted to a cAMP responsive phenotype.[140] The molecular basis for the $V_{max}$ phenotype is not understood, but may have resulted from an epigenetic suppression of enzyme synthesis or activity.

A second class of mutants, Ka mutants, had protein kinases which exhibited full activity when stimulated maximally with cAMP but which exhibited reduced affinity for the cyclic nucleotide. The Ka mutants resembled the Kin mutants isolated from Y1 cells (vide supre) and represented a large fraction of the cyclic nucleotide-resistant clones arising after mutagenesis of S49 cells with agents causing missense mutations.[141] In these mutants, cAMP resistance resulted from mutations in the regulatory subunit of the type 1 cAMP-dependent protein kinase, the predominant isozyme in S49 cells.[142-144] Several lines of evidence supported this hypothesis. Purified $R^I$ subunits from the Ka mutants conferred cAMP resistance upon holoenzymes reconstituted with wild-type catalytic subunits.[143] $R^I$ subunits from the Ka mutants were structurally different from the wild-type subunit as evidenced by their different isoelectric points.[142] Most definitively, McKnight and co-workers[145] isolated $R^I$ cDNA clones from two of the S49 Ka mutants and showed by sequence analysis that each contained a single amino acid substitution in the first and second cyclic binding domain respectively. When incorporated into an expression vector and transfected into Y1 mouse adrenocortical tumor cells, these cDNA clones conferred resistance to the growth inhibitory and steroidogenic effects of the cyclic nucleotide. Steinberg[140] observed some complex interactions between mutant and wild-type forms of $R^I$. In the Ka mutants, wild-type and mutants forms of $R^I$ were synthesized in equal amounts; however, the wild-type $R^I$ contributed negligibly to the cAMP-dependent protein kinase activity.[140] Apparently, mutant subunits were incorporated preferentially into the holoenzyme complex while most of the wild-type $R^I$ was in a ''free'' subunit pool complexed with cAMP. The wild-type $R^I$ subunits which found their way into the holoenzyme complex exhibited mutant-like activity. These observations indicated that the mutant subunit in a hybrid holoenzyme complex interacted with and inhibited the activity of the wild-type $R^I$ subunit.[140] Possibly, the interaction and competition between mutant and wild-type subunits contributed to the dominant nature of the mutant phenotype seen in mutant selection and cell hybridization.[140,146] In addition, wild-type $R^I$ subunits were poorly phosphorylated in Ka mutants whereas mutant subunits largely existed in the phosphorylated form.[142] From these data one might infer that phosphorylation of $R^I$ depends upon its incorporation into holoenzyme complexes. Fine structure peptide mapping of mutated $R^I$ indicated that the Ka mutations were clustered in the first and second cAMP binding domains of the protein.[140,147] Surprisingly, some of these mutations seemed to influence the interaction of $R^I$ with the catalytic subunit rather than the interaction of $R^I$ with cAMP.[140,144] Reversion of the Ka mutation was accompanied by recovery of wild-type, cAMP-dependent protein kinase activity.[148] In a few cases, reversion appeared to result from mutations which restored wild-type activity to the mutant $R^I$ subunit. More frequently, the revertants lost the capacity to synthesize the mutant $R^I$ and only expressed the wild-type gene product. These revertants were cAMP responsive and functionally hemizygous for the $R^I$ gene. As noted by Steinberg,[140] new cAMP-resistant mutants which behave recessively and map to other domains of $R^I$ may be selectable from this functionally hemizygous revertant.

A third class of S49 mutants, Kin⁻, lacked detectable protein kinase activity over a wide range of cAMP concentrations.[138,149] These mutants occurred much less frequently than did mutants from the other two classes, though their formation was favored somewhat by treatment of S49 cells with the frame-shift mutagen ICR-191.[141] The Kin⁻ phenotype did not arise from the generation of an inhibitor of protein kinase activity nor did it arise from mutations in the structural genes encoding R or C (the catalytic subunit of the cAMP-dependent protein kinase). Rather, Kin⁻ may have resulted from a *trans*-acting dominant mutation which effectively abolished the synthesis of C.[149,150] The Kin⁻ mutants also contained much less $R^I$ than normally seen in S49 cells,[149] prompting an evaluation of the factors governing $R^I$ synthesis in these mutants. Steinberg and colleagues demonstrated that treatment of wild-type S49 cells with agents which increased cAMP levels promoted the dissociation of R and C subunits and accelerated $R^I$ degradation.[151] In the Kin⁻ mutants, the rate of degradation of $R^I$ increased, and approached that seen in wild-type cells under conditions where R was dissociated from C. These results suggested that the decreased levels of $R^I$ seen in Kin⁻ mutants were secondary to reduced synthesis of C and resulted from enhanced degradation of free subunits.

A fourth mutant was isolated during a selection of a oubain resistant mutant from thymidine kinase-deficient S49 cells.[149] This subclone harbored a mutation in $R^I$ at the amino-terminal end and near the C binding domain of the protein.[149,152] The mutation was functionally silent; it rendered the protein more basic on two-dimensional gel electrophoresis, but did not appear to adversely influence the modulation of protein kinase activity.[149] This mutation has provided an S49 cell line with two distinct and functional $R^I$ alleles, and has been of particular value during analyses of forward and back mutational events affecting protein kinase activity.[147,149]

The Kin mutants of S49 cells have been used to demonstrate the importance of the cAMP-dependent protein kinase in the cAMP-mediated inhibition of growth,[131,138] inhibition of ornithine and S-adenosylmethionine decarboxylase activities[132] and induction of cAMP phosphodiesterase activity.[133,138,149] Kin⁻ mutants progress through the cell cycle with the same kinetics as parental S49 cells, indicating that cAMP's action is not an obligatory regulator of cell proliferation.[131] The various Kin mutants also have been used to identify which protein phosphorylation reactions are under the control of the cAMP-dependent protein kinase.[66,153,154] Whereas all cAMP-induced phosphorylation reactions required an intact protein kinase,[66] TPA-induced phosphorylations were divided into several distinct groups:[153,154] those that were cAMP-independent; those that were cAMP-dependent and secondary to an increase in adenylate cyclase activity; those that were inhibited by cAMP-dependent protein kinase; and those that required both TPA and an active cAMP-dependent protein kinase.

The detailed analysis of Kin mutations in S49 cells has identified hotspots for mutations in the $R^I$ gene, determined how these mutations influence the metabolism of $R^I$ and identified a putative trans-acting regulatory element required for the expression of C. In addition, these studies have provided the conceptual and experimental framework for analyses of Kin mutations in many other cell types. With the availability of expression vectors bearing cDNA clones of the mutant $R^I$ gene,[145] it will be possible to transfer Ka mutations to other systems where the roles of cAMP and the protein kinase are less well defined.

## C. Adenylate Cyclase Mutants

Guided by the successful isolation of cAMP-resistant, protein kinase defective mutants,[2] Tomkins, Gilman and their co-workers isolated a second group of mutants that were defective in the adenylate cyclase system. Since this work has been reviewed extensively elsewhere,[155-157] it will be treated here briefly. S49 cells accumulate cAMP when treated with cholera toxin, prostaglandin $E_1$, forskolin, or β-adrenergic agonists such as isoproterenol.[106,158] In addition, adenylate cyclase activity in S49 membranes is stimulated by sodium fluoride, and GMPP(NH)P (guanylyl-5'-imidodiphosphate).[159] Treatment of S49 cells with β-adrenergic agonists or with cholera toxin increased the endogenous levels of cAMP sufficiently to cause cytolysis in responsive S49 cells and thus permitted the isolation of resistant mutants. The isolation of resistant mutants was less efficient when using β-adrenergic agonists as selective agents, possibly because S49 cells become refractory to the β-adrenergic agonists during selection.[158,160,161] Adenylate cyclase-defective mutants arose spontaneously and with a rather high frequency $(1 \times 10^{-5}$ per cell per generation).[160] In three of the mutants recoverd from these selections—Cyc⁻, Unc, and H21a—[158-160] the defects were traced to recessive mutations affecting the α subunit of Gs. The Cyc⁻ mutant had an adenylate cyclase which was insensitive to β-adrenergic agonists, prostaglandin $E_1$, cholera toxin, GMPP(NH)P, or sodium fluroide;[158] however, the catalytic subunit of adenylate cyclase was present in these mutants and could be stimulated by manganese ions[162] or by the diterpene, forskolin.[106] The Cyc⁻ mutation resulted from defective synthesis of the α subunits of Gs and was correlated with virtually undetectable levels of α subunit mRNA.[163] Addition of α subunit to membranes from the Cyc⁻ mutants repaired the defective adenylate cyclase, and restored the enzyme's ability to respond to catecholamines, cholera toxin, sodium fluoride, and guanyl nucleotides.[17] In the mutants Unc and H21a, the α subunits of Gs were present at the same level as in wild-type S49 cells,[160,164] but were unable to complement the defective adenylate cyclase of Cyc⁻ mutants in cell fusion experiments[165] or in biochemical reconstitution studies.[155,160] Furthermore, in the Unc mutant, the α subunit was structurally altered and exhibited charge-modified forms on isoelectric focusing gels.[164] The α subunit of the Unc mutant was specifically uncoupled from cell surface receptors such that adenylate cyclase activity in this mutant was unresponsive to β adrenergic agonists and prostaglandin $E_1$. In the Unc mutant, however, adenylate cyclase activity was responsive to cholera toxin, sodium fluoride, and GMPP(NH)P.[159] The α subunit of the H21a mutant was able to interact with the β adrenergic receptor, but was unable to interact with the catalytic subunit of adenylate cyclase so that the enzyme responded poorly to the various agonists.[160]

The Cyc⁻ mutant has contributed significantly to our understanding of the adenylate cyclase system and the mechanism of its regulation. The successful reconstitution of adenylate cyclase activity in this mutant using extracts from responsive cells[166] eventually led to the purification and characterization of Gs.[167] In addition, the responsiveness of the Cyc⁻ mutant to forskolin helped determine the relative importance of Gs and the catalytic subunit of adenylate cyclase in the diterpene's actions. Most recently, Cyc⁻ has been used to identify cDNA clones encoding the α Gs subunit.[163] Ultimately these cDNA clones will help map the subunits of Gs to specific chromosomes, define the molecular defects responsible for the Cyc⁻, Unc, and H21a phenotypes, and identify the domains on the α Gs polypeptide which interact with hormone receptors and with the catalytic subunit of adenylate cyclase.

## D. Other S49 Mutants

Other mutants isolated from S49 cells include mutants deficient in β-adrenergic receptors,[161] mutants which secrete cAMP at an enhanced rate[168] and mutants with elevated cyclic nucleotide phosphodiesterase activity.[160] The phosphodiesterase mutant, K30a, was isolated following the selective growth of S49 cells in the presence of cholera toxin.[160] In K30a cells, adenylate cyclase and cAMP-dependent protein kinase activities appeared normal; cAMP phosphodiesterase activity was increased five to 10-fold. The cyclic nucleotide phosphodiesterase from the K30a mutant was markedly different from the predominant enzyme found in parental S49 cells.[169] The enzyme from the K30a mutant was larger, exhibited a higher affinity for cAMP, and had a different substrate specificity. Whereas the phosphodiesterase from the parent hydrolyzed only cAMP, the enzyme from the mutant hydrolyzed both cAMP and cGMP with high affinity. The K30 phosphodiesterase may represent a mutated form of the wild-type enzyme, or it may represent an amplification of one of the forms of phosphodiesterase normally found in S49 cells in low abundance.

## IV. MUTANTS OF THE CHINESE HAMSTER OVARY CELL LINE (CHO)

### A. General Properties of CHO Cells

The origin, properties, and much of the molecular genetics of CHO cells have been reviewed recently.[170] Briefly, fibroblasts from a CHO were introduced into culture and eventually underwent a transformation event, giving rise to a permanent cell line capable of anchorage independent growth and tumor formation in nude mice and in the hamster cheek pouch.[171] The cell line currently used is aneuploid with a modal chromosome number of 21, a plating efficiency approaching 100%, an average doubling time of approximately 12 hr and a high degree of functional hemizygosity.[171,172] These characteristics have made the CHO line a popular choice for genetic analysis of somatic cells.[170] A large number of auxotrophic and drug-resistant mutants have been isolated from CHO cells and characterized, and several of the affected genes have been assigned to specific CHO chromosomes.[173]

cAMP and its analogs bring about a number of morphological, enzymatic, and growth-related changes in CHO cells. Upon treatment with cAMP analogs, CHO cells change from compact, randomly growing, triangular cells into ordered, well-stretched, fibroblast-like elements which display contact inhibition.[174] Puck[171,174] has suggested that these effects of cAMP on growth and morphology essentially serve to reverse the transformed phenotype and may involve actions of cAMP on the cells' microtubular network. Consistent with this view, cAMP analogs effectively inhibit the growth of CHO cells in semisolid media such as soft agar, providing the basis for the isolation of cAMP-resistant mutants.[175] Other effects of cAMP in CHO cells include inhibition of glucose and amino acid transport[176] and stimulation of gap junction formation[177] and of ornithine decarboxylase,[178] transglutaminase,[179] cAMP-dependent protein kinase,[180] and cAMP phosphodiesterase[175] activities. Cholera toxin stimulates adenylate cyclase activity in these cells, causing a sustained accumulation of cAMP and effectively mimics the effects of the cAMP analogs on morphology and growth inhibition.[180,181] Prostaglandin $E_1$, human chorionic gonadotropin, and follicle stimulating hormone also stimulate adenylate cyclase activity; however, the hormones only transiently increase cAMP levels in CHO cells.[180,182]

### B. Cyclic AMP-Resistant Mutants

Gottesman and co-workers[181] isolated a variety of cAMP-resistant mutants from mutagenized CHO cells on the basis of their resistance to growth inhibition by cholera toxin or 8BrcAMP. Some mutants apparently were isolated in an enrichment process from suspension cultures, while others were selected in a single step by cloning in soft agar. cAMP-resistant mutants were recovered from CHO cells with a frequency of approximately 3 per $10^5$ cells, and the majority exhibited defective cAMP-dependent protein kinase activities. Most of the mutants behaved dominantly in cell fusion studies with the cAMP-sensitive parent; however, three mutants behaved recessively and divided into two different complementation groups.[175] Two dominant cyclic nucleotide-resistant mutants, 10215 and 10248, were characterized in greatest detail. They were isolated following mutagenesis by selective growth from suspensions in the presence of cholera toxin. In some respects, the two mutants, 10215 and 10248 were phenotypically similar. Whereas extracts from parental CHO cells contained equal amounts of type 1 and type 2 cAMP-dependent protein kinase activity, extracts from the two mutants exhibited only a type 1 protein kinase with reduced affinity for activation by cAMP. Neither mutant exhibited much type 2 protein kinase activity though both contained appreciable amounts of $R^{II}$ subunit.[5,183] The mutation in clone 10215 was associated with an altered activity of the C subunit.[5] The C subunit from mutant 10215 had a higher Km for substrate ATP and a reduced capacity to phosphorylate acidic acceptor proteins. Gottesman and co-workers[5] speculated that the mutation in clone 10215 resulted from a defect in the C subunit which selectively increased its affinity for $R^I$; as a result, the C subunit could not form complexes with $R^{II}$ and higher concentrations of cAMP were required to dissociate and activate the type 1 enzyme. The cAMP-resistant phenotype of clone 10248 was ascribed to a defect in $R^I$.[183] In this mutant, $R^I$ subunits existed in holoenzyme complexes with C and in a "free" pool. The $R^I$ subunits recovered from the mutant holoenzyme complex had a markedly reduced affinity for cAMP (approx. 200-fold), whereas the $R^I$ subunits recovered from the "free" pool bound cAMP normally; $R^{II}$ and C subunits exhibited normal kinetic properties. Gottesman and co-workers[183] suggested that clone 10248 contained both a mutated and a wild-type form of $R^I$. The mutated $R^I$ subunit may have bound the C subunit with high affinity and reduced the amount of C subunit available for complex formation with normal $R^I$ and $R^{II}$ subunits. In protein kinase mutants from Y1 adrenal and S49 lymphoma cells, it was possible to assign the mutation to a specific enzyme subunit by reconstituting mutant holoenzymes using isolated R and C subunits,[50,144] and by demonstrating charge-modifications in the affected protein on isoelectric focusing gels.[50,142] Similar experiments may have strengthened the assignment of mutations to R and C in the CHO mutants 10248 and 10215. Unfortunately, charge modifications in the affected subunits were not detected, and the C subunit was unstable in extracts of CHO cells,[5] so that reconstitution experiments were not possible. Genomic DNA isolated from the mutant clones 10215 and 10248 was able to transform wild-type CHO cells to a cAMP-resistant phenotype.[184,185] In each case the protein kinase activities in the transformants resembled the protein kinase activities of the respective mutants. These gene transfer experiments helped establish the genetic nature of the cAMP-resistant phenotype in CHO mutants, and the linkage of cAMP resistance to altered cAMP-dependent protein kinase activity. Transformants generated using genomic DNA from the putative $R^I$ mutant, 10248, acquired an increased number of $R^I$ genes together with the cAMP-resistant phenotype, supporting the view that the mutation in 10248 was linked to the $R^I$ gene.[184]

In all cases examined to date, the CHO mutants defective in cAMP-dependent protein kinase activity, were resistant to the various cellular effects of cAMP. Mutant clones did not undergo the characteristic morphological changes[186] or the increases in electrically cou-pled gap junctions[177] induced by the cyclic nucleotide, nor did they increase the activities of ornithine decarboxylase,[178] transglutaminase,[179] or cAMP phosphodiesterase[175] in response to agonists of the cAMP pathway. The inhibition of glucose and amino acid transport normally seen in parental CHO cells in response to cAMP was not seen in the protein kinase-defective clones.[176] These results argue for an obligatory role of the cAMP-dependent protein kinase in these actions of cAMP on CHO cells.

The CHO mutants also have been effective in identifying control mechanisms which were independent of cAMP. Ornithine decarboxylase activity in wild-type CHO cells was increased by TPA as well as by cAMP analogs; however, in cAMP-resistant CHO mutants, the induction of ornithine decarboxylase activity by TPA was only partially impaired.[178] These observations suggested that a major portion of TPA's action was independent of the cAMP-dependent pathway in CHO cells. Transglutaminase activity also was regulated, in part, by a cAMP-independent process. The growth of wild-type CHO cells to saturation density increased the activity of the enzyme transglutaminase.[179] Under these conditions, cAMP levels increased as well. Therefore, the cAMP-resistant CHO mutants were analyzed to determine if cAMP played a role in the density-dependent increase in transglutaminase activity. The density-dependent increase in transglutaminase activity was unimpaired in protein kinase defective CHO mutants, suggesting that cAMP was not a component of this regulatory process.[179] Gottesman and co-workers also have used the cAMP-resistant CHO mutants to demonstrate a cAMP-independent pathway for sodium butyrate's actions on growth and morphology.[181,186] In wild-type CHO cells, dibutyryl cAMP behaved like other cAMP analogs, inhibiting growth and changing cell shape.[187] Sodium butyrate, a degradation product of dibutyryl cAMP, increased cAMP levels slightly, and brought about cAMP-like changes in growth and morphology.[187] Interestingly, the CHO mutants described above, were responsive to the growth inhibitory and morphological effects of sodium butyrate and dibutyryl cAMP.[181,186] These results suggested that dibutyryl cAMP affected growth and morphology by a mechanism not involving cAMP and cautioned against the use of dibutyryl derivatives in the selection of cAMP-resistant mutants.[186]

## V. OTHER MUTANT CELL LINES

Clones harboring defects in cAMP-dependent pathways have been isolated from several other differentiated cell lines. In most instances, the defects have been less well defined in these clones than in the mutants described above, and the involvement of a single genetic locus has not been established. Because of these uncertainties, the defective clones often have been identified as variants of the cAMP-dependent pathway rather than mutants. Nevertheless, the lesions in these variants have been useful in evaluating the role of cAMP in the regulation of various cellular processes. Variants in this group include protein kinase-defective mouse neuroblastoma cells,[3] adenylate cyclase- and protein kinase-defective mouse macrophage-like tumor cells,[4] cAMP-resistant and cAMP-dependent mouse melanoma cells,[188,189] protein kinase- and phosphodiesterase-defective canine kidney cells,[7,190] protein kinase-defective porcine kidney cells,[8] protein kinase-defective rat pheochromocytoma cells,[9] and adenylate cyclase-defective rat pituitary tumor cells.[6] Only the properties of the variant mouse macrophage and canine kidney cells are summarized here.

### A. Variants of the Macrophage Cell Line, J774.2

J774.2 cells were established in culture from a murine reticulum cell sarcoma by Ralph and Nakoinz.[191] The cell line exhibited several macrophage-like characteristics in vitro including antibody-dependent phagocytosis, lysozyme synthesis and secretion, and expression of Fc receptors.[191,192] Muschel et al.,[192] isolated variants from J774.2 on the basis of their inability to phagocytize antibody-coated erythrocytes containing the toxic drug, tubercidin, and demonstrated that 8BrcAMP was able to restore phagocytic activity in the defective variants. They also showed that 8BrcAMP was capable of stimulating antibody-mediated phagocytosis in parental J774.2 cells, provided that phagocytosis first was restricted by limiting the amount of antibody in the reaction or by treating the cells with insulin.[193] Taken together these results suggested that cAMP was a potential regulator of macrophage-like functions in the cell line. In order to establish the extent of involvement of the cAMP-dependent pathway in macrophage function, additional variants were isolated from J774.2 cells by selective growth in the presence of cholera toxin or 8BrcAMP.[194] Variants resistant to the growth inhibitory effects of cholera toxin were isolated from J774.2 cells in a single step without mutagenesis and at a high frequency (approximately $3 \times 10^{-4}$). In these variants, adenylate cyclase activity became markedly insensitive to a number of effector molecules including cholera toxin, $\beta$ adrenergic agonists, prostaglandin $E_1$, and sodium fluoride. The isolation of variants resistant to 8BrcAMP was more difficult and required mutagenesis and a multi-step selection process. In these variants, the type 2 cAMP-dependent protein kinase isozyme was lost and the type 1 enzyme exhibited a lower affinity for activation by cAMP. As seen in studies of CHO cells (*vide supra*) this cAMP-resistant phenotype could be associated with lesions affecting either $R^I$ or C. In both macrophage variants, unrestricted antibody-mediated phagocytosis was not markedly diminished. In the protein kinase variants, antibody-restricted phagocytosis was unresponsive to 8BrcAMP.[194] These results suggested that cAMP was not an obligatory regulator of the unrestricted phagocytic process, or, alternatively, only small levels of cAMP and cAMP-dependent protein kinase were required for the antibody-mediated phagocytic process.[194] The adenylate cyclase and protein kinase variants of J774.2 also were used to evaluate the roles of cAMP and the protein kinase in some of interferon's actions on these cells.[195] In parental J774.2 cells, interferon increased intracellular levels of cAMP, stimulated phagocytosis, inhibited viral replication and inhibited cell growth. In both the adenylate cyclase and protein kinase defective variants, the phagocytic and growth inhibitory responses to interferon were impaired, while the antiviral action of interferon was unaffected. These observations suggested that the antiviral actions of interferon involved a cAMP-independent process whereas the effects on cell growth and phagocytosis were cAMP-dependent. In confirmation of these observations, Schenck et al.[195] were able to reisolate the adenylate cyclase variant from parental J774.2 cells by selective growth in the presence of interferon. The adenylate cyclase and protein kinase variants also have been used to implicate cAMP and cAMP-dependent protein kinase in the regulation of lipoprotein lipase activity[196] and transcobalamin II production[197] in the macrophage-like cell line.

## B. Variants of the Canine Kidney Cell Line, MDCK

The MDCK cell line was established from the kidney of a female cockerspaniel, is pseudodiploid and retains some features characteristic of normal kidney epithelia. One of the morphological features of MDCK cells is their ability to form hemicysts or "domes" in monolayer culture, indicative of their capacity for vectorial salt and water transport.[198] In this cell line, prostaglandin $E_1$ is a potent stimulator of cell proliferation, and is part of a hormonal supplement which can be used in place of serum in growth medium.[199] In addition to its growth promoting activity, prostaglandin $E_1$ also dramatically stimulates dome formation,[199] and increases salt transport.[200] The growth requirement for prostaglandin $E_1$ can be fulfilled by other agents which increase the intracellular concentration of cAMP in these cells, including glucagon, dibutyryl cAMP, and 3-isobutyl-1-methylxanthine. Taub et al.[190,201] isolated MDCK variants which continued to grow in the absence of prostaglandin $E_1$. These variants had much less cAMP phosphodiesterase activity than did parental MDCK cells, and consequently, had higher basal levels of cAMP. Presumably, the higher basal levels of cAMP were sufficient to support growth in the absence of prostaglandin $E_1$. In these phosphodiesterase-deficient variants, prostaglandin $E_1$ and dibutyryl cAMP inhibited growth and stimulated dome formation, suggesting that growth control by cAMP-dependent mechanisms was biphasic—low levels of the cyclic nucleotide promoted growth whereas pharmacological levels of cAMP were inhibitory to growth. In contrast, dome formation was stimulated over a wider range of cyclic nucleotide concentrations. Surprisingly, glucagon stimulated the growth of these phosphodiesterase-deficient variants,[190] leading to the hypothesis that glucagon acted via two distinct mechanisms, one of which was independent of the cyclic nucleotide. Variants with defective cAMP-dependent protein kinase activity also were isolated from MDCK cells following their selective growth in the presence of high concentrations of dibutyryl cAMP.[200] In the cyclic nucleotide-resistant variants, protein kinase activity measured with maximally effective concentrations of cAMP was reduced approximately 50%; the affinity of the enzyme for cAMP was unaffected. The cyclic nucleotide-resistant variants showed normal growth responses to prostaglandin $E_1$; however, their capacity for prostaglandin-stimulated dome formation and salt transport were impaired. These observations implicated cAMP and cAMP-dependent protein kinase in dome formation and salt transport. Furthermore, they suggested that residual protein kinase activity was sufficient to support the growth promoting activity of prostaglandin $E_1$.

## VI. SUMMARY AND PROSPECTS

Several significant and fundamental observations have emerged from studies of cell lines harboring defects in the pathways of cAMP metabolism and action. These studies have established obligatory roles for cAMP and the cAMP-dependent protein kinase in the actions of a variety of effector molecules on a large number of end-responses. In a few instances cAMP-dependent mechanisms have been exluded. These genetic studies have led to the identification, isolation and characterization of a family of guanyl nucleotide-binding regulatory proteins involved in signal transduction processes, and they have provided new information on the regulation, interaction, and turnover of subunits of the cAMP-dependent protein kinase. One can anticipate that future research directions will include the isolation of the specific genes affected by mutation for analyses of structure function relationships, and for transfer to other differentiated systems where the roles of cAMP and the cAMP-dependent protein kinase are poorly understood. As noted above, investigations already have been initiated along these lines.[114,115,145,184,185]

Other important issues also may be amendable to resolution by genetic analyses. The adenylate cyclase system may be far more complex than currently appreciated. Although four components of the adenylate cyclase system have been identified—hormone/drug receptor, two guanyl nucleotide-binding regulatory proteins, and catalytic subunit—other proteins including ADP-ribosylation factors,[202] and receptor kinases[203] have been implicated in the regulation of this enzyme. The relative importance and specific functions of the various cAMP phosphodiesterase isozymes remains to be solved. Unique roles for the type 1 and type 2 cAMP-dependent protein kinase isozymes have yet to be established, and distinct functions for the regulatory subunits of protein kinase apart from regulating the activity of the catalytic subunit have been proposed but not proven. The important substrates of the cAMP-dependent protein kinases in most instances have not been identified; however, mutations in the pathways of cAMP action beyond the protein kinase likely will be required for these studies. The traditional somatic cell genetic approach involving mutagenesis, selection, and characterization of mutant clones likely will have to be supplemented with newer techniques of gene isolation, in vitro mutagenesis, and DNA-mediated gene transfer to resolve these outstanding issues.

## ACKNOWLEDGMENTS

The author thanks Drs. I. Abraham, B. R. Bloom, M. M. Gottesman, G. S. McKnight, R. A. Steinberg, and M. Taub for reprints and preprints of their recent work. Unpublished work and work in press from this laboratory were supported by grants from the Medical Research Council of Canada and the National Cancer Institute of Canada.

## REFERENCES

1. **Schimmer, B. P.,** Phenotypically variant adrenal tumor cell cultures with biochemical lesions in the ACTH-stimulated steroidogenic pathway, *J. Cell. Physiol.,* 74, 115, 1969.
2. **Daniel, V., Litwack, G., and Tomkins, G. M.,** Induction of cytolysis of cultured lymphoma cells by adenosine 3′:5′-cyclic monophosphate and the isolation of resistant variants, *Proc. Natl. Acad. Sci., U.S.A.,* 70, 76, 1973.
3. **Simantov, R. and Sachs, L.,** Temperature sensitivity of cyclic adenosine 3′:5′-monophosphate-binding proteins and the regulation of growth and differentiation in neuroblastoma cells, *J. Biol. Chem.,* 250, 3236, 1975.
4. **Muschel, R. J., Rosen, N., and Bloom, B. R.,** Isolation of variants in phagocytosis of a macrophage-like continuous cell line, *J. Expt. Med.,* 145, 175, 1977.
5. **Evain, D., Gottesman, M., Pastan, I., and Anderson, W. B.,** A mutation affecting the catalytic subunit of cyclic AMP-dependent protein kinase in CHO cells, *J. Biol. Chem.,* 254, 6931, 1979.
6. **Martin, T. F. J. and Ronning, S. A.,** Multiple mechanisms of growth inhibition by cyclic AMP derivatives in rat GH₁ pituitary cells: Isolation of an adenylate cyclase-deficient variant, *J. Cell. Physiol.,* 190, 289, 1981.

7. **Devis, P. E., Grohol, S. H., and Taub, M.,** Dibutyryl cyclic AMP resistant MDCK cells in serum free medium have reduced cyclic AMP dependent protein kinase activity and a dimished effect of $PGE_1$ on differentiated function, *J. Cell. Physiol.*, 125, 23, 1985.

8. **Jans, D. A. and Hemmings, B. A.,** LLC-PK$_1$ cell mutants in cAMP metabolism respond normally to phorbol esters, *FEBS Lett.*, 205, 127, 1986.

9. **Van Buskirk, R., Corcoran, T., and Wagner, J. A.,** Clonal variants of PC12 pheochromocytoma cells with defects in cAMP-dependent protein kinases induce ornithine decarboxylase in response to nerve growth factor but not to adenosine agonists, *Mol. Cell. Biol.*, 5, 1984, 1985.

10. **Sutherland, E. W. and Robinson, G. A.,** The role of cyclic AMP in responses to catecholamines and other hormones, *Pharmacol. Rev.*, 18, 145, 1966.

11. **Robison, G. A., Butcher, R. W., and Sutherland, E. W.,** *Cyclic AMP,* Academic Press, New York, 1971.

12. **Kuo, J. F. and Greengard, P.,** An adenosine 3′,5′-monophosphate-dependent protein kinase from *Escherichia coli, J. Biol. Chem.*, 244, 3417, 1969.

13. **Schimmer, B. P.,** Cyclic nucleotides in hormonal regulation of adrenocortical function, *Adv. Cyclic Nucleotide Res.*, 13, 181, 1980.

14. **Exton, J. H., Cherrington, A. D., Blackmore, P. F., Dehaye, J. -P., Stickland, W. G., Jordan, J. E., and Chrisman, T. D.,** Hormonal regulation of liver glycogen metabolism, in *Protein Phosphorylation: Cold Spring Harbor Conferences On Cell Proliferation,* Vol. 8, Book A, Rosen, O. M., and Krebs, E. G., Eds., Cold Spring Harbor Laboratory, New York, 1981, 513.

15. **Wakelam, M. J. O., Murphy, G. J., Hruby, V. J., and Houslay, M. D.,** Activation of two signal transduction systems in hepatocytes by glucagon, *Nature,* 323, 68, 1986.

16. **Daly, J. W.,** Forskolin, adenylate cyclase and cell physiology: an overview, *Adv. Cyclic Nucleotide Protein Phosphorylation Res.*, 17, 81, 1984.

17. **Smigel, M., Kitada, T., Northup, J. K., Bokoch, G. M., Ui, M., and Gilman, A. G.,** Mechanisms of guanine nucleotide-mediated regulation of adenylate cyclase activity, *Adv. Cyclic Nucleotide Protein Phosphorylation Res.*, 17, 1, 1984.

18. **Strada, S. J. and Thompson, W. J.,** Multiple forms of cyclic nucleotide phosphodiesterases: Anomalies or biologic regulators?, *Adv. Cyclic Nucleotide Res.*, 9, 265, 1978.

19. **Weiss, B. and Levin, R. M.,** Mechanism for selectively inhibiting the activation of cyclic nucleotide phosphodiesterase and adenylate cyclase by antipsychotic agents, *Adv. Cyclic Nucleotide Res.*, 9, 285, 1978.

20. **Miller, J. P., Sigman, C. C., Johnson, H. L., Novinson, T., Springer, R. H., Senga, K., O'Brien, D. E., and Robins, R. K.,** Inhibition of cyclic AMP phosphodiesterases by cyclic nucleotide analogs and nitrogen heterocycles, *Adv. Cyclic Nucleotide Protein Phosphorylation Res.*, 16, 277, 1984.

21. **Thompson, W. J., Pratt, M. L., and Strada, S. J.,** Biochemical properties of high-affinity cyclic AMP phosphodiesterases, *Adv. Cyclic Nucleotide Protein Phosphorylation Res.*, 17, 137, 1984.

22. **Barber, R. and Butcher, R. W.,** The egress of cyclic AMP from metazoan cells, *Adv. Cyclic Nucleotide Res.*, 13, 119, 1983.

23. **Krebs, E. G.,** The phosphorylation of proteins: a major mechanism for biological regulation, *Biochem. Soc. Trans.*, 13, 813, 1985.

24. **Pastan, I. and Perlman, R. L.,** Regulation of gene transcription in *Escherichia coli* by cyclic AMP, *Adv. Cyclic Nucleotide Res.*, 1, 11, 1972.

25. **Weber, I. T., Takio, K., Titani, K., and Steitz, T. A.,** The cAMP-binding domains of the regulatory subunit of cAMP-dependent protein kinase and the catabolite gene activation protein and homologs, *Proc. Natl. Acad. Sci. U.S.A.*, 79, 7679, 1982.

26. **Constantinou, A. I., Squinto, S. P., and Jungmann, R. A.,** The phosphoform of the regulatory subunit RII of cyclic AMP-dependent protein kinase possesses intrinsic topoisomerase activity, *Cell,* 42, 429, 1985.

26a. **Shabb, J. B. and Granner, D. K.,** Separation of topoisomerase 1 activity from the regulatory subunit of type II cyclic adenosine monophosphate dependent protein kinase, *Mol. Endocrinol.*, 2, 324, 1988.

27. **Nagamine, Y. and Reich, E.,** Gene expression and cyclic AMP, *Proc. Natl. Acad. Sci. U.S.A.*, 82, 4606, 1985.

28. **Takai, Y., Kikkawa, U., Kaibuchi, K., and Nishizuka, Y.,** Membrane phospholipid metabolism and signal transduction for protein phosphorylation, *Adv. Cyclic Nucleotide Protein Phosphorylation Res.*, 18, 119, 1984.

29. **Flockhart, D. A. and Corbin, J. D.,** Regulatory mechanisms in the control of protein kinases, *Crit. Rev. Biochem.*, 12, 133, 1982.

30. **Corbin, J. D., Keely, S. L., and Park, C. R.,** The distribution and dissociation of cAMP-dependent protein kinase in adipose, cardiac and other tissues, *J. Biol. Chem.*, 250, 218, 1975.

31. **Corbin, J. D. and Keely, S. L.,** Characterization and regulation of heart adenosine 3′:5′-monophosphate-dependent protein kinase isozymes, *J. Biol. Chem.*, 252, 910, 1977.

32. **Walter, U., Uno, I., Liu, A. Y.-C., and Greengard, P.,** Study of autophosphorylation of isoenzymes of cyclic AMP-dependent protein kinases, *J. Biol. Chem.,* 252, 6588, 1977.

33. **Hofmann, F., Beavo, J. A., Bechtel, P. J., and Krebs, E. G.,** Comparison of cAMP-dependent protein kinase from rabbit skeletal and bovine heart muscle, *J. Biol. Chem.,* 250, 7795, 1975.

34. **Rosen, O. M., Rangel-Aldao, R., and Erlichman, J.,** Soluble cyclic AMP-dependent protein kinases: Review of the enzyme isolated from bovine cardiac muscle, *Curr. Topics Cell. Reg.,* 12, 39, 1977.

35. **Zoller, M. J., Kerlavage, A. R., and Taylor, S. S.,** Structural comparisons of cAMP-dependent protein kinases I and II from porcine skeletal muscle, *J. Biol. Chem.,* 254, 2408, 1979.

36. **Rosen, O. M., Erlichman, J., and Rubin, C. S.,** Molecular structure and characterization of bovine heart protein kinase, *Adv. Cyclic Nucleotide Res.,* 5, 253, 1975.

37. **Taylor, S. S., Lee, C.-Y., Swain, L., and Stafford, P. H.,** Cyclic AMP-dependent protein kinase: purification of the holoenzyme by affinity chromatography, *Anal. Biochem.,* 76, 45, 1976.

38. **Miyamoto, E., Petzold, G. L., Kuo, J. F., and Greengard, P.,** Dissociation and activation of adenosine 3′,5′-monophosphate-dependent protein kinases by cyclic nucleotides and by substrate proteins, *J. Biol. Chem.,* 248, 179, 1973.

39. **Erlichman, J., Sarkar, D., Fleischer, N., and Rubin, C. S.,** Identification of two subclasses of type II cAMP-dependent protein kinases, *J. Biol. Chem.,* 255, 8179, 1980.

40. **Beebe, S. J. and Corbin, J. D.,** Rat adipose tissue cAMP-dependent protein kinase: a unique form of type II, *Mol. Cell. Endocrinol.,* 36, 67, 1984.

41. **Jahnsen, T., Lohmann, S. M., Walter, U., Hedin, L., and Richards, J. S.,** Purification and characterization of hormone-regulated isoforms of the regulatory subunit of type II cAMP-dependent protein kinase from rat ovaries, *J. Biol. Chem.,* 260, 15980, 1985.

42. **Corbin, J. D., Sugden, P. H., Lincoln, T. M., and Keely, S. L.,** Compartmentalization of adenosine 3′:5′-monophosphate and adenosine 3′:5′-monophosphate-dependent protein kinase in heart tissue, *J. Biol. Chem.,* 252, 3854, 1977.

43. **Dreyfuss, G., Schwartz, K. J., and Blout, E. R.,** Compartmentalization of cyclic AMP-dependent protein kinases in human erythrocytes, *Proc. Natl. Acad. Sci., U.S.A.,* 75, 5926, 1978.

44. **Rannels, S. R. and Corbin, J. D.,** Studies of functional domains of the regulatory subunit from cAMP-dependent protein kinase isozyme I, *J. Cyclic Nucleotide Res.,* 6, 201, 1980.

45. **Taylor, S. S., Kerlavage, A. R., Zoller, M. J., Nelson, N. C., and Potter, R. L.,** Nucleotide-binding sites and structural domains of cAMP-dependent protein kinases, in, *Protein Phosphorylation: Cold Spring Harbor Conferences on Cell Proliferation,* Vol. 8, Book A, Rosen, O. M., and Krebs, E. G., Eds., Cold Spring Harbor Laboratory, New York, 1981, 3.

46. **Hashimoto, E., Takio, K., and Krebs, E. G.,** Studies on the site in the regulatory subunit of type I cAMP-dependent protein kinase phosphorylated by cGMP-dependent protein kinase, *J. Biol. Chem.,* 256, 5604, 1981.

47. **Corbin, J. D., Rannels, S. R., Flockhart, D. A., Robinson, A. M., and Atkins, P. D.,** Cyclic nucleotide-binding sites of protein kinases, in, *Protein Phosphorylation: Cold Spring Harbor Conferences On Cell Proliferation,* Vol. 8, Book A, Rosen, O. M., and Krebs, E. G., Eds., Cold Spring Harbor Laboratory, New York, 1981, 45.

48. **Fleischer, N., Rosen, O. M., and Reichlin, M.,** Radioimmunoassay of bovine heart protein kinase, *Proc. Natl. Acad. Sci., U.S.A.,* 73, 54, 1976.

49. **Schimmer, B. P., Rae, P. A., Gutmann, N. S., Watt, V. M., and Tsao, J.,** Genetic dissection of ACTH action in adrenal tumor cells, in, *Hormones and Cell Culture: Cold Spring Harbor Conferences On Cell Proliferation,* Vol. 6, Book A, Sato, G. H., and Ross, R., Eds., Cold Spring Harbor Laboratory, New York, 1979, 281.

50. **Doherty, P. J., Tsao, J., Schimmer, B. P., Mumby, M. C., and Beavo, J. A.,** Alteration of the regulatory subunit of type 1 cAMP-dependent protein kinase in mutant Y1 adrenal cells resistant to 8-bromoadenosine 3′:5′-monophosphate, *J. Biol. Chem.,* 257, 5877, 1982.

51. **Rangel-Aldao, R. and Rosen, O. M.,** Dissociation and reassociation of the phosphorylated and non-phosphorylated forms of adenosine 3′:5′-monophosphate-dependent protein kinase from bovine cardiac muscle, *J. Biol. Chem.,* 251, 3375, 1976.

52. **Titani, K., Sasagswa, T., Ericsson, L. H., Kumar, S., Smith, S. B., Krebs, E. G., and Walsh, K. A.,** Amino acid sequence of the regulatory subunit of bovine type I adenosine cyclic 3′,5′-phosphate dependent protein kinase, *Biochemistry,* 23, 4193, 1984.

53. **Takio, K., Smith, S. B., Krebs, E. G., Walsh, K. A., and Titani, K.,** Primary structure of the regulatory subunit of type II cAMP-dependent protein kinase from bovine cardiac muscle, *Proc. Natl. Acad. Sci. U.S.A.,* 79, 2544, 1982.

54. **Shoji, S., Parmelee, D. C., Wade, R. D., Kumar, S., Ericsson, L. H., Walsh, K. A., Neurath, H., Long, G. L., Demaille, J. G., Fischer, E. H., and Titani, K.,** Complete amino acid sequence of the catalytic subunit of bovine cardiac muscle cycle AMP-dependent protein kinase, *Proc. Natl. Acad. Sci., U.S.A.,* 78, 848, 1981.

55. **Lee, D. C., Carmichael, D. F., Krebs, E. G., and McKnight, G. S.,** Isolation of a cDNA clone for the type I regulatory subunit of bovine cAMP-dependent protein kinase, *Proc. Natl. Acad. Sci. U.S.A.,* 80, 3608, 1983.

56. **Jahnsen, T., Hedin, L., Kidd, V. J., Beattie, W. G., Lohmann, S. M., Walter, U., Durica, J., Schulz, T. Z., Schiltz, E., Browner, M., Lawrence, C. B., Goldman, D., Ratoosh, S. L., and Richards, J. S.,** Molecular cloning, cDNA structure, and regulation of the regulatory subunit of type II cAMP-dependent protein kinase from rat ovarian granulosa cells, *J. Biol. Chem.,* 261, 12352, 1986.

57. **Uhler, M. D., Carmichael, D. F., Lee, D. C., Chrivia, J. C., Krebs, E. G., and McKnight, G. S.,** Isolation of cDNA clones coding for the catalytic subunit of mouse cAMP-dependent protein kinase, *Proc. Natl. Acad. Sci. U.S.A.,* 83, 1300, 1986.

58. **Walsh, D. A., Ashby, C. D., Gonzalez, C., Calkins, D., Fischer, E. H., and Krebs, E. G.,** Purification and characterization of a protein inhibitor of adenosine 3′,5′-monophosphate-dependent protein kinases, *J. Biol. Chem.,* 246, 1977, 1971.

59. **Szmigielski, A., Guidotti, and Costa, E.,** Endogenous protein kinase inhibitors. Purification, characterization, and distribution in different tissues, *J. Biol. Chem.,* 252, 3848, 1977.

60. **Demaille, J. G., Peters, K. A., and Fischer, E. H.,** Isolation and properties of the rabbit skeletal muscle protein inhibitor of adenosine 3′,5′-monophosphate dependent protein kinases, *Biochemistry,* 16, 3080, 1977.

61. **Beavo, J. A., Bechtel, P. J., and Krebs, E. G.,** Mechanisms of control for cAMP-dependent protein kinase from skeletal muscle, *Adv. Cyclic Nucleotide Res.,* 5, 241, 1975.

62. **Walter, U., De Camilli, P., Lohmann, S. M., Miller, P., and Greengard, P.,** Regulation and cellular localization of cAMP-dependent and cGMP-dependent protein kinases, in *Protein Phosphorylation: Cold Spring Harbor Conferences On Cell Proliferation,* Vol. 8, Book A, Rosen, O. M. and Krebs, E. G., Eds., Cold Spring Harbor Laboratory, New York, 1981, 141.

63. **Koide, Y., Beavo, J. A., Kapoor, C. L., Spruill, W. A., Huang, H. -L., Levine, S. N., Ong, S. -L., Bechtel, P. J., Yount, W. J., and Steiner, A. L.,** Hormonal effects on the immunocytochemical location of 3′,5′-cyclic adenosine monophosphate-dependent protein kinase in rat tissues, *Endocrinology,* 109, 2226, 1981.

64. **Feramisco, J. R., Glass, D. B., and Krebs, E. G.,** Optimal spatial requirements for the location of basic residues in peptide substrates for the cyclic AMP-dependent protein kinase, *J. Biol. Chem.,* 255, 4240, 1980.

65. **Garrison, J. C., Borland, M. K., Moylan, R. D., and Ballard, B. J.,** The role of $Ca^{++}$ ion and cyclic-nucleotide-independent protein kinases in the control of hepatic carbohydrate metabolism, in *Protein Phosphorylation: Cold Spring Harbor Conferences On Cell Proliferation,* Vol. 8, Book A, Rosen, O. M. and Krebs, E. G., Eds., Cold Spring Harbor Laboratory, New York, 1981, 529.

66. **Steinberg, R. A.,** Cyclic-AMP-dependent protein phosphorylation in intact cultured cells, in *Protein Phosphorylation: Cold Spring Harbor Conferences On Cell Proliferation,* Vol. 8, Book A, Rosen, O. M. and Krebs, E. G., Eds., Cold Spring Harbor Laboratory, New York, 1981, 179.

67. **Yasumura, Y., Buonassisi, V., and Sato, G.,** Clonal analysis of differentiated function in animal cell cultures. I. Possible correlated maintenance of differentiated function and the diploid karyotype, *Cancer Res.,* 26, 529, 1966.

68. **Schimmer, B. P.,** The adrenocortical tumor cell line, Y1, in *Functionally Differentiated Cell Lines,* Sato, G., Ed., Alan R. Liss, New York, 1981, 61.

69. **Schimmer, B. P., Ueda, K., and Sato, G. H.,** Site of action of adrenocorticotropic hormone (ACTH) in adrenal cell cultures, *Biochem. Biophys. Res. Commun.,* 32, 806, 1968.

70. **Lefkowitz, R. J., Roth, J., Pricer, W., and Pastan, I.,** ACTH receptors in the adrenal: Specific binding of ACTH-[125]I and its relation to adenyl cyclase, *Proc. Natl. Acad. Sci. U.S.A.,* 65, 745, 1970.

71. **Taunton, O. D., Roth, J., and Pastan, I.,** Studies on the adrenocorticotropic hormone-activated adenyl cyclase of a functional adrenal tumor, *J. Biol. Chem.,* 244, 247, 1969.

72. **Londos, C., Salomon, Y., Lin, M. C., Harwood, J. P., Schramm, M., Wolff, J., and Rodbell, M.,** 5′-Guanylylimidodiphosphate, a potent activator of adenylate cyclase systems in eukaryotic cells, *Proc. Natl. Acad. Sci. U.S.A,* 71, 3087, 1974.

73. **Schimmer, B. P. and Zimmerman, A. E.,** Steroidogenesis and extracellular cAMP accumulation in adrenal tumor cell cultures, *Mol. Cell. Endocrinol.,* 4, 263, 1976.

74. **Gutman, N. S., Rae, P. A, and Schimmer, B. P.,** Altered cyclic AMP-dependent protein kinase activity in a mutant adrenocortical tumor cell line, *J. Cell. Physiol.,* 97, 451, 1978.

75. **Pierson, R. W., Jr.,** Metabolism of steroid hormones in adrenal cortex tumor cultures, *Endocrinology,* 81, 693, 1967.

76. **Kowal, J. and Fiedler, R.,** Adrenal cells in tissue culture, I. Assay of steroid products; steroidogenic responses to peptide hormones, *Arch. Biochem. Biophys.,* 128, 406, 1968.

77. **Masui, H. and Garren, L. D.,** Inhibition of replication in functional mouse adrenal tumor cells by adrenocorticotropic hormone mediated by adenosine 3':5'-cyclic monophosphate, *Proc. Natl. Acad. Sci. U.S.A.,* 68, 3206, 1971.

78. **Gill, G. N. and Weidman, E. R.,** Hormonal regulation of initiation of DNA synthesis and of differentiated function in Y-1 adrenal cortical cells, *J. Cell. Physiol.,* 92, 65, 1977.

79. **Weidman, E. R. and Gill, G. N.,** Differential effects of ACTH or 8-Br-cAMP on growth and replication in a functional adrenal tumor cell line, *J. Cell. Physiol.,* 90, 91, 1977.

80. **Kowal, J., Frenkel, R., and Angee, I.,** Adrenal cells in tissue culture. IX: The site of ACTH stimulation of glucose metabolism, *Endocrinology,* 91, 1219, 1972.

81. **Faust, J. R., Goldstein, J. L., and Brown, M. S.,** Receptor-mediated uptake of low density lipoprotein and utilization of its cholesterol for steroid synthesis in cultured mouse adrenal cells, *J. Biol. Chem.,* 252, 4861, 1977.

82. **Roos, B. A.,** ACTH and cAMP stimulation of adrenal ribosomal protein phosphorylation, *Endocrinology,* 93, 1287, 1973.

83. **Stollar, V., Buonassisi, V., and Sato, G.,** Studies on hormone secreting adrenocortical tumor in tissue culture, *Exp. Cell Res.,* 35, 608, 1964.

84. **Kowal, J., Simpson, E. R., and Estabrook, R. W.,** Adrenal cells in tissue culture. V. On the specificity of the stimulation of 11B-hydroxylation by adrenocorticotropin, *J. Biol. Chem.,* 245, 2438, 1970.

85. **Nambi, P., Aiyar, N. V., Roberts, A. N., and Sharma, R. K.,** Relationship of calcium and membrane guanylate cyclase in adrenocorticotropin-induced steroidogenesis, *Endocrinology,* 111, 196, 1982.

86. **Widmaier, E. P. and Hall, P. F.,** Protein kinase C in adrenal cells: Possible role in regulation of steroid synthesis, *Mol. Cell. Endocrinol.,* 43, 181, 1985.

87. **Sato, G., Zaroff, L., and Mills, S. E.,** Tissue culture populations and their relation to the tissue of origin, *Proc. Natl. Acad. Sci. U.S.A.,* 46, 963, 1960.

88. **Sato, G. H., Rossman, T., Edelstein, L., Holmes, S., and Buonassisi, V.,** Phenotypic alterations in adrenal tumor cultures, *Science,* 148, 1733, 1965.

89. **Schimmer, B. P.,** Adenylate cyclase activity in adrenocorticotropic hormone-sensitive and mutant adrenocortical tumor cell lines, *J. Biol. Chem.,* 247, 3134, 1972.

90. **Wolff, J. and Cook, G. H.,** Choleragen stimulates steroidogenesis and adenylate cyclase in cells lacking functional hormone receptors, *Biochim. Biophys. Acta,* 413, 283, 1975.

91. **Rae, P. A., Tsao, J., and Schimmer, B. P.,** Evaluation of receptor function in ACTH-responsive and ACTH-insensitive adrenal tumor cells, *Can. J. Biochem.,* 57, 509, 1979.

92. **Schimmer, B. P.,** unpublished observations.

93. **Wishnow, R. M. and Feist, P.,** The effect of cholera enterotoxin on steroidogenesis in cultured adrenal tumor cells, *J. Infect. Dis.,* 129, 690, 1974.

94. **Donta, S.,** Differentiation between the steroidogenic effects of cholera enterotoxin and adrenocorticotropin through use of a mutant adrenal cell line, *J. Infect. Dis.,* 129, 728, 1974.

95. **Watt, V. M. and Schimmer, B. P.,** Association of a 68,000-dalton protein with adrenocorticotropin-sensitive adenylate cyclase activity in Y1 adrenocortical tumor cells, *J. Biol. Chem.,* 256, 11365, 1981.

96. **Schimmer, B. P.,** Adenylate cyclase activity and steroidogenesis in phenotypic revertants of an ACTH-insensitive adrenal tumour cell line, *Nature,* 259, 482, 1976.

97. **Buonassisi, V., Sato, G., and Cohen, A. I.,** Hormone-producing cultures of adrenal and pituitary origin, *Proc. Natl. Acad. Sci. U.S.A.,* 48, 1184, 1962.

98. **Rae, P. A., Gutmann, N. S., Tsao, J., and Schimmer, B. P.,** Mutations in cyclic AMP-dependent protein kinase and corticotropin (ACTH)-sensitive adenylate cyclase affect adrenal steroidogenesis, *Proc. Natl. Acad. Sci. U.S.A.,* 76, 1896, 1979.

99. **Schimmer, B. P., Tsao, J., and Knapp, M.,** Isolation of mutant adrenocortical tumor cells resistant to cyclic nucleotides, *Mol. Cell. Biol.,* 8, 135, 1977.

100. **Kudlow, J. E., Rae, P. A., Gutmann, N. S., Schimmer, B. P., and Burrow, G. N.,** Regulation of ornithine decarboxylase activity by corticotropin in adrenocortical tumor cell clones: roles of cyclic AMP and cyclic AMP-dependent protein kinase, *Proc. Natl. Acad. Sci. U.S.A.,* 77, 2767, 1980.

101. **Watt, V. M. and Schimmer, B. P.,** Clonal variation in adrenocorticotropin-induced desensitization of adenylate cyclase in Y1 adrenocortical tumor cells, *J. Biol. Chem.,* 257, 1684, 1982.

102. **Schimmer, B. P., Robinson, R., Tsao, J., and Watt, V. M.,** A 68,000 dalton protein genetically associated with corticotropin-sensitive adenylate cyclase activity. Purification and preliminary characterization using a specific antiserum, *Can. J. Biochem. Cell Biol.,* 62, 601, 1984.

103. **Schimmer, B. P. and Tsao, J.,** Isolation of forskolin-resistant adrenal cells defective in the adenylate cyclase system, *J. Biol. Chem.,* 259, 5376, 1984.

104. **Schimmer, B. P., Tsao, J., Collie, G., Wong, M., and Schulz, P.,** Analysis of the mutation to forskolin-resistance in Yl adrenocortical tumor cells, *Endocrine Res.,* 10, 365, 1984-85.

104a. **Schimmer, B. P., Tsao, J., Borenstein, R., and Endrenyi, L.,** Forskolin-resistant Y1 mutants harbor defects associated with the guanyl nucleotide-binding regulatory protein, G$_s$, *J. Biol. Chem.,* 262, 15521, 1987.

105. **Seamon, K. B. and Daly, J. W.,** Forskolin: a unique diterpene activator of cyclic AMP-generating systems, *J. Cyclic Nucleotide Res.,* 7, 201, 1981.

106. **Seamon, K. B. and Daly, J. W.,** Activation of adenylate cyclase by the diterpene forskolin does not require the guanine nucleotide regulatory protein, *J. Biol. Chem.,* 256, 9799, 1981.

107. **Birnbaumer, L., Stengel, D., Desmier, M., and Hanoune, J.,** Forskolin regulation of liver membrane adenylyl cyclase, *Eur. J. Biochem.,* 136, 107, 1983.

108. **Zahler, W. L.,** Evidence for multiple interconvertible forms of adenylate cyclase detected by forskolin activation, *J. Cyclic Nucleotide Protein Phosphorylation Res.,* 9, 221, 1983.

109. **Smigel, M. D.,** Purification of the catalyst of adenylate cyclase, *J. Biol. Chem.,* 261, 1976, 1986.

110. **Schimmer, B. P. and Schulz, P.,** The roles of cAMP and cAMP-dependent protein kinase in forskolin's actions on Y1 adrenocortical tumor cells, *Endocrine Res.,* 11, 199, 1985.

111. **Seamon, K. B. and Daly, J. W.,** Forskolin, cyclic AMP and cellular physiology, *Trends Pharmacol. Sci.,* 4, 120, 1983.

112. **Williams, S. A. and Schimmer, B. P.,** mRNA from mutant Y1 adrenal cells directs the synthesis of altered regulatory subunits of type 1 cAMP-dependent protein kinase, *J. Biol. Chem.,* 258, 10215, 1983.

113. **Schimmer, B. P., Horney, S. J., Williams, S. A., Aitchison, W. A., and Doherty, P. J.,** Recovery of cyclic nucleotide regulation in protein-kinase-defective adrenal cells through somatic cell fusion, *J. Cell. Physiol.,* 121, 483, 1984.

114. **Schimmer, B. P., Wong, M. W., O'Brien, D., and Schulz, P.,** Recovery of hormonal regulation in protein kinase defective adrenal cells through DNA-mediated gene transfer, *J. Cell. Physiol.,* 126, 77, 1986.

115. **Wong, M. W., O'Brien, D., and Schimmer, B. P.,** The roles of cAMP and cAMP-dependent protein kinase in the regulation of adrenocortical functions: analysis using DNA-mediated gene transfer, *Biochem. Cell Biol.,* 64, 1066, 1986.

116. **Wigler, M., Pellicer, A., Silverstein, S., and Axel, R.,** Biochemical transfer of single-copy eucaryotic genes using total cellular DNA as donor, *Cell,* 14, 725, 1978.

117. **Wigler, M., Pellicer, A., Silverstein, S., Axel, R., Urlaub, G., and Chasin, L.,** DNA-mediated transfer of the adenosine phosphoribosyltransferase locus into mammalian cells, *Proc. Natl. Acad. Sci. U.S.A.,* 76, 1373, 1979.

118. **Doherty, P. J., Tsao, J., Schimmer, B. P., Mumby, M. C., and Beavo, J. A.,** cAMP-dependent protein kinase and regulation of adrenocortical functions: A genetic evaluation, in *Protein Phosphorylation: Cold Spring Harbor Conferences On Cell Proliferation,* Vol. 8, Book A, Rosen, O. M., and Krebs, E. G., Eds., Cold Spring Harbor Laboratory, New York, 1981, 211.

119. **Duch, D. S., Woolf, J. H., Edelstein, M. P., Viveros, O. H., Abou-Donia, A., and Nicol, C. A.,** Regulation of tetrahydrobiopterin biosynthesis in cultured adrenal cortical tumor cells by adrenocorticotropin and adenosine 3',5'-cyclic monophosphate, *Endocrinology,* 118, 1897, 1986.

120. **Seelig, S. and Sayers, G.,** Isolated adrenal cortex cells: ACTH agonists, partial agonists, antagonists; cyclic AMP and corticosterone production, *Arch. Biochem. Biophys.,* 154, 230, 1973.

121. **Moyle, W. R., Kong, Y. C., and Ramachandran, J.,** Steroidogenesis and cyclic adenosine 3',5'-monosphosphate accumulation in rat adrenal cells. Divergent effects of adrenocorticotropin and its o-nitrophenyl sulfenyl derivative, *J. Biol. Chem.,* 248, 2409, 1973.

122. **Rae, P. A., Zinman, H., Ramachandran, J., and Schimmer, B. P.,** Responses of Y1 adrenocortical tumor cells to o-nitrophenyl sulfenyl ACTH, *Mol. Cell. Endocrinol.,* 17, 171, 1980.

123. **Estensen, R. D., Zustiak, K., Chuang, A., Schultheiss, P., and Ditmanson, J.,** Action of 12-O-tetradecanoylphorbol-13-acetate on Y1 adrenal cells apparently requires the regulatory subunit of type 1 cyclic AMP dependent protein kinase, *J. Exp. Pathol.,* 1, 49, 1983.

124. **Castagna, M., Takai, Y., Kaibuchi, K., Sano, K., Kikkawa, U., and Nishizuka, Y.,** Direct activation of calcium-activated phospholipid-dependent protein kinase by tumor-promoting phorbol esters, *J. Biol. Chem.,* 257, 7847, 1982.

125. **Watanabe, Y., Horn, F., Bauer, S., and Jakobs, K. H.,** Protein kinase C interferes with Ni-mediated inhibition of human platelet adenylate cyclase, *FEBS Lett.,* 192, 23, 1985.

126. **Temple, R. and Wolff, J.,** Stimulation of steroid secretion by antimicrotubular agents, *J. Biol. Chem.,* 248, 2691, 1973.

127. **Kotani, M., Koizumi, Y., Yamada, T., Kawasaki, A., and Akabane, T.,** Increase of cyclic adenosine 3':5'-monophosphate concentration in transplantable lymphoma cells by Vinca alkaloids, *Cancer Res.,* 38, 3094, 1978.

128. **Rudolph, S. A., Hegstrand, L. R., Greengard, P., and Malawista, S. E.,** The interaction of colchicine with hormone-sensitive adenylate cyclase in human leukocytes, *Mol. Pharmacol.,* 16, 805, 1979.

129. **Sackett, D. L. and Wolff, J.,** Cyclic AMP-independent stimulation of steroidogenesis in Y-1 adrenal tumor cells by antimitotic agents, *Biochim. Biophys. Acta,* 888, 163, 1986.

130. **Horibata, K. and Harris, A. W.,** Mouse myelomas and lymphomas in culture, *Exp. Cell Res.,* 60, 61, 1970.

131. **Coffino, P., Gray, J. W., and Tomkins, G. M.,** Cyclic AMP, a nonessential regulator of the cell cycle, *Proc. Natl. Acad. Sci. U.S.A.,* 72, 878, 1975.

132. **Insel, P. A. and Fenno, J.,** Cyclic AMP-dependent protein kinase mediates a cyclic AMP-stimulated decrease in ornithine and S-adenosylmethione decarboxylase activities, *Proc. Natl. Acad. Sci. U.S.A.,* 75, 862, 1978.

133. **Bourne, H. R., Tomkins, G. M., and Dion, S.,** Regulation of phosphodiesterase synthesis: Requirement for cyclic adenosine monophosphate-dependent protein kinase, *Science,* 181, 952, 1973.

134. **Bourne, H. R., Coffino, P., and Tomkins, G. M.,** Somatic genetic analysis of cyclic AMP action: Characterization of unresponsive mutants, *J. Cell. Physiol.,* 85, 611, 1975.

135. **Gehring, U. and Coffino, P.,** Independent mechanisms of cyclic AMP and glucocorticoid action, *Nature,* 268, 167, 1977.

136. **Yamamoto, K. R., Gehring, U., Stampfer, M. R., and Sibley, C. H.,** Genetic approaches to steroid hormone action, *Recent Prog. Hormone Res.,* 32, 3, 1976.

137. **Coffino, P., Bourne, H. R., and Tomkins, G. M.,** Somatic genetic analysis of cyclic AMP action: selection of unresponsive mutants, *J. Cell. Physiol.,* 85, 603, 1975.

138. **Insel, P. A., Bourne, H. R., Coffino, P., and Tomkins, G. M.,** Cyclic AMP-dependent protein kinase: pivotal role in regulation of enzyme induction and growth, *Science,* 190, 896, 1975.

139. **Bourne, H. R., Coffino, P., Melmon, K. L., Tomkins, G. M., and Weinstein, Y.,** Genetic analysis of cyclic AMP in a mammalian cell, *Adv. Cyclic Nucleotide Res.,* 5, 771, 1975.

140. **Steinberg, R. A.,** Molecular approaches to the study of cyclic AMP action, in *Biochemical Actions of Hormones,* Vol. 11, Litwack, G., Ed., Academic Press, New York, 1984, 25.

141. **Friedrich, U. and Coffino, P.,** Mutagenesis in S49 mouse lymphoma cells: Induction of resistance to ouabain, 6-thioguanine, and dibutyryl cyclic AMP, *Proc. Natl. Sci. U.S.A.,* 74, 679, 1977.

142. **Steinberg, R. A., O'Farrell, P. H., Freidrich, U., and Coffino, P.,** Mutations causing charge alterations in regulatory subunits of the cAMP-dependent protein kinase of cultured S49 lymphoma cells, *Cell,* 10, 381, 1977.

143. **Hochman, J., Insel, P. A., Bourne, H. R., Coffino, P., and Tomkins, G. M.,** A structural gene mutation affecting the regulatory subunit of cyclic AMP-dependent protein kinase in mouse lymphoma cells, *Proc. Natl. Acad. Sci. U.S.A.,* 72, 5051, 1975.

144. **Hochman, J., Bourne, H. R., Coffino, P., Insel, P. A., Krasny, L., and Melmon, K. L.,** Subunit interaction in cyclic AMP-dependent protein kinase of mutant lymphoma cells, *Proc. Natl. Acad. Sci. U.S.A.,* 74, 1167, 1977.

145. **Clegg, C. H., Correll, L. A., and McKnight, G. S.,** Cloning and expression of wildtype and mutant regulatory subunit genes of cAMP dependent protein kinase, *J. Cell. Biochem.,* Suppl. 10D, 97, 1986.

146. **Lemaire, I. and Coffino, P.,** Coexpression of mutant and wild type protein kinase in lymphoma cells resistant to dibutyryl cyclic AMP, *J. Cell. Physiol.,* 92, 437, 1977.

147. **Murphy, C. S. and Steinberg, R. A.,** Hotspots for spontaneous and mutagen-induced lesions in regulatory subunit of cyclic AMP-dependent protein kinase in S49 mouse lymphoma cells, *Somat. Cell Mol. Genet.,* 11, 605, 1985.

148. **van Daalen Wetters, T. and Coffino, P.,** Reversion of an S49 cell cyclic AMP-dependent protein kinase structural gene mutant occurs primarily by functional elimination of mutant gene expression, *Mol. Cell. Biol.,* 3, 250, 1983.

149. **Steinberg, R. A., van Daalen Wetters, T., and Coffino, P.,** Kinase-negative mutants of S49 mouse lymphoma cells carry a trans-dominant mutation affecting expression of cAMP-dependent protein kinase, *Cell,* 15, 1351, 1978.

150. **van Daalen Wetters, T., Murtaugh, M. P., and Coffino, P.,** Revertants of a trans-dominant S49 mouse lymphoma mutant that affects expression of cAMP-dependent protein kinase, *Cell,* 35, 311, 1983.

151. **Steinberg, R. A. and Agard, D. A.,** Turnover of regulatory subunit of cyclic AMP-dependent protein kinase in S49 mouse lymphoma cells, *J. Biol. Chem.,* 256, 10731, 1981.

152. **Steinberg, R. A.,** Sites of phosphorylation and mutation in regulatory subunit of cyclic AMP-dependent protein kinase from S49 mouse lymphoma cells: mapping to structural domains, *J. Cell Biol.,* 97, 1072, 1983.

153. **Kiss, Z. and Steinberg, R. A.,** Phorbol ester-mediated protein phosphorylations in S49 mouse lymphoma cells, *Cancer Res.,* 45, 2731, 1985.

154. **Kiss, Z. and Steinberg, R. A.,** Interactions between cyclic AMP- and phorbol ester-dependent phosphorylation systems in S49 mouse lymphoma cells, *J. Cell. Physiol.,* 125, 200, 1985.

155. **Gilman, A. G., Sternweis, P. C., Howlett, A. C., and Ross, E. M.,** Biochemical and genetic resolution of components of the S49 lymphoma adenylate cyclase system, in, *Hormones and Cell Culture: Cold Spring Harbor Conferences On Cell Proliferation,* Vol. 6, Book A, Sato, G. H., and Ross, R., Eds., Cold Spring Harbor Laboratory, New York, 1979, 299.

156. **Farfel, Z., Salomon, M. R., and Bourne, H. R.,** Genetic investigation of adenylate cyclase: mutations in mouse and man, *Annu. Rev. Pharmacol. Toxicol.,* 21, 251, 1981.

157. **Bourne, H. R., Casperson, G. F., van Dop, C., Abood, M. E., Beiderman, B. B., Steinberg, F., and Walker, N.,** Mutations of adenylate cyclase in yeast, mouse, and man, *Adv. Cyclic Nucleotide Protein Phosphorylation Res.,* 17, 199, 1984.

158. **Bourne, H. R., Coffino, P., and Tomkins, G. M.,** Selection of a variant lymphoma cell deficient in adenylate cyclase, *Science,* 187, 750, 1975.

159. **Haga, T., Ross, E. M., Anderson, H. J., and Gilman, A. G.,** Adenylate cyclase permanently uncoupled from hormone receptors in a novel variant of S49 mouse lymphoma cells, *Proc. Natl. Acad. Sci. U.S.A.,* 74, 2016, 1977.

160. **Salomon, M. R. and Bourne, H. R.,** Novel S49 lymphona variants with aberrant cyclic AMP metabolism, *Mol. Pharmacol.,* 19, 109, 1981.

161. **Johnson, G. L., Bourne, H. R., Gleason, M. K., Coffino, P., Insel, P. A., and Melmon, K.,** Isolation and characterization of S49 lymphoma cells deficient in β-adrenergic receptors: relation of receptor number to activation of adenylate cyclase, *Mol. Pharmacol.,* 15, 16, 1979.

162. **Ross, E. M., Howlett, A. C., Ferguson, K. M., and Gilman, A. G.,** Reconstitution of hormone-sensitive adenylate cyclase activity with resolved components of the enzyme, *J. Biol. Chem.,* 253, 6401, 1978.

163. **Harris, B. A., Robishaw, J. D., Mumby, S. M., and Gilman, A. G.,** Molecular cloning of complementary DNA for the alpha subunit of the G protein that stimulates adenylate cyclase, *Science,* 229, 1274, 1985.

164. **Schleifer, L. S., Garrison, J. C., Sternweis, P. C., Northup, J. K., and Gilman, A. G.,** The regulatory component of adenylate cyclase from uncoupled S49 lymphona cells differs in charge from the wild type protein, *J. Biol. Chem.,* 255, 2641, 1980.

165. **Bourne, H. R., Beiderman, B., Steinberg, F., and Brothers, V. M.,** Three adenylate cyclase phenotypes in S49 lymphoma cells produced by mutations of one gene, *Mol. Pharmacol.,* 22, 204, 1982.

166. **Ross, E. M. and Gilman, A. G.,** Reconstitution of catecholamine-sensitive adenylate cyclase activity: interaction of solubilized components with receptor-replete membranes, *Proc. Natl. Acad. Sci. U.S.A.* 74, 3715, 1977.

167. **Northup, J. K., Sternweis, P. C., Smigel, M. D., Schleifer, L. S., Ross, E. M., and Gilman, A. G.,** Purification of the regulatory component of adenylate cyclase, *Proc. Natl. Acad. Sci. U.S.A.,* 77, 6516, 1980.

168. **Steinberg, R. A., Steinberg, M. G., and van Daalen Wetters, T.,** A variant of S49 mouse lymphoma cells with enhanced secretion of cyclic AMP, *J. Cell. Physiol.,* 100, 579, 1979.

169. **Brothers, V. M., Walker, N., and Bourne, H. R.,** Increased cyclic nucleotide phosphodiesterase activity in mutant S49 lymphoma cells, *J. Biol. Chem.,* 257, 9349, 1982.

170. **Gottesman, M. M.,** *Molecular Cell Genetics,* John Wiley & Sons, New York, 1985.

171. **Puck, T. T.,** Development of the Chinese hamster ovary (CHO) cell for use in somatic cell genetics, in *Molecular Cell Genetics,* Gottesman, M. M., Ed., John Wiley & Sons, New York, 1985, 37.

172. **Siminovitch, L.,** On the nature of hereditable variation in cultured somatic cells, *Cell,* 7, 1, 1976.

173. **Siciliano, M. J., Stallings, R. L., and Adair, G. M.,** The genetic map of the Chinese hamster and the genetic consequences of chromosomal rearrangements in CHO cells, in *Molecular Cell Genetics,* Gottesman, M. M., Ed., John Wiley & Sons, New York, 1985, 95.

174. **Hsie, A. W. and Puck, T. T.,** Morphological transformation of Chinese hamster cells by dibutyryl adenosine cyclic 3′:5′-monophosphate and testosterone, *Proc. Natl. Acad. Sci. U.S.A.,* 68, 358, 1971.

175. **Gottesman, M. M.,** Genetics of cyclic-AMP-dependent protein kinases, in *Molecular Cell Genetics,* Gottesman, M. M., Ed., John Wiley & Sons, New York, 1985, 711.

176. **LeCam, A., Gottesman, M. M., and Pastan, I.,** Mechanism of cyclic AMP effect on nutrient transport in Chinese hamster ovary cells, *J. Biol. Chem.,* 255, 8103, 1980.

177. **Wiener, E. C. and Loewenstein, W. R.,** Correction of cell-cell communication defect by introduction of a protein kinase into mutant cells, *Nature,* 305, 433, 1983.

178. **Lichti, U. and Gottesman, M. M.,** Genetic evidence that a phorbol ester tumor promoter stimulates ornithine decarboxylase activity by a pathway that is independent of cyclic AMP-dependent protein kinases in CHO cells, *J. Cell. Physiol.,* 113, 433, 1982.

179. **Milhaud, P. G., Davies, P. J. A., Pastan, I., and Gottesman, M. M.,** Regulation of transglutaminase activity in Chinese hamster ovary cells, *Biochim. Biophys. Acta,* 630, 476, 1980.

180. **Li, A. P., O'Neill, P., Kawashima, K., and Hsie, A. W.,** Correlation between changes in intracellular level of cyclic AMP, activation of cyclic AMP-dependent protein kinase, and the morphology of Chinese hamster ovary cells in culture, *Arch. Biochem. Biophys.,* 182, 181, 1977.

181. **Gottesman, M. M., LeCam, A., Bukowski, M., and Pastan, I.,** Isolation of multiple classes of mutants of CHO cells resistant to cyclic AMP, *Somat. Cell Genet.,* 6, 45, 1980.
182. **Evain, D. and Anderson, W. B.,** Gonadotropin stimulation of cyclic AMP levels in Chinese hamster ovary cells in culture, *J. Cell Physiol.,* 99, 153, 1979.
183. **Singh, T. J., Hochman, J., Verna, R., Chapman, M., Abraham, I., Pastan, I. H., and Gottesman, M. M.,** Characterization of a cyclic AMP-resistant Chinese hamster ovary cell mutant containing both wild-type and mutant species of type 1 regulatory subunit of cyclic AMP-dependent protein kinase, *J. Biol. Chem.,* 260, 13927, 1985.
184. **Abraham, I., Brill, S.,, Hyde, J., Fleischmann, R., Chapman, M., and Gottesman, M. M.,** DNA-mediated gene transfer of a mutant regulatory subunit of cAMP-dependent protein kinase, *J. Biol. Chem.,* 260, 13934, 1985.
185. **Abraham, I., Brill, S., Chapman, M., Hyde, J., and Gottesman, M.,** DNA-mediated transfer of cAMP resistance in CHO cells, *J. Cell. Physiol.,* 127, 89, 1986.
186. **Gottesman, M.,** Using mutants to study cAMP-dependent protein kinase, *Methods Enzymol.,* 99, 197, 1983.
187. **Storrie, B., Puck, T. T., and Wenger, L.,** The role of butyrate in the reverse transformation reaction in mammalian cells, *J. Cell. Physiol.,* 94, 69, 1978.
188. **Pawelek, J., Sansone, M., Koch, N., Christie, G., Halaban, R., Hendee, J., Lerner, A. B., and Varga, J. M.,** Melanoma cells resistant to inhibition of growth by melanocyte stimulating hormone, *Proc. Natl. Acad. Sci. U.S.A.,* 72, 951, 1975.
189. **Pawelek, J., Halaban, R., and Christie, G.,** Melanoma cells which require cyclic AMP for growth, *Nature,* 258, 539, 1975.
190. **Taub, M., Saier, M. H. Jr., Chuman, L., and Hiller, S.,** Loss of the PGE$_1$ requirement for MDCK cell growth associated with a defect in cyclic AMP phosphodiesterase, *J. Cell. Physiol.,* 114, 153, 1983.
191. **Ralph, P. and Nakoinz, I.,** Phagocytosis and cytolysis by a macrophage tumour and its cloned cell line, *Nature,* 257, 393, 1975.
192. **Muschel, R. J., Rosen, N., and Bloom, B. R.,** Isolation of variants in phagocytosis of a macrophage-like continuous line, *J. Expt. Med.,* 145, 175, 1977.
193. **Muschel, R. J., Rosen, N., Rosen, O. M., and Bloom, B. R.,** Modulation of Fc-mediated phagocytosis by cyclic AMP and insulin in a macrophage-like cell line, *J. Immunol.,* 119, 1813, 1977.
194. **Rosen, N., Piscitello, J., Schneck, J., Muschel, R. J., Bloom, B. R., and Rosen, O. M.,** Properties of protein kinase and adenylate cyclase-deficient variants of a macrophage-like cell line, *J. Cell. Physiol.,* 98, 125, 1979.
195. **Schneck, J., Rager-Zisman, B., Rosen, O. M., and Bloom B. R.,** Genetic analysis of the role of cAMP in mediating effects of interferon, *Proc. Natl. Acad. Sci. U.S.A.,* 79, 1879, 1982.
196. **Melmed, R. M., Friedman, G., Chajek-Shaul, T., Stein, O., and Stein, Y.,** Lipoprotein lipase activity in cultured macrophage cell line, J774$_2$ and its increase in variants deficient in adenylate cyclase and cyclic AMP-dependent protein kinase, *Biochim. Biophys. Acta,* 762, 58, 1983.
197. **Melmed, R. N., Rachmilewitz, B., Schneider, A., and Rachmilewitz, M.,** The modulation of trans-cobalamin II (TC-II) production by cyclic adenosine 3′,5′-monophosphate in the murine macrophage cell line J774: relationship to growth behavior, *J. Cell. Physiol.,* 126, 430, 1986.
198. **McRoberts, J. A., Taub, M., and Saier, M. H., Jr.,** The Madin Darby canine kidney (MDCK) cell line, in *Functionally Differentiated Cell Lines,* Sato, G., Ed., Alan R. Liss, New York, 1981, 117.
199. **Taub, M., Chuman, L., Saier, M. H., Jr., and Sato, G.,** Growth of Madin-Darby canine kidney epithelial cell (MDCK) line in hormone-supplemented, serum-free medium, *Proc. Natl. Acad. Sci. U.S.A.,* 76, 3338, 1979.
200. **Devis, P. E., Grohol, S. H., and Taub, M.,** Dibutyryl cyclic AMP resistant MDCK cells in serum free medium have reduced cyclic AMP dependent protein kinase activity and a diminished effect of PGE$_1$ on differentiated function, *J. Cell. Physiol.,* 125, 23, 1985.
201. **Taub, M., Devis, P. E., and Grohol, S. H.,** PGE$_1$-independent MDCK cells have elevated intracellular cyclic AMP but retain the growth stimulatory effects of glucagon and epidermal growth factor in serum-free medium, *J. Cell. Physiol.,* 120, 19, 1984.
202. **Kahn, R. A. and Gilman, A. G.,** Purification of a protein cofactor required for ADP-ribosylation of the stimulatory regulatory component of adenylate cyclase by cholera toxin, *J. Biol. Chem.,* 259, 6228, 1984.
203. **Stadel, J. M., Nambi, P., Shorr, R. G. L., Sawyer, D. F., Caron, M. G., and Lefkowitz, R. J.,** Catecholamine-induced desensitization of turkey erythrocyte adenylate cyclase is associated with phosphorylation of the β-adrenergic receptor, *Proc. Natl. Acad. Sci. U.S.A.* 80, 3173, 1983.

Chapter 14

# AMINO ACID ANALOGS

**A. Elizabeth L. Cairney and Irene L. Andrulis**

## TABLE OF CONTENTS

I.    Introduction ........................................................................212

II    Proteins Overproduced in Drug-Resistant Cell Lines ...........................212
      A.    Mutations Affecting Amino Acid Biosynthetic Enzymes ................212
            1.    Aspargine Synthetase Overexpressing Lines .....................212
                  a.    Single-Step β-AHA$^r$ and Alb$^R$ Mutants ..................213
                  b.    Multistep β-AHA$^r$ and Alb$^R$ Lines ......................215
                  c.    Gene Amplification in Alb$^R$ Lines ........................216
            2.    Glutamine Synthetase Overproducers ...........................216
                  a.    Methionine Sulfoximine-Resistant Lines .................216
                  b.    Albizziin-Resistant Lines ...............................217
            3.    Canavanine-Resistant Lines with Elevated Levels of
                  Argininosuccinate Synthetase .................................218
                  a.    Isolation of Mutant Lines ...............................219
                  b.    Molecular Studies .......................................219
            4.    Pyrroline-5-Carboxylate Synthetase Overproducers ..............220
            5.    Methionine Adenosyl Transferase Overexpressors ...............222
      B.    Aminoacyl-tRNA Synthetase Overproducers ..........................223
            1.    Histidinol-Resistant Lines ...................................223
            2.    Tyrosinol-Resistant Lines ....................................223
            3.    Borrelidin-Resistant Lines ...................................224
      C.    Amino Acid Transport Mutants .....................................224
            1.    "A" System Mutants ..........................................224
                  a.    Isolation of Alanine-Resistant Lines ....................225
                  b.    Increase in "A"System Transport ........................225
            2.    ASC System Mutants ..........................................226
            3.    "L" System Mutants ..........................................226
                  a.    Substrate Mediated Regulation ..........................227
                  b.    "L" System Overproduction ..............................227
                  c.    Decreased "L" System Transport .........................228
                  d.    Melphalan Resistance ...................................228

III.   Summary ..........................................................................228

Acknowledgments ......................................................................228

References .............................................................................229

# I. INTRODUCTION

Until recently studies on the regulation of expression of enzymes involved in basic eukaryotic cellular metabolism relied on genetic and biochemical approaches. In the past few years the scope has been widened for a number of housekeeping enzymes by taking advantage of genetic systems to obtain molecular probes for such analysis. In this chapter we will concentrate on those proteins which are overexpressed in somatic cell lines resistant to various amino acid analogs. Such analogs have been used as inhibitors of amino acid biosynthetic enzymes, aminoacyl-tRNA synthetases, and amino acid transport proteins in prokaryotic and lower eukaryotic cells. Since these processes are common to higher eukaryotic cells as well, a number of investigators have utilized specific amino acid analogs to isolate resistant mammalian cell lines with alterations in the level of activity of the affected proteins (Table 1).[1-22]

There are a number of different types of mutations which could give rise to resistance to amino acid analogs. These include defects in transport and structural genes and changes in expression due to alterations in regulatory regions or gene amplification. Although we mention the various types of mutations where appropriate, we have concentrated on examples where resistance to an amino acid analog is associated with elevated levels of the target protein. In several systems described in this chapter the enzyme and mRNA overproduction facilitated the cloning of the gene and the increased expression has been shown to be due to gene amplification.

Gene amplification has been observed in numerous other cell lines where drug resistance results from overproduction of the target protein.[23,24] These drug resistant cell lines share common properties such as selection in multiple steps, codominance in hybrids, increase in the level of RNA and protein, and presence of the amplified copies of the gene either chromosomally as homogeneously staining regions (HSRs) or extra-chromosomally as double minutes. Mutant cell lines which contain amplified genes as HSRs are generally found to be stable in the absence of selection, whereas cell lines with double minutes often show an unstable phenotype. Most of the amino acid analog-resistant cell lines exhibit some, if not all, of these features and we will point these out where they have been examined. There is wide variation in the extent of characterization of amino acid analog-resistant mutants, therefore we described the progress made at the level which has been analyzed (i.e., biochemical, genetic, or molecular).

# II. PROTEINS OVERPRODUCED IN DRUG-RESISTANT CELL LINES

## A. Mutations Affecting Amino Acid Biosynthetic Enzymes

Cultured mammalian cells are prototropic for a limited number of amino acids since they express only a fraction of amino acid biosynthetic enzymes. Amino acid analogs have been used successfully to inhibit enzymes involved in the biosynthesis of the nonessential amino acids, asparagine,[1-4] glutamine,[5-7] arginine,[8,9] and proline.[10-13]

### 1. Asparagine Synthetase Overexpressing Lines

Asparagine is a nonessential amino acid for most mammalian cells since they express a basal level of AsnSyn activity. However, certain tumor cells lack this activity and rely on their external nutrients for asparagine.[25,26] They are thus sensitive to the chemotherapeutic agent L-asparaginase which removes the exogenous source of asparagine.[27] In order to find other inhibitors of AsnSyn which might be used in combination with L-asparaginase for therapy a number of other drugs have been tested. Horowitz and Meister examined analogs of glutamine and aspartic acid, the substrates of the reaction and showed that 10 different glutamine analogs and 19 aspartate analogs were capable of inhibiting AsnSyn activity.[28]

**Table 1**
**ISOLATION OF MUTANT CELL LINES**
**RESISTANT TO AMINO ACIDS AND THEIR**
**ANALOGS**

| Amino acid or amino acid analog | Function overproduced | Ref. |
|---|---|---|
| β-Aspartyl hydroxamate | Asparagine synthetase | 1,2 |
| Albizziin | Asparagine synthetase | 3,4 |
| Albizziin | Glutamine synthetase | 5 |
| Methionine sulfoximine | Glutamine synthetase | 6,7 |
| Canavanine | Argininosuccinate synthetase | 8,9 |
| L-Azetidine-2-carboxylic acid | Pyrroline-5-carboxylate synthetase | 10-13 |
| Cycloleucine | Methionine adenosyl transferase | 14,15 |
| Histidinol | Histidyl-tRNA synthetase | 16 |
| Tyrosinol | Tyrosyl-tRNA synthetase | |
| Borrelidin | Threonyl-tRNA synthetase | 17,18 |
| Alanine | "A" system transport | 19,20 |
| 2-Methylaminoisobutyric acid | "ASC" system transport | 21 |
| Leucine | "L" system transport | 22 |

Several of these analogs were tested for drug sensitivity in Chinese hamster ovary (CHO) cells and two analogs were found to be toxic at low concentrations, an aspartic acid analog, β-(β-AHA),[1,2] and a glutamine analog, albizziin (Alb).[3,4] β-AHA and Alb were initially chosen as selective agents because they were analogs (Figure 1) of the two substrates of the reaction and mutations affecting various sites of the enzyme were anticipated. However, both acted as competitive inhibitors of AsnSyn with respect to glutamine, and mutants selected for resistance to one drug were cross-resistant to the other.[4] Cell lines resistant to β-AHA and Alb were selected in medium lacking asparagine by two methods. One employed only a single drug selection step in order to obtain structural gene mutations. The other involved multiple rounds of subculture of the cells in gradually increasing concentrations of the drug. This protocol had been useful for the isolation of gene amplification mutants which are drug resistant due to an overproduction of the target enzyme.[23,24] The phenotypes of the β-AHA[r] and Alb[R] cell lines successfully isolated were very different and their characteristics are compared in Table 2.

### a. Single-Step β-AHA[r] and Alb[R] Mutants

Single-step β-AHA[r] mutants obtained from CHO cells at a frequency of approximately $10^{-6}$ were only two- to threefold more resistant to the drug than parental cells[1,2] whereas Alb[R] lines isolated at the same frequency were tenfold more resistant than parental cells.[4] The level of resistance was determined from their $D_{10}$s (the concentration of the drug necessary to reduce the plating efficiency to 10%) as shown for Alb[R] lines in Figure 2. Both β-AHA[r] and Alb[R] single-step mutants were able to escape selection in the drug by overexpressing AsnSyn activity, with the β-AHA[r] lines showing up to 6-fold elevations in enzyme activity and the Alb[R] lines had up to 11-fold increases over parental levels. From studies of the hybrids of drug resistant X parental cells it was shown that the β-AHA resistant phenotype was recessive for 80% of the mutants, while all of the Alb resistant mutations were codominant in hybrids.

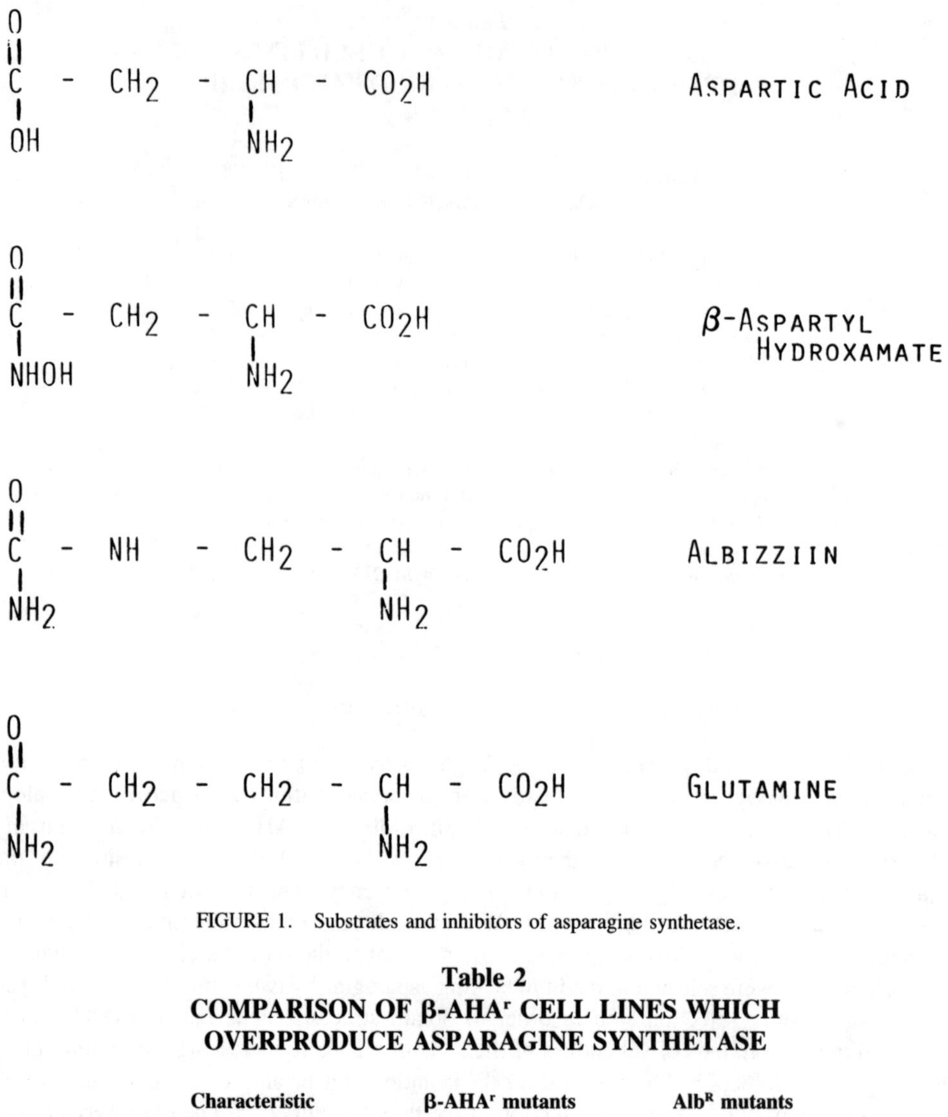

$$O$$
$$\|$$
$$C - CH_2 - CH - CO_2H$$
$$| \qquad\qquad |$$
$$OH \qquad\quad NH_2$$

ASPARTIC ACID

$$O$$
$$\|$$
$$C - CH_2 - CH - CO_2H$$
$$| \qquad\qquad |$$
$$NHOH \qquad NH_2$$

$\beta$-ASPARTYL HYDROXAMATE

$$O$$
$$\|$$
$$C - NH - CH_2 - CH - CO_2H$$
$$| \qquad\qquad\qquad |$$
$$NH_2 \qquad\qquad\quad NH_2$$

ALBIZZIIN

$$O$$
$$\|$$
$$C - CH_2 - CH_2 - CH - CO_2H$$
$$| \qquad\qquad\qquad |$$
$$NH_2 \qquad\qquad\quad NH_2$$

GLUTAMINE

FIGURE 1. Substrates and inhibitors of asparagine synthetase.

## Table 2
### COMPARISON OF β-AHAʳ CELL LINES WHICH OVERPRODUCE ASPARAGINE SYNTHETASE

| Characteristic | β-AHAʳ mutants | Albᴿ mutants |
|---|---|---|
| Competitive inhibitor of Asn Syn with respect to | Glutamine | Glutamine |
| Analogue of | Asparatic acid | Glutamine |
| Single step mutation frequency | $1 \times 10^{-6}$ | $1 \times 10^{-6}$ |
| Behavior in hybrids | Recessive (80%) Codominant (20%) | Codominant |
| Increase in Asn Syn activity | | |
| Single-step | 5- to 8-fold | 8- to 17-fold |
| Multistep | 20-fold | up to 300-fold |
| Karyotype | | |
| Single-step | Wild-type | Breaks and rearrangements affecting 1 q |
| Multistep | Wild-type | HSRs, usually on 1 q |
| High level of resistance due to | Structural alterations | Gene amplification |

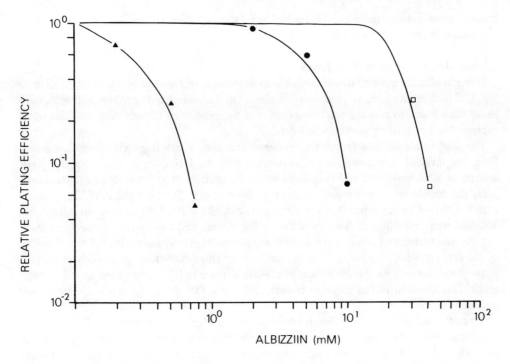

FIGURE 2.   Dose-response curves for CHO parental cells (▲), a single-step AlbR mutant (●), and a multi-step AlbR cell line (□).

### b. Multistep β-AHA$^r$ and Alb$^R$ Lines

The differences in phenotypes were even greater in the cell lines derived from multiple selection steps. CHO lines highly resistant to Alb (Figure 2) were obtained after several months of subculturing and found to be up to 100-fold more resistant to the drug.[3] However, even after 9 months of adapting β-AHA-resistant mutants to progressively increasing concentrations of the drug, the most resistant lines exhibited $D_{10}$s only 10-fold greater than the parental line.[2] These differences were correlated with the modest increases in AsnSyn activity observed in the β-AHA$^r$ mutistep lines (20-fold) vs. the high levels of expressions in the Alb$^R$ multistep lines (up to 300-fold). From the biochemical analysis of the enzyme from the drug resistant cell lines it was shown that β-AHA$^r$ multi-step lines probably contained a structural mutation, such that the enzyme differed from the parental AsnSyn in kinetic constants for glutamine and β-AHA.[2] However, only one of the Alb$^R$ lines appeared to have an alteration in the structural gene for AsnSyn.[4]

Because of the high levels of AsnSyn protein in the Alb$^R$ lines, these cells provided a good source of purified enzyme to generate antibodies to CHO AsnSyn.[29] The multistep Alb$^R$ cell lines were also found to have increased mRNA for AsnSyn and this was used to prepare and isolate nonoverlapping cDNAs for CHO AsnSyn.[27] Recently, the complete CHO (Andrulis et al, in preparation) and human (Andrulis et al, submitted) cDNAs have been obtained. The human AsnSyn cDNAs expressed functional enzymatic activity when they were transfected into asparagine-requiring Jensen rat sarcoma cells and selection for prototrophy was applied. The corresponding CHO (Andrulis et al, in preparation) and human (unpublished results) genomic sequences have been isolated from phage libraries. Restriction enzyme analysis of the phage DNA and comparisons with patterns from Southern blots indicated that in CHO and human cells there was a single functional gene for AsnSyn. However, in human cells there were additional pseudogenes detected as well. A number of questions are now being examined with these probes including the molecular basis for the lesions in the various mutants, the normal regulation of AsnSyn activity, and the lack of expression in certain tumor cells.

### c. Gene Amplification in Alb^R Lines

Using molecular probes it was possible to determine that overproduction of AsnSyn in the Alb^R mutants was due to gene amplification. On the other hand, β-AHA^r cell lines have never been found to contain amplified copies of the gene even though these mutants over-express AsnSyn activity (unpublished data).

The Alb^R cell lines have properties similar to a number of cell lines with amplified genes. First, the level of drug resistance is correlated with the DNA copy number of the gene, amount of RNA produced and enzymatic activity (Andrulis et al, unpublished data). However, the correlation is not exact for most of the mutants. For example Alb^R52, a mutant with a 100-fold increase in DNA copy number, exhibits a 100-fold increase in mRNA but 300-fold overproduction of AsnSyn activity. The mutant cell lines produce AsnSyn constitutively and therefore have lost the normal regulation of AsnSyn activity,[30-32] as controlled by the concentration of asparagine in the medium.[2,4] This constitutive expression of enzyme activity may account for the discrepancy between increase in DNA copy number and AsnSyn level. This question is amenable to investigation now that the molecular tools have been obtained.

Secondly, the mutation is codominant in hybrids as discussed previously. Thirdly, there are characteristic chromosomal abnormalities associated with the resistant phenotype. Single-step Alb^R CHO cell lines show breaks and rearrangements affecting the long arm of chromosome 1 and multistep lines have homogeneously staining region (HSRs) at the breakpoints of translocations again affecting chromosome 1. HSRs have been shown to be the sites of amplified genes in other systems. In CHO cells HSRs have been found at the site of the native gene for dihydrofolate reductase in methotrexate-resistant cell lines.[33] The chromosomal alterations which affect the long arm of chromosome 1 may indicate that this is the site of the native AsnSyn gene.

### 2. Glutamine Synthetase Overproducers

Glutamine represents one of the most versatile amino acids since it is necessary not only for protein synthesis but also acts as a nitrogen donor for the production of purines, pyrimidines, and amino sugars and is involved in detoxification.[34] The regulation of the biosynthetic enzyme glutamine synthetase (GS) has consequently been the subject of extensive investigations in prokaryotes and eukaryotes using a number of amino acid analogs which inhibit GS activity.

### a. Methionine Sulfoximine-Resistant Lines

One of the most potent of these drugs was found to be methionine sulfoximine (Msx) which was first detected as the agent causing seizures in dogs fed flour bleached with nitrogen trichloride.[35] Although structurally Msx is a methionine and glutamine analog (Figure 3), it competes for attachment to GS by acting as a glutamic acid antagonist. In the presence of GS, ATP, and metal ions Msx is phosphorylated and binds tightly to the enzyme causing irreversible inhibition of GS activity.[36]

Wilson took advantage of the properties of Msx to select CHO mutants in the absence of glutamine which were 40-fold more resistant than the parental line and expressed 10-fold more GS activity than the parental cells constitutively.[6] The drug resistant phenotype was codominant in hybrids.[6] Upon further selection in increasing concentrations of Msx more highly resistant cells were isolated which exhibited greater than 500-fold elevations in GS activity.[7,37] In one cell line approximately 30% of the soluble protein was GS.[7] What is perhaps most striking about this system is that at very high levels of the drug one line was

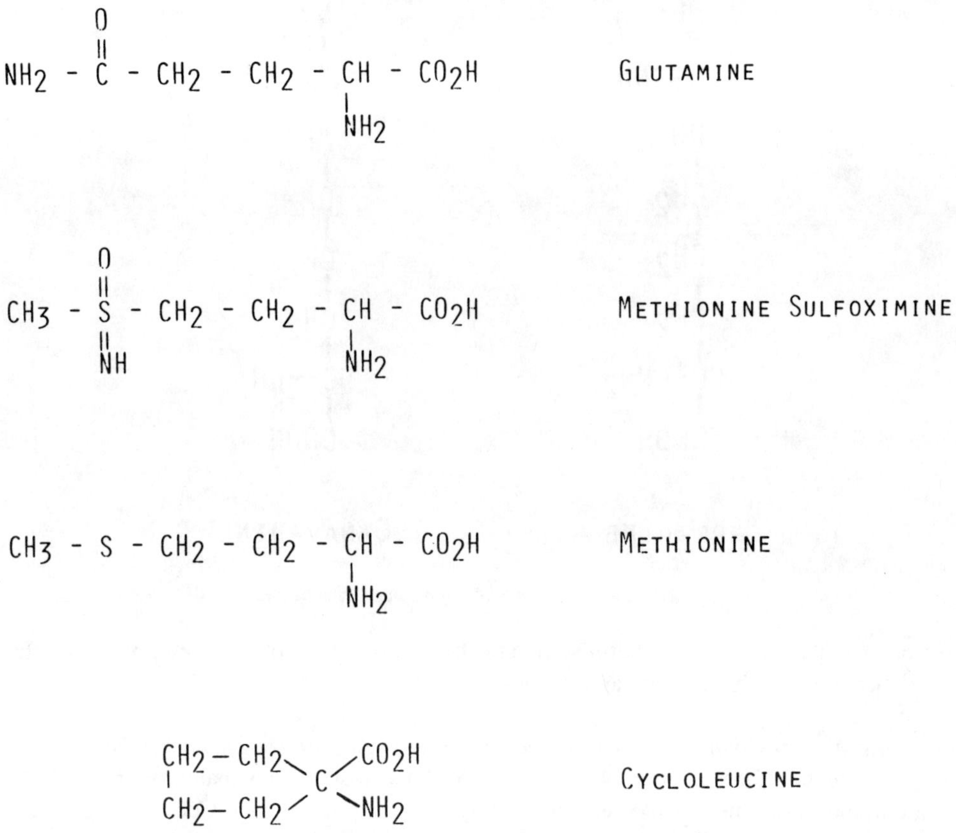

$$NH_2 - \overset{\overset{\displaystyle O}{\|}}{C} - CH_2 - CH_2 - \underset{\underset{\displaystyle NH_2}{|}}{CH} - CO_2H \qquad \text{GLUTAMINE}$$

$$CH_3 - \overset{\overset{\displaystyle O}{\|}}{\underset{\underset{\displaystyle NH}{\|}}{S}} - CH_2 - CH_2 - \underset{\underset{\displaystyle NH_2}{|}}{CH} - CO_2H \qquad \text{METHIONINE SULFOXIMINE}$$

$$CH_3 - S - CH_2 - CH_2 - \underset{\underset{\displaystyle NH_2}{|}}{CH} - CO_2H \qquad \text{METHIONINE}$$

$$\begin{matrix} CH_2 - CH_2 \\ | \qquad\qquad \\ CH_2 - CH_2 \end{matrix} C \begin{matrix} CO_2H \\ \\ NH_2 \end{matrix} \qquad \text{CYCLOLEUCINE}$$

FIGURE 3. Structures of methionine sulfoximine and cycloleucine, analogs of glutamine and methionine.

partially dependent upon Msx for growth. Presumably cellular metabolism did not function efficiently when this crucial enzyme was expressed to such an extent. Msx resistance was found to be unstable in the absence of selection which may be related to this latter property as well.

Unlike the methodology previously described where cDNAs have been isolated from the overproducing cell lines, Sanders and Wilson used the fact that the DNA in the overproducing lines was almost certainly amplified to clone the genomic sequences for GS.[7] They have obtained at least a portion, if not all of the gene, on an 8.2 kb Bg1 II DNA fragment which is amplified in the highly resistant lines. This piece of DNA most likely contains the gene for GS since it could be used to hybrid select an mRNA which was translated in vitro into a protein which comigrated with purified GS on SDS-PAGE. The amplified unit was found to be at least 50 kb. The highly resistant cells did not exhibit any karyotypic abnormalities associated with gene amplification which Sanders and Wilson suggest may be due to the small size of the amplification unit.[7]

### b. Albizziin-Resistant Lines

As mentioned previously, most Alb[R] cell lines were isolated in medium lacking asparagine (but containing 2 m$M$ glutamine) and overexpressed AsnSyn.[3] However when the selections were performed in medium which contained reduced concentrations of glutamine (0.2 m$M$) other overproducers were obtained as well.[5] In order to obtain Alb[R] lines which specifically overexpressed GS, parental cells were grown in medium containing asparagine with reduced glutamine. Alb[R] cell lines isolated in this manner exhibited elevations in GS activity up to

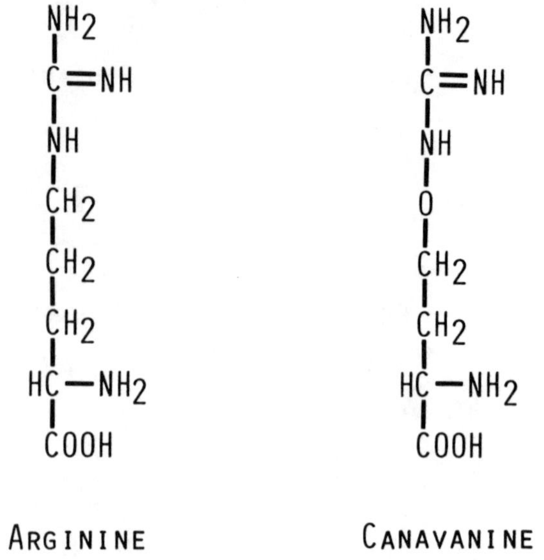

$$
\begin{array}{ccc}
NH_2 & & NH_2 \\
| & & | \\
C=NH & & C=NH \\
| & & | \\
NH & & NH \\
| & & | \\
CH_2 & & O \\
| & & | \\
CH_2 & & CH_2 \\
| & & | \\
CH_2 & & CH_2 \\
| & & | \\
HC-NH_2 & & HC-NH_2 \\
| & & | \\
COOH & & COOH
\end{array}
$$

ARGININE                    CANAVANINE

FIGURE 4.    Structures of arginine and canavanine.

20-fold over parental levels (Andrulis, unpublished data). It has not been determined whether these increases are due to gene amplification.

### 3. Canavanine-Resistant Lines with Elevated Levels of Argininosuccinate Synthetase

L-Canavanine (Can), 2-amino-4-(guanidinooxy)butyric acid is an analog of arginine, differing in the substitution of oxygen for a methylene group (Figure 4). Cells are sensitive to canavanine because arginyl-tRNA synthetase cannot discriminate adequately between canavanine and arginine. This results in the incorporation of canavanine into protein in place of arginine, leading to structural and functional abnormalities. The analog interferes with both DNA and RNA synthesis, believed to be due to the formation of abnormal proteins involved in DNA replication and transcription.

Canavanine was found to exhibit some antitumor activities, both against L1210 leukemia cells in mice, and a colon tumor in rats.[38,39] It was also effective in enhancing the cytotoxic effects of gamma rays on a human colon adenocarcinoma.[40] Growth in sublethal doses of canavanine either before or after radiation, resulted in a marked increase in cell killing at all radiation doses. The mechanisms by which canavanine causes tumor toxicity and enhancement of radiation effects are unknown, but the toxic effects are seen preferentially in rapidly dividing cells, suggesting alterations in proteins required for cell proliferation.

Most cell types are able to synthesize arginine from citrulline and aspartate, although most tissues lack the full urea cycle found in liver cells. Arginine synthesis involves argininosuccinate synthetase (AS), which catalyzes the formation of argininosuccinate from citrulline and aspartate, and argininosuccinate lyase (AS lyase), producing fumarate and arginine from argininosuccinate (Figure 5). Both AS and AS lyase enzyme activity are present in most tissues, with the highest levels being found in liver. In some cell types, AS activity is regulated by the concentration of arginine in the medium. The basal level of activity found in lymphoblasts is considerably less than that found in the liver. However, human lymphoblasts transferred from arginine supplemented to citrulline supplemented medium show a greater than 50-fold increase in AS activity, but no change in AS lyase activity.[41] This effect is specifically mediated by the arginine concentration; incubation with both arginine and citrulline produces no change in As activity.[41]

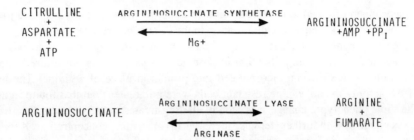

FIGURE 5.   Pathway of arginine biosynthesis.

### a. Isolation of Mutant Lines

Jacoby obtained canavanine resistant variants of human lymphoblastoid cells by selection in arginine deficient medium containing citrulline and canavanine, in an attempt to isolate human cell variants with altered expression of one of the urea cycle enzymes.[8] After 4 to 8 weeks, resistant cells which grew in 12 $\mu M$ canavanine were isolated and found to be resistant to up to 60 $\mu M$ canavanine, compared to the parental line which was inhibited by 6 $\mu M$ canavanine. A number of canavanine-resistant clones were selected, all with the same phenotype. The phenotype was stable in the absence of drug for at least 100 generations, and the karyotype of the resistant cells was indistinguishable from the parental line.

AS activity was elevated in the resistant cells, suggesting that the resistance to canavanine in these cells was due to their ability to synthesize sufficient arginine to compete with canavanine and prevent its toxicity. The resistant cells showed the same degree of AS increase when grown in citrulline, citrulline and canavanine, or arginine. AS levels in the resistant cells were 4- to 5-fold greater than those of the parental cells grown in arginine deficient conditions, and more than 200-fold higher than the basal levels of parental cells grown in medium containing arginine. The activity of AS in resistant cells showed no repression, even in high (12 $\mu M$) concentrations of arginine, in striking contrast to the repression caused by 0.6 m$M$ arginine in normal lymphoblasts. Consistent changes in argininosuccinate lyase activity were not seen, suggesting that AS is the rate limiting step in lymphoblasts, as it is believed to be in liver and other tissues. The higher levels of AS activity observed in the resistant cells was within the range of activity found in normal liver.[9]

Su, Beaudet, and O'Brien selected similar resistant lines from a human squamous cell carcinoma line, by culturing cells in medium lacking arginine but containing citrulline, and with stepwise increases in canavanine concentration.[9] AS activity in one resistant clone (Can$^r$1) was increased 180-fold, another (Can$^r$2) 50-fold over basal levels in parental cells. Again, the resistant phenotype was stable without selection, and metabolite regulation was absent in resistant cells. The increase in activity seen in the resistant cells was comparable to the increase in antigenic material, indicating that increased amounts of a normal AS enzyme were present in the resistant cells.[9]

### b. Molecular Studies

As demonstrated by in vitro translation, the Can$^r$ cells isolated by Su et al. contained increased translatable poly(A)$^+$ mRNA for AS. The latter was used to construct a human cDNA library from which cDNAs for AS were isolated.[42] Using the longest cDNA as a probe for a northern blot, Su et al. confirmed that the level of mRNA expression correlated with the level of enzyme activity, for wild-type cells grown either in arginine or citrulline, and for Can$^r$ cells. Thus the changes in As due to metabolite regulation correlated with the levels of mRNA.

Despite a 180-fold increase in the amount of AS mRNA in the Can$^r$1 cells, and more than a 200-fold increase in the canavanine resistant lymphoblasts, there was no evidence that the mechanism of enzyme overproduction in either of these systems was due to DNA amplification.[42,43] The absence of amplification in the canavanine resistant cells can probably be attributed to a number of characteristics of this latter system in contrast to other drug resistant systems, in which amplification is observed. Canavanine is not a direct inhibitor of As, but rather is toxic when incorporated into protein in place of arginine. The highest levels of AS activity in canavanine resistant cells were no greater than that found in normal liver. The same phenotypic change was seen in all drug-treated cells, and no increase in AS activity was obtained with further stepwise increases in canavanine concentration. Karyotypic changes were not detected in the canavanine resistant lymphoblasts, and the resistant variants were stable when grown in the absence of drug for long periods of time.

In order to delineate the mechanism of mRNA overproduction in these cells, further studies of the AS gene regulation have been performed. Based on evidence from a canavanine resistant lymphoblast line derived from a patient heterozygous for a mutant AS gene, Freytag and colleagues suggested that a *trans*-acting mechanism might be involved in the activity of the resistant cells.[44] In the patient's cells, both the normal and mutant AS mRNA were present in equally increased amounts, although the mutant nonfunctional allele would not be subjected to direct selection pressure.

Despite this evidence, studies using a series of chloramphenicol acetyltransferase (CAT) minigenes under the transcriptional control of the human AS promoter were unable to demonstrate such *trans* induction.[44,45] While the CAT gene was subject to arginine-mediated repression when placed into parental cells, when it was transfected into Can^r1 cells CAT expression was relatively unchanged from that seen with the parental line. Even when the CAT gene was integrated into parental cells which were then selected for canavanine resistance, the endogenous A gene became expressed at greatly elevated levels, but no change was seen in CAT expression.[44]

The canavanine-resistant variants show the same expression of the integrated CAT gene when grown in either arginine or citrulline, similar to the lack of regulation of the AS gene in resistant cells. However, when canavanine resistant cells with the integrated CAT gene were subjected to deprivation for both arginine and citrulline, while no change in endogenous AS activity was seen, increased expression of the AS promoter controlled CAT gene occurred.[45] This suggested that intracellular arginine depletion was necessary for the substrate-mediated regulation of the CAT gene, and that Can^r cells retain the *trans*-acting components necessary for this regulation.

The mechanism for overproduction of AS mRNA in canavanine resistant cells remains unknown at this time, but may be analogous to that involved in the high expression of AS in hepatocytes. Further studies will help elucidate the molecular basis of the regulation of this system.

*4. Pyrroline-5-Carboxylate Synthetase Overproducers*

L-Azetidine-2-carboxylic acid (AZCA) is an analog of proline (Figure 6) that is toxic to mammalian cells because of its incorporation into protein in place of proline, leading to cytotoxicity due to the resulting altered protein structures. In mammalian cells, proline is synthesized either from glutamic acid or from ornithine (Figure 7).

A number of AZCA resistant lines have been selected in mammalian systems. Wasmuth and Caskey selected Chinese hamster lung (CHL) fibroblasts resistant to AZCA in a single step after mutagenesis, and these were shown to be 3- to 3.5-fold more resistant to AZCA than parental cells.[10] No karyotypic changes were apparent. In two resistant clones, more rapid conversion of glutamic acid to proline, leading to overproduction of proline was detected, and the conversion of glutamic acid to proline was not inhibited by AZCA as it was in the parental cells.

Subsequently, Hooper et al selected AZCA resistant variants of a Chinese hamster cell

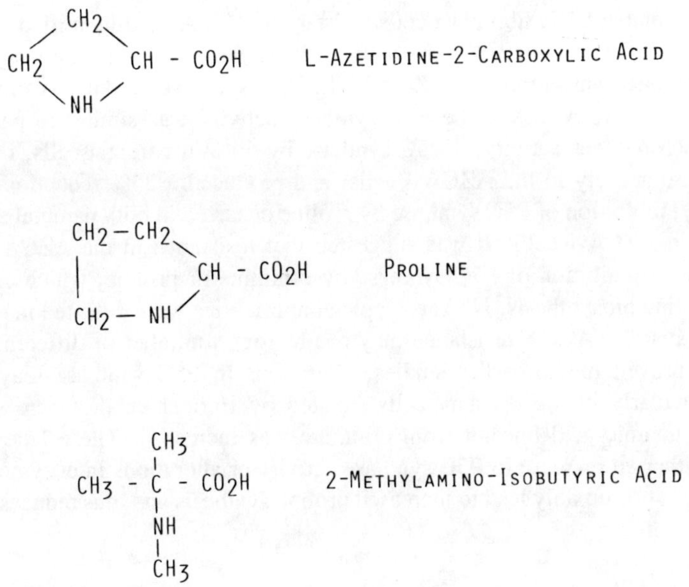

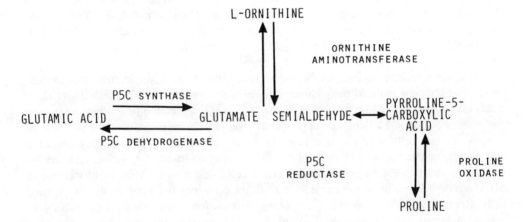

FIGURE 6.    Structures of L-azetidine-2-carboxylic acid and 2-methylamino-iso-butyric acid, analogues of proline.

FIGURE 7.    Pathways of proline biosynthesis and degradation in mammalian cells. [Pyrroline-5-carboxylate(P5C)]

line.[11] AZCA[R] cells were obtained using a multistep selection procedure, and cells isolated after three selection steps were more than 100-fold more resistant to AZCA than parental cells. These AZCA[R] cells were shown to be cross resistant to other proline analogues which competed for incorporation into protein (e.g., 3,4-dehydroproline), but not to 4-thioproline which competes with proline for uptake. The synthesis of proline from glutamic acid was increased significantly in the AZCA[R] cells, while the synthesis from ornithine was unchanged. Karyotypic changes were detected in the AZCA[R] cells, including the addition of two marker chromosomes, and extra chromosomal material on one homolog each of three chromosomes. Preliminary studies suggested that the resistant phenotype showed partial dominance in cell X cell hybridization. Although the exact mechanism of resistance was undefined, these findings might suggest amplification of the gene for the enzyme pyrroline-5-carboxylate (P5C) synthase involved in the conversion of glutamic acid to glutamate — semialdehyde.

Smith et al. isolated CHL fibroblast cells resistant to AZCA, and identified alterations in P5C synthase in resistant cells.[12,13] Two mutant clones were selected in a single step after mutagenesis. In one resistant clone, AZCA[r]1, the P5C synthase activity was increased 30-fold, while in another, AZCA[r]4, the P5C synthase activity was similar to parental cells. Ornithine, which reduces activity of P5C synthase by 50% in parental cells, had no effect on P5C synthase activity in the AZCA[r]4 cells, and produced a 25% reduction in AZCA[r]1 cells. Similarly, inhibition of P5C synthase by proline occurred in both parental and AZCA[r]1 cells, but not in AZCA[r]4 cells. It was suggested that resistance in the AZCA[r]4 cells was due to the lack of inhibition of P5C synthase by ornithine or proline, which could lead to accelerated proline biosynthesis. No karyotypic abnormalities were detected in either clone.

Thus it appears that AZCA-resistance may result from a number of different mutations. Although not proven in the earlier studies, alterations in P5C synthase may have been involved, particularly in the resistant cells isolated by Hooper et al. where synthesis of proline from glutamic acid but not from ornithine was increased. These latter alterations may involve either an increase in P5C synthase activity or alterations in enzyme regulation. All these changes presumably lead to increased proline synthesis and thus reduces the toxicity of AZCA.

### 5. Methionine Adenosyl Transferase Overexpressors

Cycloleucine is an analog of methionine (Figure 3), and a competitive inhibitor of methionine adenosyltransferase (MAT), the enzyme which catalyzes the formation of S-adenosylmethionine from methionine and ATP. A number of human tumor cell lines have been found to be methionine dependent, and the use of different methionine analogs, including cycloleucine, for chemotherapeutic purposes has been suggested. Using cycloleucine, inhibition of cell growth has been shown to correlate with inhibition of S-adenosylmethionine biosynthesis.[46]

Cycloleucine resistant cells have been obtained. After finding single step selection unsuccessful, Caboche isolated baby hamster kidney cells resistant to this analogue by alternately exposing cells to 3 to 4 day cycles of growth first in low methionine medium containing cycloleucine, then in methionine supplemented medium lacking cycloleucine.[14] After 10 selective cycles, cells were plated at low cell density in the same methionine/cycloleucine concentrations and resistant clones isolated. This selection resulted in stable cycloleucine resistance, about threefold greater than parental cells, and a two- to threefold increase in MAT activity. The Km of the enzyme in resistant cells was the same as that in parental cells. Regulation of MAT activity in resistant cells by low methionine concentrations remained demonstrable, although very high methionine concentrations, which have little effect on the parental cells, decreased the MAT specific activity in the resistant cells. Karyotypic abnormalities were present in the resistant cells, primarily an increase in chromosome number.

Caboche and Mulsant subsequently isolated single step cycloleucine-resistant CHO cells,[15] at a frequency which was not affected by mutagenesis. Cycloleucine-resistant lines were stable when grown without selection, and showed a codominant phenotype in cell X cell hybridization studies. Cells were found to be cross-resistant to selenomethionine and S-isobutyladenosine, both inhibitors of MAT activity. Up to eightfold increases in S-adenosylmethionine concentrations were seen in the resistant cells, which correlated with increased MAT activity in resistant cells. Addition of cycloleucine to the medium, which does not significantly affect MAT activity in parental cells, resulted in a superinduction of the enzyme in cycloleucine resistant cells.

Although further characterization of the mechanism of cycloleucine resistance in these cells has not been reported, these studies do suggest overproduction and perhaps altered regulation of MAT in response to the amino acid analog.

## B. Aminoacyl-tRNA Synthetase Overproducers

Aminoacyl-tRNA synthetases are crucial housekeeping enzymes since they catalyze the first committed reactions in protein synthesis. In order to obtain mutants which overproduced aminoacyl-tRNA synthetases investigators have used protein synthesis inhibitors such as macrolides and amino alcohols which specifically affect aminoacylation of tRNA. Lobban, Murialdo, and Siminovitch tested a number of amino alcohols for cytotoxicity on CHO cells (personal communication). Of these only histidinol and tryrosinol proved to be effective at low drug concentrations.

### 1. Histidinol-Resistant Lines

The histidine analog, histidinol, was particularly useful since it does not affect the transport of histidine, does not itself become acylated to tRNA and consequently incorporated into protein, and yet it reversibly inhibits protein synthesis at low concentrations.[47] Histidinol is produced during histidine biosynthesis in prokaryotes and lower eukaryotes, but this pathway is not functional in mammalian cells. Recently histidinol has been tested in combination chemotherapy since it arrests the growth of normal cells but not of tumor cells. It was found to enhance the effectiveness of other agents such as ara-C and 5-FU, which require proliferation for toxicity.[48,49]

Mutant lines resistant to histidinol have been isolated in single and multiple steps.[16] Single step HisOH[R] cell lines are approximately four-fold more resistant to the drug than the parental cell line. This slight increase in drug resistance was greatly increased by growing the cells in gradually increasing concentrations of the amino alcohol. HisOH[R] cell lines with increases in drug resistance of almost 300-fold have been obtained by this method.[16]

Unlike the previously described overproducers (e.g., Alb[R] and Msx[R] cell lines) where extremely high levels of enzyme activity were correlated with the high level of resistance, Tsui et al. found that the highly resistant multistep HisOH[R] lines exhibited at most a 30-fold increase in HisRS activity.[16] The defect in the HisOH[R] mutants did not appear to be in the structural gene for the histidyl-tRNA synthetase since biochemical properties of the enzyme, such as $K_m$ and $K_i$, remained unaffected.[16] The HisOH[R] lines have also been used to show that HisRS contains phosphoserine.[50]

The increased level of HisRS activity was correlated with an increase in mRNA and this enriched source was used to prepare a cDNA probe for HisRS. Using this probe Tsui et al. found that the gene for HisRS was amplified in the HisOH[R] line and that the increases in DNA copy number correlated directly with the level of mRNA and amount of HisRS protein.[16]

### 2. Tyrosinol-Resistant Lines

Tyrosinol has been shown to inhibit CHO tyrosyl-tRNA synthetase with respect to tyrosine (Andrulis and Siminovitch, unpublished observations), however, the specific mechanism of action of tyrosinol has not been characterized. Tyrosinol-resistant (TyrOH[R]) CHO cell lines were isolated by the same protocol used to obtain HisOH[R] mutants and the properties of the TyrOH[R] and HisOH[R] mutants were quite similar. In the initial steps of selection TyrOH[R] cell lines exhibited only twofold increases in D10 over the parental line and Six- to tenfold elevations in specific activity of TyrRS (Andrulis and Siminovitch, unpublished data).

Because the selection protocol was designed to obtain gene amplification mutants and the highly resistant cell lines overproduced enzymatic activity, it was possible that these lines had other properties associated with gene amplification, such as karyotypic alterations. In fact, years ago Worton et al. had detected a chromosome containing a translocation and a lightly staining region in one of the original single-step TyrOH[R] mutants.[51]

On examination of the karyotypes, the TyrOH[R] cell lines were found to contain specific chromosomal abnormalities affecting the CHO chromosome Z2 (Worton, Duff, Siminovitch, and Andrulis, unpublished observations). This chromosome is equivalent to the Chinese hamster chromosome 2 with an interstitial deletion of some material.[51] It was particularly interesting that some of the TyrOH[R] cell lines have extensive HSRs even at low levels of drug resistance (Plate 4*). Thus TyrOH-resistance is unlike other gene amplification systems where HSRs are detected only in the highly resistant cell lines. The HisOH[R] cell lines also have karyotypic alterations which affect the Chinese hamster chromosome 2. In some cases there is a multiple chromosome 2 and in other resistant lines HSRs (unpublished observations). It is likely that the genes for HisRS and TyrRS are located on Chinese hamster chromosome 2 and it is interesting that another aminoacyl-tRNA synthetase, LeuRS, maps to this chromosome as well. Further studies remain to be performed in order to verify that this is indeed the location of the TyrRS and HisRS genes.

### 3. Borrelidin-Resistant Lines

Drugs other than amino alcohols have also been useful for the selection of mutants which overproduce aminoacyl-tRNA synthetases. An example is the macrolide antibiotic, borrelidin, which specifically inhibits threonyl-rRNA synthetase (ThrRS). To obtain mutants of mammalian cells Gantt et al. selected single-step mutants of CHO cells resistant to borrelidin in medium containing reduced threonine.[17] The cell line isolated in this manner was only threefold more resistant to borrelidin than the parental line and exhibited only a threefold increase in ThrRS activity. The single-step mutant was recessive in hybrids and most likely was not due to gene amplification.

On the other hand, when Gerken and Arfin used a multistep selection protocol they were able to isolate a borrelidin-resistant line which was greater than 1000-fold more resistant than the parental line.[18] These cells contained 60 to 100-fold more ThrRS protein as determined by immunoblotting and immunoprecipitation with anti-ThrRS serum, yet they expressed only a 10- to 20-fold increase in ThrRS specific activity. There did not appear to be a structural change in the protein which could account for this since no alterations were observed in thermostability and $K_M$s. This does not, however, rule out a mutation leading to a catalytically less efficient enzyme which was overproduced. The latter possibility appears to be less likely since it requires two alterations. Gerken and Arfin[18] offer other possibilities for the discrepancy between the increase in protein and specific activity of ThrRS. They suggest that since some aminoacyl-tRNA synthetase exist in complexes the activity of the enzyme may differ when it is not involved with the complex. The other explanation is that since ThrRS has been shown to contain phosphoserine the specific activity of the enzyme might be regulated by the level of phosphorylation.[53]

### C. Amino Acid Transport Mutants

Amino acids and their analogs have been useful for the selection of resistant mutant lines with alterations in one or several amino acid transport systems. In most cases these mutants have been isolated from parental lines with increased requirement for a particular amino acid. The selection schemes have utilized high concentrations of an amino acid or analogue which competes for the same transport mechanism, or growth conditions deficient in the required amino acid. These mutants provide an opportunity to define the amino acid transport systems (A, ASC, and L, as described below) and the mechanisms of substrate-mediated control.

### 1. "A" System Mutants

The A or alanine-preferring system of amino acid transport is sodium dependent and transports mainly the amino acids with short, polar, or linear side chains, such as alanine, glycine, and proline. The function of system A is usually assayed by measurement of that

---

\* See Plate 4 following p.24.

part of the uptake of a test amino acid in a sodium-containing buffer that is inhibited by 2-methylaminoisobutyric acid (MeAIB, Figure 6), a nonmetabolizable analog.[54] The transport activity of the A system is repressed by high intracellular concentrations of substrate amino acids. Under conditions of amino acid starvation, the velocity of amino acid transport through the A system increases markedly.[19,55] This de-repression is prevented by incubation with either actinomycin-D or cycloheximide, suggesting that transcription of mRNA and subsequent protein synthesis is required for the increase in A system activity.

### a. Isolation of Alanine-Resistant Lines

Using a Chinese hamster ovary line CHO-K1 which is a proline auxotroph, Moffett et al selected alanine-resistant mutants with increased velocity of proline transport.[19,20] In the parental CHO-Kl line, growth is strongly inhibited by amino acids which are transported by the A system. These amino acids competitively inhibit transport of proline, which is required for growth of procells. Mutant lines were derived in a single step following EMS mutagenesis by selection in a low concentration of proline (0.05 m$M$) and a high concentration of alanine (25 m$M$). Subsequently, it was shown that EMS mutagenesis increased the frequency of isolation of alanine-resistant (ala$^r$) clones by more than 50-fold. Resistant clones were tested to exclude reversion to the pro$^+$ phenotype. The remaining pro$^-$, ala$^r$ clones were shown to survive due to increases in one or more of the systems transporting proline, so that in the presence of a competing amino acid, sufficient proline enters the cell to allow near normal intracellular proline concentrations and permit protein synthesis and growth.

### b. Increase in "A" System Transport

Three resistant clones (ala$^r$2, 4 and ala$^R$3), selected by this means were characterized, and shown to have elevated rates of proline transport through the A system. Using kinetic studies of proline transport in these clones it was shown that the mutations in ala$^r$2 and ala$^r$4 resulted in an increase in the $V_{max}$ with no significant change in the $K_m$, while that in ala$^R$3 resulted in changes in both $K_m$ and $V_{max}$. A similar increase in the transport of MeAIB suggested that the changes in the alanine resistant lines were not confined to the transport of proline alone, but rather were changes in the A system affecting the transport of other related amino acids. In addition, these mutants also showed an increase in amino acid transport through two other sodium-dependent systems, the ASC and proline (P) systems.

Moffett and Englesberg found that CHO-K1 cells exhibited a 6.5-fold increase in proline transport when exposed to starvation conditions for 24 hr.[19] Under similar derepression conditions, ala$^r$2, which had twice the basal level of proline transport, also showed an increase in activity to the derepressed level seen in CHO-K1 cells, while ala$^R$3 cells which express a twofold increase in A system activity under repressed conditions, exceeded the level of transport of CHO-K1 cells by two fold when grown under amino acid starvation conditions. In contrast, the ala$^r$4 cells, with five times the velocity of proline transport under repressed conditions, showed no change in activity with depression.

In cell X cell hybridization studies, both ala$^r$2 and ala$^r$4 behaved recessively, while the phenotype of ala$^R$3 appeared to be codominant. Ala$^r$2 and ala$^R$3 were stable phenotypically when grown in the absence of selection for at least 2 months. When CHO-K1 cells were derepressed by starvation, then exposed to proline, the A system activity dropped rapidly by 40% over the first 30 min, then declined slowly thereafter.[19] This initial rapid drop, which was coincident with the maximum uptake of proline, was reversible by subsequent starvation in the presence of cycloheximide, suggesting the rapid decrease was due to *trans*-inhibition, while the slow decline was attributed to proline induced inactivation of the A system carrier. Both *trans*-inhibition and inactivation occurred in the ala$^r$2 and ala$^R$3 cells, while the initial rapid 40% decrease in activity was seen in the ala$^r$4 cells, but no further decline was observed over a 6-hr period. This suggested that *trans*-inhibition still occurred in the ala$^r$4 mutant, but the cells were resistant to proline induced inactivation.[20]

From these studies, Moffett and Englesberg proposed the following mechanisms of altered proline transport for each of these mutants. Ala$^r$2 was believed to be a partial constitutive mutant, with twice the rate of proline transport under repressive conditions, and behaved like the parental line under derepressive conditions. Ala$^r$4 was proposed to be a fully constitutive mutant for the A system, being completely derepressed under conditions that repress the parental cell. Ala$^R$3, however, behaved like a structural mutation with double the A system activity, since (1) it had twice the velocity of proline transport during both repressed and derepressed conditions, (2) it showed an increase in both $V_{max}$ and $K_m$, and (3) it behaved codominantly in hybrids.

From the alterations seen in these mutants, the above authors proposed a model for the regulation of the A system in CHO-K1 cells.[19] Under this model, the A system is considered to be a repressible system under negative control of a regulatory gene, whose product is also able to inactivate an A system carrier protein. The concomitant increase in transport of proline through the ASC and P systems seen with all three mutants suggests that there are common elements to all three systems. In the case of ala$^r$2 and ala$^r$4 this would involve a common regulatory protein, but in ala$^R$3 perhaps it would involve some protein shared by the A, ASC, and P systems. Further work with these and other mutants will be necessary to characterize the genes involved in transport through these systems.

*2. ASC System Mutants*

The ASC system is also a sodium dependent transport system. However, it is not inhibited by MeAIB, and shows a preference for alanine, serine, and cysteine. Serine is primarily transported by the ASC system in CHO-K1 cells, and inhibition of amino acid transport by serine has been used to determine transport by the ASC system in these cells.[20]

Ertsey and Englesberg used the CHO-K1 pro-cells to select mutants for the ASC system, using MeAIB, which inhibits uptake specifically through the A system.[21] This permitted selection for mutations with increased proline transport by other than the A system. Mutant cells were again selected in a single step following EMS mutagenesis, by exposure to limiting proline (0.05 m$M$), and a concentration of MeAIB (5 m$M$) causing 95% inhibition of growth in the parent line.

A MeAIB resistant clone, MeAIB$^r$22 was isolated and characterized. This line was significantly more resistant to MeAIB than the parent, and showed cross-resistance to other amino acids which inhibit proline transport, such as serine, methionine, and aminoisobutyric acid. When grown in nonselective media, 75% of the resistance was maintained over a one month period. MeAIB$^r$22 cells had a 1.6-fold increase in the rate of proline transport compared to the parental line. This increase was due to a 5.4-fold increase in the transport of proline through the ASC system, usually a minor system involved in proline transport. The increase in the ASC system fully accounted for the resistance of MeAIB$^r$22 cells to MeAIB. The $K_m$ and $V_{max}$ for serine transport through the ASC system of MeAIB$^r$22 cells were found to be 1.8- and 6-fold greater than in the parent CHO-K1 cells. Cell × cell hybridization studies indicated that MeAIB$^r$22 behaved recessively, suggesting that the increase in the ASC system was due to a mutation in a regulatory gene specific for the ASC system. Mutations in a regulatory transacting repressor could lead to increased production of an ASC carrier.

*3. "L" System Mutants*

The L or leucine-preferring system is sodium independent, and transports primarily the branched chain and aromatic amino acids, such as leucine, isoleucine, valine, and phenylalanine. The L system has usually been assayed by the uptake of an amino acid in sodium-free buffer which is subject to inhibition by 10 m$M$ 2-aminobicyclo[2,2,1]heptane-2-carboxylic acid.[54]

### a. Substrate Mediated Regulation

Substrate mediated regulation of the L system has been shown using a CHO cell line CHO-tsH1, which has a temperature sensitive defect in leucyl-tRNA synthetase.[56] At a marginally permissive temperature (38°C or 38.5°C), the rate of growth of CHO-tsH1cells decreased to 10% of that seen at the permissive temperature (34°C). Increased concentrations of leucine in the medium reversed the temperature sensitivity of growth of CHO-tsH1 cells by increasing the transport of leucine, resulting in greater intracellular leucine pools.[57] Similarly, in the parental line, CHO-S, growth in a limited leucine concentration (0.1 m$M$ or less), caused an increased in L-system transport. Under these conditions, other amino acids transported by the L system (isoleucine, valine, phenylalanine) exhibited increased transport, while no change was observed in the transport of amino acids by the A or ASC systems. Cycloheximide rapidly suppressed the temperature dependent transport enhancement in CHO-tsH1 cells, while actinomycin-D produced no significant inhibition until 4 hr. after addition. This suggested that transcription was not necessary for the increased in L system activity and that regulation of this system occurred at the level of translation.

The regulation of the L system was shown to depend on the level of aminoacylation of tRNA, rather than the size of the intracellular pool of L system amino acids. Enhancement of L system transport was observed when the leucyl-tRNA synthetase mutant was grown at a concentration of leucine sufficient to repress transport in the parental cells.[58] Further support for leucine-mediated regulation of L system activity was shown in CHO-K1 cells, using extensively dialyzed fetal calf serum and lower levels of leucine supplementation.[58]

### b. "L" System Overproduction

In order to obtain mutant lines with increased L system transport, Shotwell et al. placed CHO-tsH1 cells under increased selection.[22] Cells were initially mutagenized with MNNG, then plated in 0.4 m$M$ leucine and grown at 38°C. Subsequently, the temperature was increased to 39°C, a nonpermissive temperature for growth of the parental line. Cells were then selected further in decreasing concentrations of leucine. Three clones with the greatest increase in leucine transport were selected for further characterization.

The uptake of leucine at 34°C was two- to threefold higher in these revertants than in the parental line, with a concomitant increase in the $V_{max}$ of leucine uptake. Whereas the parental line showed a two- to threefold increase in leucine transport at 38.5°C compared to the values at 34°C, only a small increase in transport was seen in the revertant lines. At permissive temperatures, the revertant lines also showed a 1.5 to 3-fold increase in the transport of other amino acids transported by the L system, but no change in amino acids transported by the A or ASC systems. This suggested a specific change in the activity of the L system in the revertants leading to increased intracellular concentrations of leucine and other L system amino acids. The leucyl-tRNA synthetases of the revertants were unchanged from that of the CHO-tsH1 line in terms of size distribution on sucrose gradients, or their thermolability in vitro. The revertant phenotype was found to be stable for at least 62 days under nonselecting conditions, in contrast to the substrate-mediated increases in L system activity which were rapidly reversed by a shift back to growth conditions under which leucine was not limited.[22,57] This suggested a mutation in a negative regulatory gene in the revertant lines leading to constitutively high expression of L system activity.

The CHO temperature sensitive leucyl-tRNA synthetase mutants have also proven useful for mapping a high leucine transport phenotype. Using a hybrid of another leucyl-tRNA synthetase mutant, CHO-ts025C1 X human leukocytes, Lobaton et al found that a temperature resistant phenotype could be due to retention of the human leucyl-tRNA synthetase gene, which mapped to chromosome 5, or to increased leucine transport, which segregated with chromosome 20.[59]

### c. Decreased "L" System Transport

Mutant cell lines with decreased amino acid transport have also been selected and characterized. One such line, CHY-2, was selected from the parent CHO(PEOT/1) line by growth, after EMS mutagenesis, in limited concentrations of leucine while exposed first to BrdU, then to visible light.[60] This process selected for cells with decreased leucine transport and thus decreased ability to grow and divide, making them resistant to the effects of BrdU incorporation and visible light exposure. Cells were then regrown in high concentrations of leucine. The uptake of leucine was shown to be reduced to 62% of the wild-type level in the CHY-2 cells. Similarly, uptake by the A system was reduced to 55% and that of the Ly$^+$ (lysine-preferring) system to 43%. The uptake by the ASC system was unchanged. No alterations in either the intracellular sodium concentration or the fluidity of the plasma membrane were detected, and the pleotropic nature of the mutation in these cells remains to be explained.

### d. Melphalan Resistance

The cancer chemotherapeutic agent melphalan is a nitrogen mustard analog of phenylalanine. Melphalan uptake has been shown to be mediated by the L and ASC systems, and in L1210 leukemic cells selected for resistance to melphalan the L system had previously been shown to be defective. The CHY-2 cells are particularly interesting because although they were selected for decreased amino acid transport, they were also shown to be resistant to melphalan (T11). Under conditions of sodium depletion, the mutant cells showed a threefold increase in the $D_{10}$ for melphalan compared to the parental line. Concurrent exposure to leucine or phenylalanine reduced the cytotoxicity even further, confirming the involvement of the defective L system in the melphalan resistance of the CHY-2 cells.

## III. SUMMARY

Although these various amino acid analogs affect functions ranging from amino acid biosynthesis and protein synthesis to amino acid transport, the ways they have been utilized to study the different systems have certain similarities. Most other drug resistant cell lines have been isolated in a single step to insure that the phenotype is the result of a single lesion. This allows for biochemical comparisons of properties of the target enzymes from parental and resistant cells. However, the systems that we have described have expanded on this analysis by using the genetic selection systems to isolate resistant cell lines in a series of steps in order to generate particular types of mutants. The multistep resistant cell lines are, in general, highly resistant to the selective amino acid analog and express elevated levels of the target protein. The mutations in these lines are often co-dominant in hybrids and associated with karyotypic abnormalities. For four of these systems, (Alb$^R$, Msx$^R$, CAN$^r$, and HisOH$^R$) the drug resistant cells facilitated the cloning of the target genes (asparagine synthetase, glutamine synthetase, argininosuccinate synthetase, and histidyl-tRNA synthetase, respectively). It has been shown for Alb, Msx, and HisOH resistance that the enzyme overproduction was a result of gene amplification, whereas canavanine-resistance was not due to gene amplification. Further studies on the other systems will require cloning of the genes for the overexpressed proteins and will most likely follow similar strategies.

## ACKNOWLEDGMENTS

We thank Dr. Louis Siminovitch for helpful comments on the manuscript and Dr. Ron Worton and Catherine Duff for the karyotype used for Figure 8.

# REFERENCES

1. **Gantt, J. S., Chiang, C-S., Hatfield, G. W., and Arfin, S. M.,** Chinese hamster ovary cells resistant to β-aspartyl hydroxamate contain increased levels of asparagine synthetase, *J. Biol. Chem.,* 255, 4808, 1980.
2. **Andrulis, I. L. and Siminovitch, L.,** Isolation and characterization of Chinese hamster ovary cell mutants resistant to the amino acid analog β-aspartyl hydroxamate, *Somat. Cell. Genet.,* 8, 533, 1982.
3. **Andrulis, I. L., Duff, C., Evans-Blackler, S., Worton, R., and Siminovitch, L.,** Chromosomal alterations associated with overproduction of asparagine synthetase in albizziin-resistant Chinese hamster ovary cells, *Mol. Cell Biol.,* 3, 391, 1983.
4. **Andrulis, I. L., Evans-Blackler, S., and Siminovitch, L.,** Characterization of single-step albizziin-resistant Chinese hamster ovary cell lines with elevated levels of asparagine synthetase activity, *J. Biol. Chem.,* 260, 7523, 1985.
5. **Andrulis, I. L.,** Regulation and amplification of asparagine synthetase, in *Molecular Cell Genetics,* Gottesman, M. M., Ed., John Wiley and Sons, New York, 1985, 489.
6. **Wilson, R. H.,** Methionine sulfoxiomine resistant mutants of CHO cells, *Heredity,* 46, 285, 1981.
7. **Sanders, P. G. and Wilson, R. H.,** Amplification and cloning of the Chinese hamster glutamine synthetase gene, *EMBO J.,* 3, 65, 1984.
8. **Jacoby, L. B.,** Canavanine-resistant variants of human lymphoblasts, *Genetics,* 4, 221, 1978.
9. **Su, T. S., Beaudet, A. L., and O'Brien, W. E.,** Increased translatable messenger ribonucleic acid for argininosuccinate synthetase in canavanine-resistant human cells, *Biochemistry,* p. 2956, 1981.
10. **Wasmuth, J. J. and Caskey, C. T.,** Biochemical characterization of azetidine carboxylic acid-resistant Chinese hamster cells, *Cell,* 8, 71, 1976.
11. **Hooper, M. L., Carritt, B., Goldfarb, P. S. G., and Slack, C.,** Variant Chinese hamster cells resistant to the proline analog L-Azetidine-2-carboxylic acid, *Somat. Cell. Genet.,* 3, 313, 1977.
12. **Smith, R. J., Lodato, R. F., Valle, D. L., and Kazakis, A.,** Mutant cell lines resistant to azetidine carboxylic acid: quantitative and qualitative differences in pyrroline-5-carboxylate synthetase activity, *Biochem. Biophys. Res. Commun.,* 99, 789, 1981.
13. **Lodato, R. F., Smith, R. J., Valle, D. L., and Crane, K.,** Mutant cell lines resistant to azetidine-2-carboxylic acid: alterations in the synthesis of proline from glutamic acid, *J. Cell. Physiol.,* 119, 137, 1984.
14. **Caboche, M.,** Methionine metabolism in BHK cells: the regulation of methionine adenosyltransferase, *J. Cell. Physiol.,* 92, 407, 1977.
15. **Caboche, M. and Mulsant, P.,** Selection and preliminary characterization of cycloleucine-resistant CHO cells affected in methionine metabolism, *Somat. Cell. Genet.,* 4, 407, 1978.
16. **Tsui, F. W. L., Andrulis, I. L., Murialdo, H., and Siminovitch, L.,** Amplification of the gene for histidyl-tRNA synthetase in histidinol resistant Chinese hamster ovary cells, *Mol. Cell. Biol.,* 5, 2381, 1985.
17. **Gantt, J. S., Bennett, C. A., and Arfin, S. M.,** Increased levels of threonyl-tRNA synthetase in a borrelidin-resistant Chinese hamster ovary cell line, *Proc. Natl. Acad. Sci. U.S.A.,* 78, 5367, 1981.
18. **Gerkin, S. C. and Arfin, S. M.,** Chinese hamster ovary cells resistant to borrelidin overproduce threonyl-tRNA synthetase, *J. Biol. Chem.,* 259, 9202, 1984.
19. **Moffett, J. and Englesberg, E.,** Recessive constitutive mutant Chinese hamster ovary cells (CHO-K1) with an altered A system for amino acid transport and the mechanism of gene regulation of the A system, *Mol. Cell. Biol.,* 4, 799, 1984.
20. **Moffett, J., Curriden, S., Ertsey, R., Mendian, E., and Englesberg, E.,** Alanine-resistant mutants of Chinese hamster ovary cells, CHO-K1, producing increases in velocity of proline transport through the A, ASC and P systems, *Somat. Cell Genet.,* 9, 189, 1983.
21. **Ertsey, R. and Englesberg, E.,** Recessive 2-(methylamino)-isobutyrate (MeA1B)-resistant mutant of Chinese hamster ovary cells (CHO-K1) with increased transport through ASC system, *Somat. Cell Mol. Genet.,* 10, 171, 1984.
22. **Shotwell, M. A., Collarini, E. J., Mansukhani, A., Hampel, A. E., and Oxender, D. L.,** Isolation of Chinese hamster ovary cell mutants defective in the regulation of leucine transport, *J. Biol. Chem.,* 258, 8183, 1983.
23. **Stark, G. R. and Wahl, G. M.,** Gene amplification, *Annu. Rev. Biochem.,* 53, 447, 1984.
24. **Schimke, R.,** Summary, in *Gene Amplification,* Schimke, R. T., Ed., Cold Spring Harbor Laboratory, Cold Spring Harbor, New York, 1982, 317.
25. **Horowitz, B., Madras, B. K., Meister, A., Old, L. J., Boyse, E. A., and Stockert, E.,** Asparagine synthetase activity of mouse leukemias, *Science,* 160, 533, 1968.
26. **Patterson, M. K., Jr. and Orr, G.,** L-asparagine biosynthesis by nutritional variants of the Jensen sarcoma, *Biochem. Biophys. Res. Commun.,* 26, 228, 1967.

27. **Boyse, E. A., Old, L. J., Campbell, H. A., and Mashburn, L. T.,** Suppression of murine leukemias by L-asparaginase, *J. Exp. Med.,* 125, 17, 1967.
28. **Horowitz, B. and Meister, A.,** Glutamine-dependent asparagine synthetase from leukemia cells, *J. Biol. Chem.,* 247, 6708, 1972.
29. **Ray, P. N., Siminovitch, L., and Andrulis, I. L.,** Molecullar cloning of a cDNA for Chinese hamster ovary asparagine synthetase, *Gene,* 30, 1, 1984.
30. **Arfin, S. M., Simpson, D. R., Chiang, C. S., Andrulis, I. L., and Hatfield, G. W.,** A role for asparaginyl-tRNA in the regulation of asparagine synthetase in a mammalian cell line, *Proc. Natl. Acad. Sci. U.S.A.,* 74, 2367, 1977.
31. **Andrulis, I. L., Hatfield, G. W., and Arfin, S. M.,** Asparaginyl-tRNA aminoacylation levels and asparagine synthetase expression in cultured Chinese hamster ovary cells, *J. Biol. Chem.,* 254, 10629, 1979.
32. **Gantt, J. S. and Arfin, S. M.,** Elevated levels of asparagine synthetase activity in physiologically and genetically derepressed Chinese hamster ovary cells are due to increased rates of enzyme synthesis, *J. Biol. Chem.,* 256, 7311, 1981.
33. **Nunberg, J. H., Kaufman, R. J., Schimke, R. T., Urlaub, G., and Chasin, L.,** Amplified dihydrofolate reductase genesare localized to a homogeneously staining region of a single chromosome in a methotrexate-resistant Chinese hamster ovary cell line, *Proc. Natl. Acad. Sci. U.S.A.,* 75, 5553, 1978.
34. **Stadtman, E. R.,** Introduction: a note on the significance of glutamine inintermediary metabolism, in *The Enzymes of Glutamine Metabolism,* Prusiner, S. and Stadtman, E. R., Eds., Academic Press, New York, 1973, 1.
35. **Misani, F. and Reiner, L.,** Studies on nitrogen trichloride treated prolamines. VIII. Synthesis of the toxic factor, *Arch. Biochem.,* 127, 234, 1950.
36. **Ronzio, R. A., Rowe, W. B., and Meister, A.,** Studies on the mechanism of inhibition of glutamine synthetase by methionine sulfoximine, *Biochemistry,* 8, 1066, 1969.
37. **Wilson, R. H.,** The structure and expression of the glutamine synthetase gene in CHO cells, *Heredity,* 49, 131, 1982.
38. **Green, M. H., Brooks, T. L., Mendelsohn, J., and Howell, S. B.,** Antitumor activity of L-canavanine against L1210 murine leukemia, *Cancer Res.,* 40, 535, 1980.
39. **Thomas, D. A., Rosenthal, G. A., Gold, D. V., and Dickey, K.,** Growth inhibition of rat colon tumor by L-canavanine, *Cancer Res.,* 46, 2898, 1986.
40. **Green, M. H. and Ward, J. F.,** Enhancement of human tumor cell killing by L-canavanine in combination with radiation, *Cancer Res.,* 43, 4180, 1983.
41. **Irr, J. D. and Jacoby, L. B.,** Control of argininosuccinate synthetase by arginine in human lymphoblasts, *Somat. Cell. Genet.,* 4, 111, 1978.
42. **Su, T. S., Bock, H. G. O., O'Brien, W. E., and Beaudet, A. L.,** Cloning of cDNA for argininosuccinate synthetase mRNA and study of enzyme overproduction in a human cell line, *J. Biol. Chem.,* 256, 11826, 1981.
43. **Amos, J. A., Fleming, B. C., Gusella, J. F., Jacoby, L. B.,** Relative argininosuccinate synthetase mRNA levels and gene copy number in canavanine-resistant lymphoblasts, *Biochim. Biophys. Acta,* 782, 247, 1984.
44. **Boyce, F. M., Anderson, G. M., Rusk, C. D., and Freytag, S. D.,** Human argininosuccinate synthetase minigenes are subject to arginine-mediated repression but not to trans-induction, *Mol. Cell. Biol.,* 6, 1244, 1986.
45. **Jackson, M. J., O'Brien, W. E., and Beaudet, A. L.,** Arginine-mediated regulation of an argininosuccinate synthetase minigene in normal and canavanine-resistant human cells, *Mol. Cell. Biol.,* 6, 2257, 1986.
46. **Porter, C. W., Sufrin, J. R., and Keith, D. D.,** Growth inhibition by methionine analog inhibitors of S-adenosylmethionine biosynthesis in the absence of polyamine depletion, *Biochem. Biophys. Res. Commun.,* 122, 350, 1984.
47. **Hansen, B. S., Vaughan, M. H., and Wong, L.,** Reversible inhibition by histidinol of protein synthesis in human cells at the activation of histidine, *J. Biol. Chem.,* 247, 3854, 1972.
48. **Warrington, R. C., Muzyka, T. G., and Fang, W. D.,** Histidinol-mediated improvement in the specificity of I-β-D-arabinofuranosylcytosine and 5-fluorouracil and L1210 leukemia-bearing mice, *Cancer Res.,* 44, 2929, 1984.
49. **Warrington, R. C. and Fang, W. D.,** Histidinol-mediated enhancement of the specificity of two anti cancer drugs in mice bearing leukemic bone marrow disease, *JNCI,* 74, 1071, 1985.
50. **Gerkin, S. C., Andrulis, I. L., and Arfin, S. M.,** Histidyl-tRNA synthetase of Chinese hamster ovary cells contains phosphoserine, *Biochim. Biophys. Acta,* 869, 215, 1986.
51. **Worton, R. G., Ho, C. C., and Duff, C.,** Chromosome stability in CHO cells, *Somat. Cell. Genet.,* 3, 27, 1977.

52. **Wasmuth, J. J. and Chu, L. -Y.,** Linkage in cultured Chinese hamster cells of two genes, emtB and leuS, involved in protein synthesis and isolation of cell lines with mutations in three linked genes, *J. Cell. Biol.,* 87, 697, 1980.
53. **Gerkin, S. C. and Arfin, S. M.,** Threonyl-tRNA synthetase from Chinese hamster ovary cells is phosphorylated on serine, *J. Biol. Chem.,* 259, 11160, 1984.
54. **Shotwell, M. A., Jayne, D. W., Kilberg, M. S., and Oxender, D. L.,** Neutral amino acid transport systems in Chinese hamster ovary cells, *J. Biol. Chem.,* 256, 5422, 1981.
55. **Heaton, J. H. and Gelahrter, T. D.,** Depression of amino acid transport by amino acid starvation in rat hepatoma cells, *J. Biol. Chem.,* 252, 2900, 1977.
56. **Thompson, L. H., Harkins, J. L., and Stanners, C. P.,** A mammalian cell mutant with a temperature-sensitive leucyl-transferRNA synthetase, *Proc. Natl. Acad. Sci. U.S.A.,* 70, 3094, 1973.
57. **Shotwell, M. A., Mattes, P. M., Jayne, D. W., and Oxender, D. L.,** Regulation of amino acid transport system in Chinese hamster ovary cells, *J. Biol. Chem.,* 257, 2974, 1982.
58. **Moreno, A., Lobaton, C. D., and Oxender, D. L.,** Regulation of amino acid transport system L by amino acid availability in CHO-K1 cells, *Biochim. Biophys. Acta,* 819, 271, 1985.
59. **Lobaton, C. D., Moreno, A., and Oxender, D. L.,** Characterization of a Chinese hamster-human hybrid cell line with increased system L amino acid transport activity, *Mol. Cell. Biol.,* 4, 475, 1984.
60. **Dantzig, A. H., Fairgrieve, M., Slayman, C. W., and Adelberg, E. A.,** Isolation and characterization of a CHO amino acid transport mutant resistant to melphalan (L-phenylalanine mustard), *Somat. Cell. Mol. Genet.,* 10, 113, 1984.

Chapter 15

# CARBOHYDRATE ANALOGS

**J. -P. Thirion and Brian Talbot**

## TABLE OF CONTENTS

I.    Introduction ................................................................ 234

II.   Mutants Resistant to 2-Deoxygalactose ..................................... 234
      A.    Selection of Mutants Resistant to 2-Deoxygalactose .................. 234
      B.    Mutation Rates ..................................................... 237
      C.    Physiological Characterization of the DgA$^R$ Mutants .............. 239
      D.    Galactokinase Activities in Wild-Type and Mutant Cells ............. 239
      E.    Structural Mutations as Detected by Serologically Cross-
            Reacting Material (CRM) in Null-Allele Dga$^R$ Mutants ............ 240
      F.    Recessivity of the Dga$^R$ Phenotype .............................. 241
      G.    Complementation Analysis among the Dga$^R$ Mutants ................ 241
      H.    Mapping of the Dga$^R$ Mutations ................................. 242
      I.    Application of the Dga$^R$ Trait to Study Gene Inactivation and
            Expression ........................................................ 242
      J.    Application of the Dga$^R$ Trait to the Efficient Expression of
            Genes in Mammalian Cells .......................................... 243

III.  Chinese Hamster Somatic Cell Mutants Resistant to 3-O-Methyl-D-
      Glucose ................................................................... 243

IV.   Mutants Resistant to 2-Deoxyglucose ....................................... 244

V.    Summary ................................................................... 245

Acknowledgments ............................................................... 245

References ..................................................................... 245

# I. INTRODUCTION

In somatic cells, the metabolism of D-glucose through the Emden Meyerhof pathway is essential for cell growth and cell cloning. As a result only somatic cell mutants resistant to the four carbohydrate analogs, 2-deoxygalactose (Dga), galactosamine, 3-O-methyl-D-glucose (MG), and 2-deoxyglucose (Dgu) (Figure 1), have been isolated so far since most mutations specific for the catabolic pathway of D-glucose are probably lethal.

# II. MUTANTS RESISTANT TO 2-DEOXYGALACTOSE

In living cells, UDP-Gal is an essential metabolite for growth. UDP-Gal can either be synthesized *de novo* from D-glucose to UDPG or from D-galactose through the Leloir pathways according to the following enzymatic reaction

Gal + ATP $\rightleftharpoons$ Gal-1-P (galactokinase, EC.2.7.1.6)

Gal-1-P + UDPG $\rightleftharpoons$ UDP-Gal + Glu-1-P (uridylyltransferase, EC.2.7.7.12)

UDPG $\rightleftharpoons$ UDP-Gal (UDP-glucose-4-epimerase, EC.5.1.3.2)

2-deoxygalactose (Dga) and galactosamine, two analogs of galactose are also substrates of the same enzymatic reactions.[1] In mammals, their action results in uridylate and phosphate trapping plus inhibition of glycolysis and cell growth.[2-3] Table 1 shows that the plating efficiency of Chinese hamster V79 cells decreases with increasing concentration of Dga. As expected, the addition of galactose to this medium relieves that inhibition in agreement with the theory that Dga and its derivatives are substrates of the galactose pathway. Similar results and conclusions were obtained with galactosamine except that higher concentrations of galactosamine had to be used to reach the same level of inhibition. This effect was then studied with the isolation and characterization of mutants resistant to Dga that are defective for galactokinase, the first enzyme of the galactose pathway.

## A. Selection of Mutants Resistant to 2-Deoxygalactose

Figure 2 shows the plating efficiency curves against drug concentrations of a population of mutagenized and non mutagenized wild-type cells. The increase in the number of colonies resistant to Dga after mutagenesis is suggestive of a genetic modification.[4-5]

Resistant clones were picked in 28 mM Dga and replated in the presence of 28 mM Dga. Three of them, DR2R7, DR2R22, and DR2R1610, were characterized. The inactivation curves of DR2R7 and DR2R22 are similar. They differ from the inactivation curve of DR2R1610 (not shown) whose cloning efficiency was close to 100% between 0 and 55 mM Dga. The R50s (i.e., level of Dga required for 50% inhibition of clone formation) of these three clones were greater than 11 mM Dga. They are considered to be fully resistant to Dga. Clones partially resistant to Dga were obtained using a slightly different procedure. They were selected among mutagenized wild-type cells grown for 4 weeks in the presence of 5.5 mM of Dga instead of 28 mM. Killing was slow. After 4 weeks, the survivors were then seeded at 100 cells/petri dish in the presence of 5.5 mM Dga. Two weeks later one or two clones appeared in each petri dish. Figure 2 shows the inactivation curve of cell line DR2 which is partially resistant to Dga. The R50 of DR2 is about 2.8 mM Dga while the R50 of the wild-type is only 1.1 mM Dga. The resistant mutants were cloned and grown in the absence of Dga for about 70 generations. They were found to retain their Dga resistant phenotype indicating that their resistance is a stable hereditary alteration of normal cells. To determine whether Dga-resistance (Dga[R]) is an adaptation induced by the presence of Dga or the result of a mutational event, a fluctuation test à la Luria and Delbruck,[6] and a

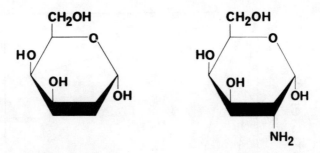

α-D-2 deoxygalactose              α-galactosamine

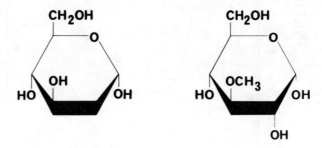

α-D-2 deoxyglucose              3-O-D-Methylglucose

FIGURE 1.   Chemical structures of the carbohydrate analogues.

## Table 1
## PLATING EFFICIENCY OF WILD-TYPE CELLS IN THE PRESENCE OF DIFFERENT CONCENTRATIONS OF GALACTOSE AND 2-DEOXYGALACTOSE

| Dga (mM) | Galactose (mM) | | | | | |
|---|---|---|---|---|---|---|
|  | 0 | 0.7 | 1.4 | 4.2 | 14 | 55 |
| 0 | 138 | 125 | 135 | 114 | 107 | 82 |
| 1.4 | 0 | 31 | 79 | 99 | 93 | 82 |
| 2.8 | 0 | 16 | 59 | 90 | 54 | 74 |
| 7 | 0 | 4 | 23 | 64 | 52 | 80 |
| 14 | 0 | 0 | 8 | 32 | 55 | 55 |

*Note*: About 170 wild-type cells were plated in 6-cm diameter petri dishes in Dulbecco's medium with 8% fetal calf serum, with 11 mM D-glucose and with different concentrations of galactose and 2-deoxygalactose (in mM). The plates were incubated until the clones were big enough (8 — 16 days), to be stained with Giemsa and enumerated.

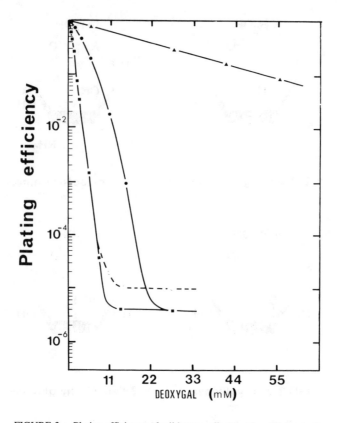

FIGURE 2. Plating efficiency of wild-type cells (■ - ■), wild-type cells mutagenized with ethyl methanesulfonate (0.01% v/v) for four hours and grown for 2 days in the absence of Dga to allow the mutations to be expressed ( ○ - ○). Partially Dga DR2 resistant cells (● - ●), and Dr2R7 subline (▲ - ▲) cells plated in the presence of Dga at the concentrations shown.

Kolmogorov-Smirnov statistical analysis were performed. The results of these tests show the genetic origin and the spontaneous random appearance of the Dga-resistant phenotype in wild-type cells.

Tables 2 and 3 show the results of two fluctuation tests performed with wild-type V79 cells and DR2, a partially resistant mutant.[7] According to Luria and Delbrück,[6] the spontaneous mutational appearance of $Dga^R$ phenotype would cause a large variance distribution for the number of resistant clones per petri dish for the "experiment" case (independent replicate cultures), whereas that number of resistant clones must follow a Poisson's distribution (variance = mean) for the "control" (sampling of the same culture). In contrast, if the phenotypic change is induced by Dga (epigenetic event), the distribution for the number of resistant clones per petri dish must follow a Poisson's law in both "experiment" and "control" cases.

Our data clearly agree with the mutational hypothesis since the ratios of the variance to the mean never exceed two for the "controls" but are always greater than six for the "experiments".

A Kolmogorov-Smirnov test was used to check the compatibility of the observed distribution with Poisson's law, using the calculated mean of each sample as an estimate. We find that all the "controls" are compatible with a Poisson's distribution ($p > 0.05$), whereas the "experiments" are not compatible at high significance levels ($p < 0.001$) with such a law. Thus, the results of fluctuation test experiments are strong evidence for the spontaneous

**Table 2**
**V79 CELL FLUCTUATION TEST FOR THE Dga[R] PHENOTYPE**

| | Experiment | Replicate-sample control |
|---|---|---|
| No. replicate cultures | 37 | 1 |
| No. samplings per culture | 1 | 20 |
| No. of replicates with N | | |
| Dga[R] colonies: | | |
| N = 0 colonies | 27 | 12 |
| 1 | 1 | 2 |
| 2 | 0 | 3 |
| 3 — 4 | 3 | 3 |
| 5 — 8 | 2 | 0 |
| 9 — 16 | 2 | 0 |
| >2000[a] | 2 | 0 |
| No. of Dga[R] colonies per replicate: | | |
| Range | 0 — 12 | 0 — 3 |
| Mean | 1.37 | 0.85 |
| Ratio, variance/mean | 7.1 | 1.6 |
| Mutation rate ($F_o$ calculation) | $1.1 \pm 0.2 \times 10^{-5}$ | |

[a] Although such high values are consistent with the expected fluctuations in a test á la Luria and Delbrück (1943), they were not used for the calculation of the range, mean and variance in order to make the statistical test more sensitive (see text).

**Table 3**
**DR2 CELLS FLUCTUATION TEST FOR THE Dga[R]**
**PHENOTYPE**

| | Experiment | Replicate-sample control |
|---|---|---|
| No. replicate cultures | 36 | 1 |
| No. samplings per culture | 1 | 20 |
| No. of replicates with N | | |
| Dga[R] colonies: | | |
| N = 0 colonies | 13 | 10 |
| 1 | 2 | 0 |
| 2 | 1 | 4 |
| 3—4 | 3 | 5 |
| 5—8 | 6 | 1 |
| 9—16 | 5 | 0 |
| 17—32 | 3 | 0 |
| 33—64 | 1 | 0 |
| 65—128 | 1 | 0 |
| >2000[a] | 1 | 0 |
| No. of Dga[R] colonies per replicate: | | |
| Range | 0 — 65 | 0 — 5 |
| Mean | 7.97 | 1.5 |
| Ratio, variance/mean | 22 | 1.8 |
| Mutation rate ($F_o$ calculation) | $3.5 \pm 0.3 \times 10^{-5}$ | |

[a] See footnote Table 2.

random appearance of cells resistant to Dga in a growing population of wild-type or partially-resistant (DR2 line) cells. This property, plus previous results,[4,8] demonstrate quite clearly that the Dga[R] phenotype results from a true mutational event rather than an epigenetic event.

## B. Mutation Rates

Although the distributions for the frequencies of dishes with a given number of resistant clones in the ''control'' are compatible with Poisson's law, their variances are slightly, but

**Table 4**
**V$_{max}$(SPECIFIC ACTIVITY) AND K$_m$ OF THE**
**WILD-TYPE AND MUTANT STRAINS[a]**

| Strains | Galactose substrate | | 2-deoxygalactose substrate | |
|---|---|---|---|---|
| | K$_m$ (m$M$) | V$_{max}$ | K$_m$ (m$M$) | V$_{max}$ |
| V6 | 0.040 | 4.1 | 1.1 | 20 |
| DR2 | 0.04 | 2.6 | 1.70 | 14.0 |
| DR2R7 | 0.030 | 1.2 | 0.4 | 2.8 |
| DR2R22 | 0.085 | 0.65 | 0.75 | 6.0 |
| DR2R1610 | — | <0.1 | — | <0.1 |
| DR11 | 0.06 | 2.3 | 1.30 | 16 |

[a]   The values in the table are the average of at least 3 experiments. The relative error was 10%.

*Note*:   V$_{max}$: the specific activity is expressed in nmole/min/mg of protein.

constantly, higher than the means (Tables 2 and 3). This suggests that a mechanism perturbs the cloning and then increases the variance of the observed distribution. A detailed analysis of the differences between the predicted theoretical Poisson's distribution and the observed distribution shows that the largest divergence occurs for the frequencies of dishes with either zero or one resistant clone. This indicates that the values of the mean used in the theoretical calculations are a slight overestimate. A simple explanation for this observation is that the manipulation of dishes during the selection procedure (especially changing the medium after three days) causes a splitting of the resistant clones and an increase in their numbers. The frequency of dishes with zero clones remains, of course, unchanged. For that reason, we used and recommend the original F$_o$ method of Luria and Delbrück to calculate the mutation rates,[6] since it is more accurate than other methods that use the means or medians of Lea and Coulson.[9]

The mutation rate for the Chinese hamster V79 cell line (Table 2) is $1.1 \pm 0.2 \times 10^{-5}$ per cell per generation which is in close agreement with the values suggested for Chinese hamster ovary (CHO) cells.[5] In contrast, for the DR2 parental cell line which is already partially resistant, we find a value of $3.5 \pm 0.3 \times 10^{-5}$ per cell per generation, which is significantly ($p > 0.05$) greater and about three times that of the wild-type. Jones and Sargent have similarly isolated mutants partially and fully resistant to 2.6 diaminopurine, deficient in the enzyme adenine phosphoribosyl transferase.[10] They concluded that their wild-type cell line was homozygous diploid ($apt^+/apt^+$), while their partially and fully resistant mutant strains were heterozygous ($apt^+/apt$) and homozygous ($apt/apt$), respectively. If a similar reasoning were applied to our Dga$^R$ cell lines, then the mutation rate of DR2 would be approximately the square root of the mutation rates for V79. This was not observed. We, therefore, propose another explanation since DR2 carries already a mutation affecting the galactose pathway (see Table 4). Using the DR2 line, mutants with fully resistant phenotype can occur through two different processes. The first one is a mutation at a site conferring full resistance to Dga. The second one is a mutation at a site conferring only partial resistance, the combination of which, with the pre-existing mutation in the DR2 cell line, results in full resistance. The expected mutation rate from DR2 to fully resistant mutants would be then slightly higher than that observed when starting from wild-type V79 cells.

In summary then, these fluctuation tests demonstrate that the phenotypic change from Dga sensitivity to resistance occurs spontaneously at random and is not induced by the selection procedure.

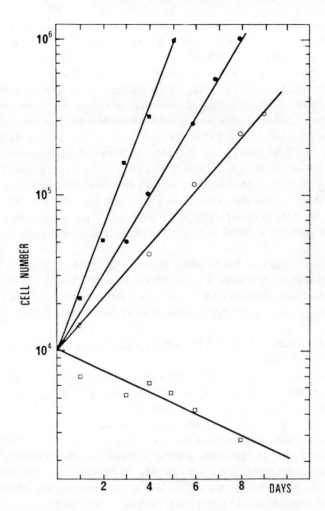

FIGURE 3.   Growth curves of wild-type cells in glucose (■ - ■), of wild-type cells in galactose (● - ●); of DR2R22 cells in galactose (○ - ○), and of DR2R1610 in galactose (□ - □).

## C. Physiological Characterization of the Dga$^R$ Mutants

V79 Chinese hamster cell lines characteristically grow and clone in medium where galactose replaces glucose. Presumably in the V79 cell line, the rate of conversion of galactose to glucose is fast enough to sustain a high rate of glycolysis which is known to be necessary for V79 to grow.[11-14] If Dga$^R$ mutants are altered in their galactose pathways, their growth in the presence of galactose should also be affected. Figure 3 shows the growth curves of the wild-type and some typical mutants in either glucose or galactose medium. As expected, the wild-type and mutant cells grow equally well in glucose with a generation time of about 18 hr. Mutants DR2 and DR11 grow as fast as wild-type in galactose with a generation time of 26 to 28 hr. Mutants DR2R7 and DR2R22 grow in galactose with a generation time of 36 and 44 hr, respectively, while mutant DR2R1610 does not grow at all in galactose. These data and the ones published by Whitfield et al.[5] indicate that some Dga resistant mutants have modified enzymes of the galactose pathway since their growth patterns are altered in galactose but not in glucose medium.

## D. Galactokinase Activities in Wild-Type and Mutant Cells

The growth curves of our mutants and of those isolated by Whitfield et al.[5] in galactose medium correlate with the galactokinase activities of the cell-free crude extracts. The fastest growing cells have the highest galactokinase specific activity. The mutants are defective for galactokinase but not for the transferase or the epimerase.[4-5] Table 4 shows values for galactokinase ranging from about 50% of the wild-type for mutants DR11 and DR2, to 10, 2%, and no detectable activity for mutants DR2R7, DR2R22, and DR2R1610, respectively. The enzyme activities of the cellular extract of the mutants, of the wild-type and of a mixture of both the wild-type and each mutant showed that these changes of specific activity did not result from the presence of inhibitors in the mutants. Moreover the enzyme activity was shown to convert galactose to Gal-1-P (not to Gal-6-P) by chromatography of the reaction product on a $0.7 \times 12$ cm Dowex-1 $\times$ 8 column (200 to 400 mesh-borate form) in borate buffer.[4] To determine whether the resistance to Dga was due to an altered form of galactokinase, the $K_m$s were determined for the wild-type and the mutants with Dga and galactose as substrates. Table 4 shows that, except for DR11, the $V_{max}$ and possibly the $K_m$ of the mutant enzymes are different from those of the wild type. This suggests that DR2, DR2R7 and DR2R22 are probably mutated in their galactokinase structural gene and that the mutations are not regulatory mutations.

Since the galactokinases of the resistant mutants have altered kinetic properties, this suggests that Dga selects for structural rather than regulatory mutations at the $galK^+$ locus. To demonstrate that such mutations exist, mutants without galactokinase activity were isolated to determine whether an inactive protein is being synthesized or not.[8]

## E. Structural Mutations as Detected by Serologically Cross-Reacting Material (CRM) in Null-Allele Dga[R] Mutants

It was initially observed that the cloning efficiency of mutants without any galactokinase activity was higher than for the other Dga[R] mutants. Such mutants were thus preferentially selected by growing mutagenized cells in 27 m$M$ Dga for 3 days and then for a further 14 to 19 days in 44 m$M$ Dga. Using this technique, about one out of every four Dga[R] mutants selected has no detectable galactokinase activity. These cell lines are called thereafter Gal K2, 3, 4, 5, 6, 7, 8, 10, 11 null-allele mutants.[4] These nine independently isolated null-allele mutants were kept and characterized further. They have (like DR2R1610 thereafter renamed GalK1) no galactokinase activity and do not incorporate any detectable tritiated-D-galactose in trichloroacetic acid-precipitable material. These mutants were then tested for the presence or the absence of an inactive galactokinase.

In the following description, the term CRM describes a protein capable of reacting with the antibody directed against purified galactokinase.[15] A precipitation inhibition assay, as described by Beaudet et al.,[16] was used to detect CRM in the cell extract (Table 5). Figure 4 shows a comparison of immune and nonimmune serum for galactokinase immunoprecipitation. The content of CRM or the antigenicity of inactive galactokinase from the Dga[R] null GalK mutants was determined quantitatively according to the arbitrary standard that 100 μℓ of extract (4 mg/mℓ) of V79 cells (wild-type) contains 100% CRM. After addition of 150 μℓ of our dialyzed galactokinase antiserum, we obtained a relative residual enzyme activity of 10% in the supernatant solution. Thus, if the mutant extract contains 100% CRM activity, then the antibody activity will be reduced to less than 10% and upon addition of the wild-type extract, the galactokinase should retain 100% of its activity. If the mutant cells contain no CRM activity, then the antibody should not be complexed and the relative enzyme activity should be inhibited to 10% or less.

All the ten Dga[R], null mutants (Galk1 to GalK11) used in this assay had no detectable galactokinase activity and did not stimulate or inhibit wild-type galactokinase. The sera used were assayed and found to be free of (and specific for) galactokinase activity. Table 5 shows that all the 10 mutants are CRM[+] and contain about the same amount of galactokinase as the wild-type cells in terms of antibody-binding capacity.[8] Thus all ten Dga[R] null GalK mutants arose from mutations at the *galK* structural gene or are defective in posttranslational

## Table 5
## DETECTION OF CRM IN Dga[R] NULL-ALLELE *gal*K MUTANTS

| Cell extract[a] | Initial galactokinase activity[b] | Serum anti-galactokinase activity[b] | Galactokinase added[c] | Final galactokinase activity in supernatants[d] | %CRM in cell extracts |
|---|---|---|---|---|---|
| None | − | + | Yes | 10 | 0 |
| V79 | + | + | Yes | 98 | 100 |
| V79 | + | + | No | 10 | 100 |
| V79 | + | −[e] | Yes | 212 | |
| GalK1 to K11 | − | + | Yes | 90—97[f] | 100 |

[a] The protein concentration in the cell extract was 4 mg/m$\ell$ and all the reaction volumes were adjusted to 400 μ$\ell$.

[b] Arbitrary activity values: +, presence of activity (V79 extract): −, absence of activity (null-mutant extract).

[c] V79 fresh cell extract equivalent to the initial V79 activity was added after the serum and cell extracts had been incubated together for 12 hr. When no extract was added at this step, the antigalactokinase serum precipitated 90% of the initial activity, i.e., it was not added in excess.

[d] Arbitrary units, with 100 signifying a V79 extract and 0 signifying a null-mutant extract.

[e] Nonimmune.

[f] The galactokinase activity had values between 90 and 97 for the ten different mutants.[4]

processing, since the phenotype shows the presence of an enzymatically inactive galactokinase protein in approximately the same concentration as in the wild-type cells.

### F. Recessivity of the Dga[R] Phenotype

Finally, it was considered important to determine (1) if the *gal*K allele is dominant or recessive to the wild-type *gal*K[+] allele and (2) the number of cistrons defined by the different mutations.

Table 6 shows the plating efficiency of some of the hybrids resulting from the fusion between the mutants and the wild-type cells (*gal*K × *gal*K[+] hybrids) and between one mutant and the other mutants (*gal*K × *gal*K hybrids). In the *gal*K[+] × *gal*K fusion, the plating efficiency of the hybrids declined to less than 0.5% as the concentration of Dga was increased from 2.5 to 25 mM. The *gal*K[+] × *gal*K[+] control hybrids showed the same behavior. These results were confirmed by Whitfield et al.[5] This indicates that the ten *gal*K mutations are recessive to the wild-type *gal*K[+] allele.[8]

The above results above were confirmed biochemically. Table 6 shows the galactokinase activity of the different hybrid combinations. As expected, the *gal*K × *gal*K[+] hybrids had about half the galactokinase specific activity of the *gal*K[+] × *gal*K[+] control hybrids and the *gal*K[+] cell lines, whereas the *gal*K × *gal*K hybrids had no detectable activity. These results establish the recessivity of the *gal*K mutations to the wild-type allele.

### G. Complementation Analysis among Dga[R] Mutants

A genetic analysis was carried out with all 10 independent null-allele *gal*K mutants. Each mutant was hybridized with each of the other null-allele *gal*K mutants and with itself. The hybrids were selected by their inability to grow in the presence of galactose (Gal[−] phenotype) in 25 m*M* galactose instead of glucose. As a control, the mutants were also hybridized with A13G9, 34A13G32, and V6IG15 which are Gal[−] mutants and defective in the electron transport system from NADH to coenzyme Q.[11] The 10 mutants analyzed did not complement each other but, as expected, complement the three Gal[−] mutants, A13G9, 34A13G32, and V6IG15.[11] These results demonstrate quite clearly that the 10 null *gal*K independent mutants are in the same complementation group and define therefore one functional genetic unit.

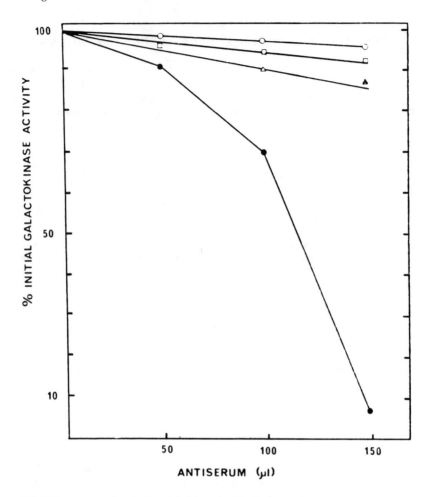

FIGURE 4. Immunoprecipitation of galactokinase. Shown is the galactokinase activity remaining in V79 cell extracts after immunoprecipitation with rabbit anti-hamster galacto-kinase serum (●) or nonimmune serum (○) and the galactokinase activity remaining in mouse LMTK cell extracts after immunoprecipitation with rabbit anti-hamster galactokinase serum (△) or nonimmune serum (□). Note that the graduations on both axes follow the pattern of a linear scale.

Thus all our Dga[R] null *gal*K mutants define one cistron and arose from mutations in the structural gene for galactokinase or are defective in posttranslational processing, since the phenotype shows the presence of an enzymatically inactive galactokinase protein in approximately the same concentration as in the wild-type cells.

### H. Mapping of the Dga[R] Mutations

The localization of the *galK*[+] locus was determined by McBride et al.[17] and McBreen et al.[18] They observed that the galactokinase locus was linked to the autosomal thymidine kinase of locus (*tyk*[+]). In human cells the regional localization is on band q21-22 of chromosome 17.[19-20] In mouse, it is on chromosome 11. Therefore, although not demonstrated here, we shall assume that the Dga[R] mutations which define the structural gene locus for galactokinase is also linked to the *tyk*[+] locus.

### I. Application of the Dga[R] Trait to Study Gene Inactivation and Expression

Resistance to Dga was used to investigate gene inactivation in somatic cells. Using a Chinese hamster ovary (CHO) cell line rather than V79, Bradley isolated two classes of cell

**Table 6**
## RECESSIVITY OF THE *Gal*K ALLELE OVER THE WILD-TYPE *Gal*K$^+$ ALLELE

| Hybrid cells | Galactokinase activity[a] | D-H$^3$ galactose incorporation (%)[b] | Plating efficiency[c] (%) at a Dga concentration of | |
|---|---|---|---|---|
| | | | 2.5 m$M$ | 25 m$M$ |
| *Gal*K$^+$ × *Gal*K$^+$ | 5.2 | 100 | 2 ± 0.5 | < 0.5 |
| *Gal*K$^+$ × *Gal*K$^d$ | 2 — 3.5[e] | 68 — 81[e] | 3 ± 0.5 | < 0.5 |
| *Gal*K × *Gal*K$^d$ | < 0.1 | 1.8 — 2.4[e] | 98 | 95 |

[a]   The values are the average of at least three experiments. The relative error was 6%. The galactokinase specific activity is expressed in micromoles of galactose-1-phosphate produced per milligram per minute at 37°C.

[b]   The values are the average of at least three experiments. The relative error was ca. 3%. The incorporations are expressed as a percentage of the *Gal*K$^+$ × *Gal*K$^+$ control hybrid.

[c]   Values represent the mean ± standard deviation.

[d]   For the different 10 mutants.

[e]   Extreme values obtained with the 10 mutants.

lines which were heterozygous at the galactokinase locus.[21] Class I was selected by plating nonmutagenized wild-type cells in 12 m$M$ Dga, a partially selective concentration which underwent subsequent mutation to the *galK/galK* genotype at low frequency. Class II heterozygotes, isolated by sib selection from mutagenized wild-type cells, had a higher spontaneous frequency of mutation to the homozygous state which was not affected by mutagenesis.

It was found that about half of the *galK/galK* mutants derived from a class II heterozygote, but not the heterozygote itself were functionally hemizygous at the syntenic thymidine kinase locus. The low frequency event may be a point mutation, but the high frequency event, in many instances, involves coordinated inactivation of a portion of a chromosome carrying the two linked alleles.

### J. Application of the Dga$^R$ Trait to the Efficient Expression of Genes in Mammalian Cells

The *galK* null allele mutants do not grow on galactose. This property is now used with great efficiency to study the expression and regulation of genes in mammalian cells after transfection.[22-24] In particular it was shown that the transformation of *galK* Chinese hamster cells increased 10- to 100-fold with the presence of enhancers in the transforming DNA.[25]

## III. CHINESE HAMSTER SOMATIC CELL MUTANTS RESISTANT TO 3-O-METHYL-D-GLUCOSE

Hexose accumulation is mediated in most tissue culture via a carrier which involves transport across the plasma membrane using facilitated diffusion and phosphorylation by hexokinase. In order to characterize the glucose transporter, Whitfield et al.[26] have sought hexose transport mutants resistant to killing by 3-O-methylglucose (MG). The results with one mutant show that the mutant cell line is 2- to 3-fold more efficient than the parent in the transport of D-glucose.

CHO cells were mutagenized with ethyl methanesulfonate and grown for 8 days for the phenotypes to be expressed. They were then plated in up to 103 m$M$ 3-O-methyl-D-glucose and 0.3 m$M$ D-glucose.

The parental CHO cells were killed on increasing 3-O-methyl-glucose concentration. In

103 m$M$, the proportion of survivors was about 0.08%. The cytotoxicity of 3-O-methylglucose was reversed by 55 m$M$ D-glucose, suggesting that it resulted from the inhibition of D-glucose transport or metabolism. One highly resistant mutant Meg$^R$24 was obtained which was almost 400-fold more resistant to 103 m$M$ 3-O-methylglucose than the parental cell line. Its phenotype was stable in the absence of selection pressure. In addition to being resistant to MG, Meg$^R$24 was resistant to 2-deoxyglucose (Dgu). At 1.5 m$M$ Dgu, the relative plating efficiency of Meg$^R$24 is approximately 12-fold higher than of the parental cell line. The cross resistance to MG and Dgu suggests a common mechanism which may be glucose transport since both substances are substrates for the glucose carrier.[27]

The kinetics of entry into the ATP-depleted mutant and wild-type cells of D-[H$^3$] glucose, was investigated using Lineweaver-Burk analysis. The apparent K$_m$ for D-glucose transport was 2.7 m$M$ for Meg$^R$24 and 8.9 m$M$ for wild-type cells while their V$_{max}$ values for D-glucose transport were not very different from one another. This suggests that D-glucose transport is three-fold more efficient in Meg$^R$24 than in wild type. These conclusions were confirmed using 3-O-methylglucose to measure D-glucose transport: the apparent K$_m$ for the uptake of 3-O-methylglucose of wild-type is twofold higher than the K$_m$ for Meg$^R$24 while their V$_{max}$ values are similar.

## IV. MUTANTS RESISTANT TO 2-DEOXYGLUCOSE

Mutants resistant to the toxicity of 2-deoxyglucose were isolated by Whitfield et al.[26] as described earlier, Meager et al.[25] and Pouyssegur et al.[28] using different procedures.

Pouyssegur et al. isolated Chinese hamster mutants defective in hexose transport and aerobic glycolysis. Mutagenized cells were incubated in the presence of 2-[$^3$H] deoxyglucose (15 to 25 Ci/mmole) for 1 hr. The cells were then frozen and stored in liquid nitrogen. After 25 days, one third of the cells that survived the tritium suicide selection were found to have less than 50% of the wild-type hexose activity. Clone D57, one of the most markedly affected clones had lost the ability to utilize glucose as a glycolytic substrate, and the production of lactic acid was barely detectable. These results suggested a glycolytic block. Indeed, when compared with the wild-type enzymes, D57 had no detectable phosphoglucose isomerase activity while the activity of other enzymes was not changed. However, because of this primary defect, D57 was also affected secondarily in its glucose transport.

Meager et al.[29] mutagenized baby hamster kidney cells (BHK 21/C13) with methyl-N-nitroso guanidine (0.5 mg/m$\ell$ of culture). The cells were then exposed to increasing concentrations of Dgu (up to 150 m$M$) in 6 m$M$ glucose. A cell line (2dG$^R$) at least 10 to 20 times more resistant to Dgu than the wild-type was isolated. However, if 2dG$^R$ cells were serially passaged in the absence of Dgu for several weeks the sensitivity to Dgu returned to the parental levels. The resistant phenotype was not stable suggesting that the cells may be variants rather than mutants.

The 2dG$^R$ cells were then characterized. The rate of uptake of $^3$H-labeled Dgu by 2dG$^R$ and normal cells was the same. Although Dgu interferes with the normal biosynthesis of BHK cellular glycoproteins,[30] the glycosylation events were equally affected by Dgu in the resistant and sensitive strains suggesting that toxicity of Dgu to normal fibroblasts was not mediated through glycosylation of cellular glycoproteins. Incorporation of radioactive glucosamine, galactose and to a lesser extent manose into glycoproteins was inhibited by Dgu to similar extents in both the wild-type and the resistant cells. However, changes induced by Dgu in the cell surface carbohydrate structure of 2dG$^R$ were detected by altered sensitivities to toxic plant lectins and by surface labeling with $^{125}$I. Three features of the iodine labeling experiment were of particular interest; (1) the apparent loss of labeling of a fraction of 250,000 mol. wt. in 2dG$^R$ cells; (2) the overall low levels of $^{125}$I-labeling; and (3) the enhanced mobility of glycoprotein species when 2dG$^R$ cells were grown in the presence of

Dgu. Without Dgu, the iodination pattern of $2dG^R$ and BHK cells was broadly similar except for the absence of the 250,000 mol. wt. glycoprotein.

## V. SUMMARY

This paper describes three classes of somatic cell mutants resistant to either 2-deoxyga-lactose, 2-deoxyglucose, or 3-O-methyl-D-glucose. Mutants resistant to Dga are the best characterized so far. They have eight important properties namely:

1. The appearance of the resistance phenotype in wild-type populations is a spontaneous and random process. Its rate is ca. $10^5$ per cell per generation.
2. The $galK^+$ locus is most probably hemizygous in the Chinese hamster V79 cell line.
3. The $Dga^R$ phenotype behaves as a recessive trait in somatic cell-cell hybrids.
4. Mutagenic treatment with ethyl methanesulfonate increases the number of resistant clones five to thirty fold in a wild-type population.
5. The $Dga^R$ phenotype is preserved from generation to generation in the absence of Dga, the selective agent.
6. One can detect a galactokinase defect in every $Dga^R$ variant.
7. $CRM^+$ material was detectable in all null-allele mutants.
8. The $galK^+$ locus is autosomal and linked to the thymidine kinase locus.

These eight properties suggest strongly that the $Dga^R$ character is the result of a genetic event at the structural locus for galactokinase.

Two classes of mutants resistant to 2-deoxyglucose have been isolated and characterized as either resistant to 3-O-methyl-D-glucose and defective in glucose transport, or resistant to tritium-suicide selection and defective for phosphoglucose isomerase.

## ACKNOWLEDGMENTS

We thank our many colleagues here and elsewhere for helpful discussions, Nicole Bernard for artful preparation of the manuscript and the MRC and the Canadian NCI for support.

## REFERENCES

1. **Starling, J. and Keppler, D. O.,** Metabolism of 2-deoxygalactose in liver induces phosphate and uridylate trapping, *Eur. J. Biochem.,* 80, 373, 1977.
2. **Smith, D. F. and Keppler, D. O.,** 2-deoxy-D-galactose metabolism in ascites. Hepatoma cells results in phosphate trapping and glycolysis inhibition. *Eur. J. Biochem.,* 73, 83, 1977.
3. **Keppler, D. O., Rudigier, J. F. M., Bischoff, E., and Decker, K.,** The trapping of uridine phosphates by galactosamine, D-glucosamine and 2-deoxygalactose. A study on the mechanism of galactosamine hepatitis, *Eur. J. Biochem.,* 17, 246, 1970.
4. **Thirion, J. P., Banville, D., and Noël, H.,** Galactokinase mutants of Chinese hamster somatic cells resistant to 2-deoxygalactose, *Genetics,* 83, 132, 1976.
5. **Whitfield, C. D., Buchsbaum, B., Bostedor, R., and Chu, E. H. Y.,** Inverse relationship between galactokinase activity and 2-deoxygalactose resistance in Chinese hamster ovary cells, *Somat, Cell Genet.,* 4, 699, 1978.
6. **Luria, S. E. and Delbrück, M.,** Mutations of bacteria from virus sensitivity to virus resistance, *Genetics,* 28, 491, 1943.
7. **Claverie, J. M., Comlan de Souza, A., and Thirion, J. P.,** Mutations of Chinese hamster somatic cells from 2-deoxygalactose sensitivity to resistance, *Genetics,* 92, 563, 1979.

8. **Talbot, B., Comlan de Souza, A., Banville, D., and Thirion, J. P.,** Immunological and genetic characterization of 2-deoxygalactose, galactokinase-deficient mutants of Chinese hamster cells: evidence for structural mutations at the *galK* locus, *Mol. Cell. Biol.,* 4, 2413, 1984.

9. **Lea, D. E. and Coulson, C. A.,** The distribution of the numbers of mutants in bacterial populations, *J. Genet.,* 49, 264, 1949.

10. **Jones, G. E. and Sargent, P. A.,** Mutants of culture Chinese hamster cells deficient in adenine phosphoribosyl transferase, *Cell,* 2, 43, 1974.

11. **Maïti, I. B., de Souza, C. A., and Thirion, J. P.,** Biochemical and genetic characterization of respiratory-deficient mutants of Chinese hamster cells with a Gal⁻ phenotype, *Somat. Cell Genet.,* 7, 567, 1981.

12. **Sun, N. C., Chang, C. C., and Chu, E. H. Y.,** Induction of auxotrophic mutations by treatment of Chinese hamster cells with 5-bromodeoxyuridine and black light. *Proc. Natl. Acad. Sci. U.S.A.,* 69, 3459, 1975.

13. **De Francesco, L., Werntz, D., and Scheffler, I. E.,** Conditionally lethal mutations in Chinese hamster cells. Characterization of a cell line with a possible defect in the Krebs cycle, *J. Cell Physiol.,* 85, 293, 1975.

14. **Soderberg, K., Mascarello, J. T., Breen, G. A. M., and Scheffler, I. E.,** Respiration-deficient Chinese hamster cell mutants: genetic characterization, *Somat. Cell Genetics,* 5, 225, 1979.

15. **Talbot, B. and Thirion, J. P.,** Isolation, purification and partial characterization of galactokinase from Chinese hamster liver, *Int. J. Biochem.,* 14, 719, 1982.

16. **Beaudet, A. L., Roufe, D. J., and Caskey, C. T.,** Mutations affecting the structure of hypoxanthine: guanine phosphoribosyltransferase in cultured Chinese hamster cells, *Proc. Natl. Acad. Sci. U.S.A.,* 70, 320, 1973.

17. **McBride, W., Burch, J. W., and Ruddle, F. R.,** Cotransfer of thymidine kinase and galactokinase genes by chromosome mediated gene transfer, *Proc. Natl. Acad. Sci. U.S.A.,* 75, 914, 1978.

18. **McBreen, P., Orkwiszewski, K. G., Chern, C. J., Mellman, W. J., and Croce, C. M.,** Synteny of the genes for thymidine kinase and galactokinase in the mouse and their assignment to mouse chromosome II, *Cytogenet. Cell Genet.,* 19, 7, 1977.

19. **Orkwiszewski, K. G., Tedesis, T. A., and Croce, C. M.,** Assignment of the human gene for galactokinase to chromosome 17, *Nature,* 252, 60, 1974.

20. **Elsevier, S. M., Kucherlapati, R. S., Nichols, E. A., Creagan, R. P., Giles, R. E., Ruddle, F. H., Willecke, K. and McDougall, J. K.,** Assignment of the gene for galactokinase to human chromosome 17 and its regional localization to band q21-22, *Nature,* 251, 633, 1974.

21. **Bradley, W. E. C.,** Mutation at autosomal loci of Chinese hamster ovary cells: involvement of a high frequency event silencing two linked alleles, *Mol. Cell. Biology,* 3, 1172, 1983.

22. **Schümperli, D., Howard, B. H., and Rosenberg, M.,** Efficient expressions of *Escherichia coli* galactokinase gene in mammalian cells, *Proc. Natl. Acad. Sci. U.S.A.,* 79, 257, 1982.

23. **Berg, P. E., Popovic, Z., and Anderson, W. F.,** Promoter dependence of enhancer activity, *Mol. Cell. Biol.,* 4, 1664, 1984.

24. **Berg, P. E., Sheffery, M., King, R. S., Gong, Y., and Anderson, W. F.,** The expression of integrated DNA depends on copy number, *Exp. Cell. Res.,* 168, 376, 1987.

25. **Berg, P. E. and Anderson, W. F.,** Correlation of gene expression and transformation frequency with the presence of an enhancing sequence in transforming DNA, *Mol. Cell. Biol.,* 4, 368, 1984.

26. **Whitfield, C. D., Hape, L. M., Nugent, C., Urbani, K., and Whitfield, H.,** Increased hexose transport in Chinese hamster ovary cells resistant to 3-0-methyl-D-glucose, *J. Biol. Chem.,* 257, 4902, 1982.

27. **Graff, J. C., Wollihueter, R. M., and Plagemann, P. Q. M.,** Deoxyglucose and 3-0-methylglucose transport in untreated and ATP-depleted Novikoff rat hepatoma cells. Analysis by a rapid kinetic technique, relationship to phosphorylation and effects of inhibitors, *J. Cell Physiol.,* 96, 171, 1978.

28. **Pouyssegur, J., Franchi, A., Salomon, J. C., and Silvestre, P.,** Isolation of a Chinese hamster fibroblast mutant defective in hexose transport and aerobic glycolysis: Its use to dissect the malignant phenotype, *Proc. Natl. Acad. Sci. U.S.A.,* 77, 2698, 1980.

29. **Meager, A., Navin, R., and Hughes, R. C.,** Properties of a baby-hamster-kidney cell line with increased resistance to 2-deoxy-glucose, *Eur. J. Biochem.,* 72, 275, 1977.

30. **Hughes, R. C., Meager, A., and Nairu, R.,** Effect of 3-deoxy-D-glucose on the cell-surface glycoproteins of hamster fibroblasts, *Eur. J. Biochem.,* 72, 265, 1977.

Chapter 16

# MISCELLANEOUS DRUGS - I

**A. K. Dudani, S. Jindal, and R. S. Gupta**

## TABLE OF CONTENTS

I.      Alanosine ...................................................................................248

II.     Auranofin ...................................................................................248

III.    6-Azauridine ...............................................................................248

IV.     Chromate ...................................................................................250

V.      6-Diazo-5-oxo-L-Norleucine .....................................................250

VI.     Glucocorticoid Hormones (Dexamethasone) ...........................250

VII.    25-Hydroxy-Cholesterol..............................................................252

VIII.   6-(p-Hydroxyphenylazo)-Uracil ................................................252

IX.     Methylglyoxal bis (Guanylhydrazone) ......................................253

X.      *N*-Phosphonoacetyl-L-Aspartate (PALA)....................................253

XI.     Phosphonoformic Acid................................................................254

XII.    Tiazofurin....................................................................................255

References.............................................................................................256

# I. ALANOSINE

The antitumor agent alanosine [L-2-amino-3-(*N*-hydroxy *N*-nitrosoamino)propionic acid] (Figure 1) is an analog of aspartic acid which inhibits de novo synthesis of AMP due to inhibition of the enzyme adenylsuccinate synthetase (ASS).[1,2] There is considerable evidence to suggest that L-alanosine is anabolized in vivo into L-alanosyl-AICOR (L-alanosyl-5-amino 4-imidazole carboxylic acid ribonucleotide) which in fact is responsible for the inhibition of ASS.[2,4] As may be expected, the growth inhibitory effects of alanosine can be alleviated by adenine but not by guanine or hypoxanthine.[1,5]

Certain leukemic tumor lines (viz., L1210 and P388) develop resistance to alanosine after being exposed to it, which persists for a long time after the drug is removed.[4,6] It was observed that DNA synthesis in sensitive cells was inhibited by 85% as compared to 20% in the resistant counterparts. In comparison to the sensitive tumor lines, the L-alanosine resistant lines were found to have significantly lower levels of the active metabolite L-alanosyl-AICOR. This reduction in L-alanosyl-AICOR seems to be a direct consequence of decreased activity of the enzyme SAICAR synthetase (5-amino-4-imidazole-*N*-succinocarboxamide ribonucleotide synthetase) which is responsible for the conjugation of L-alanosine and AICOR. In tumors resistant to alanosine, the activities of several purine salvage pathway enzymes viz., adenosine kinase, adenosine phosphorylase, inosine phosphorylase, adenine phosphoribosyl transferase, and hypoxanthine phosphoribosyl transferase were about twofold higher as compared to sensitive cells.[2,6] This increase could counteract the low level of adenine nucleotides produced as a result of the drug. Hence there appears to be two mechanisms by which cells can develop resistance to alanosine: (1) reduced accumulation of L-alanosyl-AICOR due to decreased activity of SAICAR synthetase, and (2) increased utilization of exogenous purines due to an increase in activity of the purine salvage pathway enzymes.

Stable mutants which are about 10- to 20-fold resistant to alanosine have also been isolated in Chinese hamster ovary (CHO) cells after a single-step selection.[7] These mutants show specific resistance only to alanosine and no cross resistance is observed toward other nucleoside analogs or other unrelated drugs. The drug resistant pheontype of these mutants behave codominantly in cell hybrids formed with wild-type cells.[7] However, the cellular function which is affected in these mutants has not yet been identified.

# II. AURANOFIN

Auranofin (AF) (Figure 2) is a gold compound actively used in the treatment of rheumatoid arthritis as it interferes with macrophage function.[8,9] It has been proposed that the active moiety of AF is the gold atom which interacts with sulfhydryl-containing proteins.[10] Mutants resistant to AF have been isolated from CHO cells and have been shown to accumulate metallothionein (MT) (a protein involved in detoxification of heavy metals), mRNA and protein as compared to normal cells.[11] Induction of MT by low concentrations of other metals like cadmium protected the cells against the toxic doses of AF, thus suggesting that increase in MT levels is the mechanism for resistance against gold compounds like AF.

# III. 6-AZAURIDINE

The pyrimidine analog 6-azauridine [6-AZU; (Figure 3)] inhibits the enzyme orotidine-5′-monophosphate (OMP) decarboxylase (ODCase), which catalyzes the last step in uridine monophosphate (UMP) biosynthesis.[12] In order to elicit its action, 6-AZU must first be phosphorylated to form 6-azauridine monophosphate (6-AZUMP) by uridine kinase.[12,13] Mutants resistant to 6-AZU have been isolated from L5178Y leukemia cells by exposing

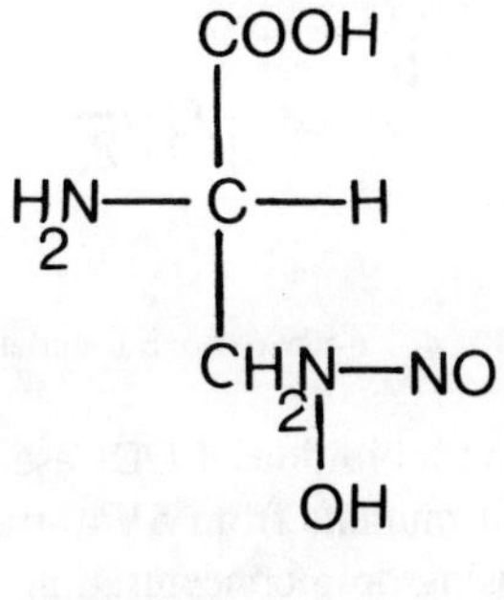

FIGURE 1. Alanosine.

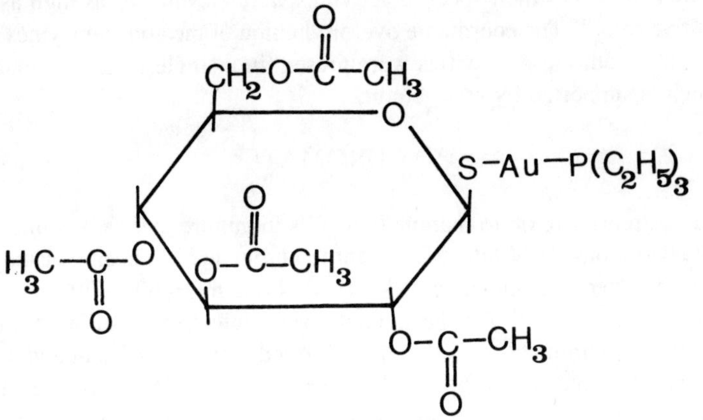

FIGURE 2. Auranofin.

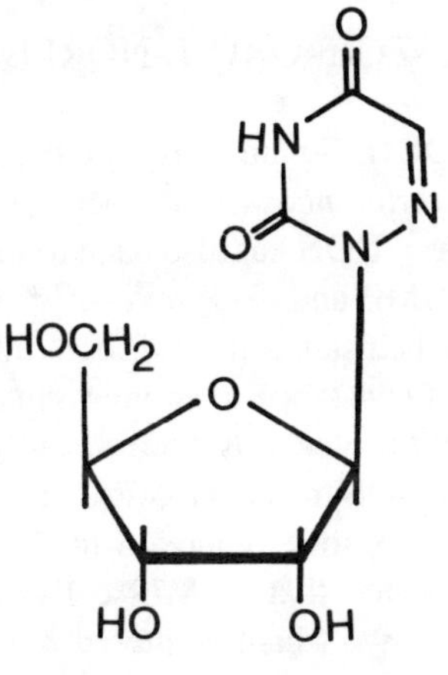

FIGURE 3. 6-Azauridine.

them to gradually increasing concentrations of the analog.[2] These mutants were found to have a defect in uridine kinase as the toxic form of the analog (viz., 6-AZUMP) was not formed. Krooth and coworkers have isolated 6-azauridine resistant mutants from the mouse cell line A9 which also exhibited cross resistance to adenosine, guanosine and thymidine.[14,15] Although the exact mechanism of resistance in these mutants is unclear, it was observed that the level of 5-phosphoribosyl-1-pyrophosphate (PRPP), the common precursor for both purine and pyrimidine synthetic pathways was elevated in these cells. Based on this observation, it has been proposed that an increase in OMP levels, due to the increased PRPP

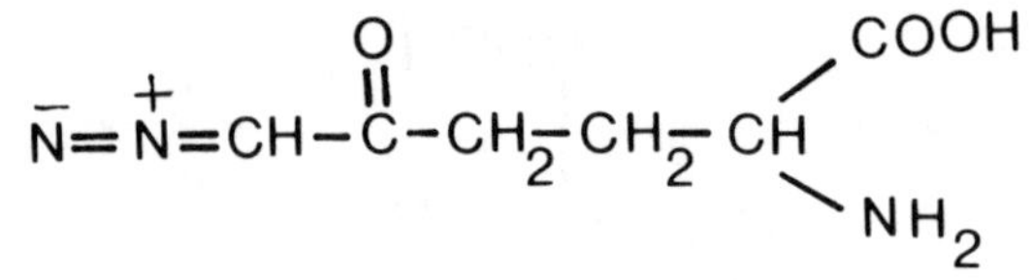

$$\overline{N}=\overset{+}{N}=CH-\overset{\overset{\textstyle O}{\|}}{C}-CH_2-CH_2-\overset{\overset{\textstyle COOH}{\diagup}}{\underset{\diagdown NH_2}{CH}}$$

FIGURE 4.    6-diazo-5-oxo-L-norleucine.

pools, could abolish or diminish the inhibition of ODCase by 6-AZUMP. Suttle and Stark[16] have isolated 6-azauridine resistant mutants from SV40 transformed Syrian hamster $BHK_{21}$ cells after exposing them to increasing drug concentration. They observed that in the mutant cells, the enzymes orotate phosphoribosyltransferase and ODCase were not only resistant to inhibition by 6-AZU but their specific activities were elevated to as high as 67 times the levels in sensitive cells.[16] The coordinate overproduction of the above enzymes in the mutant cells indicated that both these activities were present in a single multifunctional protein, an inference which is supported by other studies.[17]

## IV. CHROMATE

Chromate is extremely toxic to mammalian cells in culture and causes mitotic delay and chromosomal aberrations.[18,19] Mutants resistant to chromate have been isolated from a number of Chinese hamster cell lines like M3-1 (male bone marrow), V79 (male lung), CHO (ovarian fibroblast line), etc.[20] All the mutants were defective in sulfate transport system which is also used by chromate. In cell hybrids formed between resistant and sensitive cells, the chromate resistant phenotype behaved recessively. Genetic complementation analysis indicated that all these mutants are probably affected at a single locus which was linked to the *emt B* locus (conferring resistance to the protein synthesis inhibitor emetine) in Chinese hamster cells.[21]

## V. 6-DIAZO-5-OXO-L-NORLEUCINE

6-Diazo-5-oxo-L-norleucine (DON; Figure 4) is a glutamine analog which inhibits purine nucleotide biosynthesis due to interference with the activity of the enzyme phosphoribosyl-formyl-glycineamidine synthetase.[22] DON has also been found to inhibit guanylate synthetase activity, thereby reducing both GMP and GTP levels.[23,24] Mutants resistant to DON have been selected from V79 Chinese hamster cells.[24] These cells showed specific resistance to DON and did not show any cross resistance to another glutamine analog, O-diazoacetyl-L-serine (azaserine). The mutant phenotype was codominantly expressed in intraspecific cell hybrids. It was observed that in DON resistant cells, guanylate synthase and GTP levels were resistant to inhibition by DON in comparison to the parental cells. Based on these observations, Kaufman has suggested that in V79 cells, cytotoxicity of DON is due to inhibition of GMP synthetase activity, which is altered in the mutant cells.[24]

## VI. GLUCOCORTICOID HORMONES (DEXAMETHASONE)

The glucocorticoid hormone, dexamethasone (Figure 5), which is clinically used as an immunosuppressant and in treatment of lymphoproliferative diseases, exhibits cytotoxicity toward lymphoid cells. The mechanism of cellular action and resistance to dexamethasone has been extensively studied in murine cell lines (S49 line derived from T lymphoma, and W7 or WEH1-7, established from a thymoma) which are highly sensitive to its cytotoxic effects.[25-28] The work on cellular resistance to glucocorticoid has previously been reviewed and only a very brief summary is provided here.[25-28] The reader should refer to the above articles for further details.

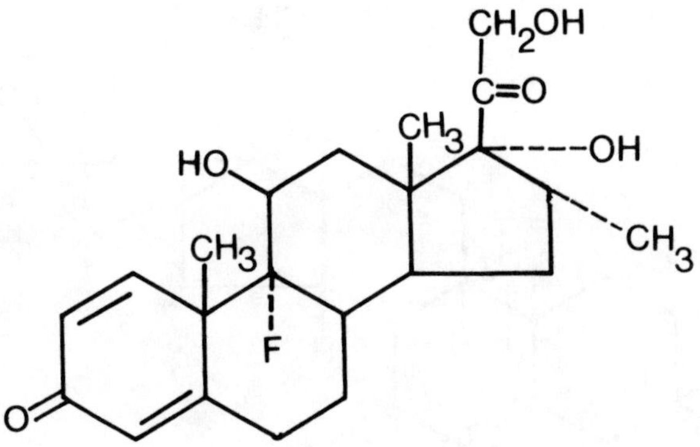

FIGURE 5.    Dexamethasone.

In S49 line, stable single-step mutants resistant to dexamethasone have been isolated at a frequency of $1 \times 10^{-5}$. Prior treatment of the cells with known chemical mutagens causes a dose-dependent increase in the frequency of the mutants.[29] Among these, four different types of mutants have been identified.[25-28] First, the majority (75 to 90%) of these mutants designated as $r^-$ show either no detectable or <25% of the glucocorticoid receptor activity in comparison to the parental cells.[25,26,30] A second group of mutants designated as $nt^-$ (nuclear transfer defective) presumably involve a defect in cytoplasmic receptors so that its nuclear translocation is affected.[26,31] A third type of mutant, in which the transfer of the steroid-receptor complex to the nucleus is increased has been designated as $nt^i$.[25,26,32] These mutants showed increased nonspecific binding of the steroid receptor complex to the chromatin. Most of the mutants of this category had a receptor of reduced molecular weight ($M_r$ 50,000 as compared to 90,000 for the parental cells).[26,28] Another category of mutants designated as $d^-$ (for deathless phenotype) contain apparently normal cytoplasmic receptors and the defect in these mutants may lie subsequent to the nuclear translocation and binding steps.[26,28]

From the W7 line, which displays slightly higher sensitivity to dexamethasone and contains twice as many receptor sites as in the S49 line, successive selection in presence of increasing concentration of dexamethasone has led to the isolation of variant lines which contain either about 50% or no detectable levels of the receptor.[27,30,33,34] The intermediate cell line containing 50% of the receptor sites is very similar to the S49 line in terms of the mutant frequency and other characteristics. This has led Bourgeois and co-workers to suggest that while the W7 line contains two functional copies of the receptor (i.e., $+/+$ genotype), the S49 line is hemizygous (i.e., $+/-$) for this allele.[27,33,34] The development of resistance to high concentration of glucocorticoid in the W7 line thus occurs in two steps ($r^+/r^+ \rightarrow r^+/ r^- \rightarrow r^-/r^-$), an inference supported by the mutation frequency and receptor contents of the lines.[27,33] Mutants resistant to dexamethasone are also obtained at a high frequency in a human leukemia cell line, CEM-C7,[35] indicating that similar to S49 cells, this cell line may also be haploid or functionally hemizygous for the gene encoding glucocorticoid receptor.[27] In cell hybrids formed with wild-type cells, the drug resistant phenotype of the $r^-$, $nt^-$, or $nt^i$ mutants behave recessively.[36] However, no complementation was observed between different types of mutants indicating that they were all affected in the same allele. Recently, the cDNA for the glucocorticoid receptor from rat liver has been cloned, and using this probe, mRNA transcripts from several of the receptor mutants have been shown to be qualitatively and quantitatively altered.[37]

Johnson et al.[38] have isolated another variant of the W7 line (selected by prolonged growth in presence of low concentrations of dexamethasone) which exhibits cross resistance to many unrelated drugs viz. puromycin, colchicine, daunomycin, gramacidin and vincristine. Sur-

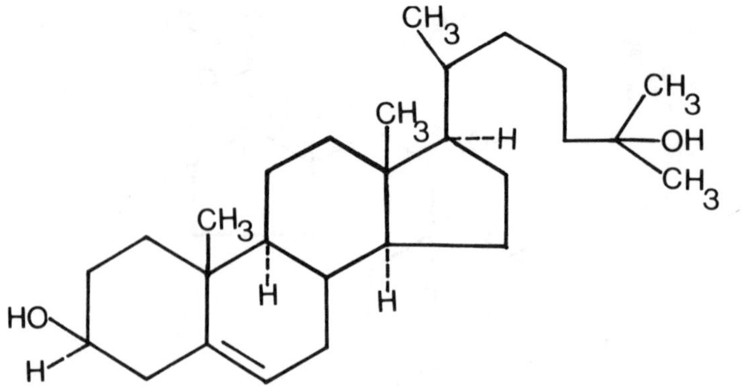

FIGURE 6.    25-Hydroxy cholesterol.

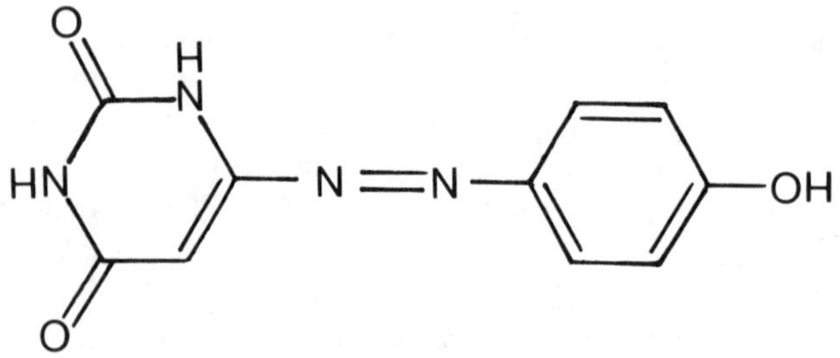

FIGURE 7.    6(p-Hydroxyphenylazo)-Uracil.

prisingly, this variant did not show any cross resistance to triamcinolone, which is structurally related to dexamethasone. The drug uptake and binding studies indicate that resistance of this variant line is due to a membrane permeability alteration.[38]

## VII. 25-HYDROXY-CHOLESTEROL

25-Hydroxy-cholesterol (Figure 6) is cytotoxic to cultured mammalian cells as it inhibits the enzyme 3-hydroxy-3-methyl-gultaryl-coenzyme A reductase (HMG-CoA reductase) responsible for synthesizing mevalonate, a key intermediate in sterol biosynthesis.[39] Mutants resistant to 25-OH-cholesterol have been isolated mainly from the CHO cell line CHO-K$_1$, as well as from a Chinese hamster lung (Dede) line.[40-42] Sinensky (1977) first isolated a 25-OH-cholesterol resistant mutant from CHO-K$_1$ cells and observed that it was defective in the regulation of cholesterol synthesis by exogenous cholesterol.[43-44] Further characterization of this mutant showed that it was most likely defective in the regulation of synthesis of HMG-CoA reductase as the resistant cells had an elevated level of the enzyme.[41] With the exception of one mutant which behaved recessively, all of the mutants resistant to 25-OH-cholesterol, which have been isolated thus far, show codominant behavior in cell hybrids formed with sensitive cells.[40-44] These results indicate that resistance to 25-OH-cholesterol may be caused by defects in more than one gene.

The mutants resistant to 25-OH-cholesterol have been reported to exhibit cross resistance to other oxygenated sterols such as 20α-hydroxy-cholesterol and 7β-hydroxy-cholesterol.[42]

## VIII. 6-(p-HYDROXYPHENYLAZO)-URACIL

Mutants resistant to 6-(p-hydroxyphenylazo)-uracil (HPUra; Figure 7), which is a specific inhibitor of DNA polymerase III in bacterial cells,[45] have been isolated in CHO cells.[46,47] One class of mutants exhibited increased resistance to bromodeoxyuridine in presence of

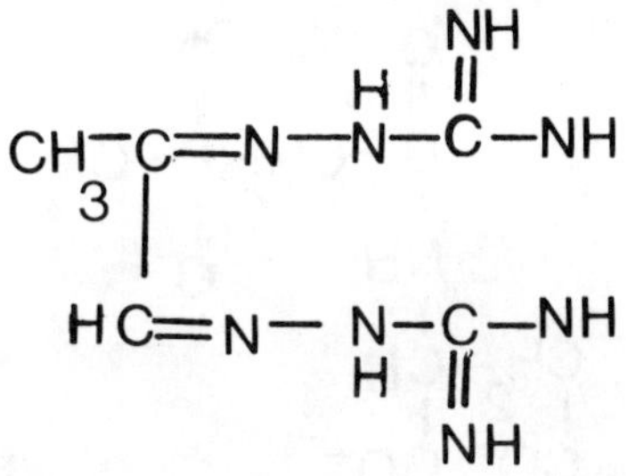

NH
CH₃—C=N—N—C—NH (with H above N, NH double bond above C)

HC=N—N—C—NH
NH

FIGURE 8.    Methylglyoxal bis(guanyl hydrazone).

thymidine, whereas the other type of mutants showed increased dependency on deoxypyrimidines for their growth, as they were unable to convert UDP to dUDP and CDP to dCDP.[46,47] This indicated that the mutants were defective in ribonucleotide reductase which carries out the above reactions, and that ribonucleotide reductase might be a direct target of HPUra.[46,47]

## IX. METHYLGLYOXAL BIS(GUANYLHYDRAZONE)

Methylglyoxal bis(guanylhydrazone) (MGBG; Figure 8) is an inhibitor of S-adenosylmethionine decarboxylase (SAM), a key enzyme involved in the biosynthesis of polyamines like spermine and spermidine.[48] MGBG also has a profound effect on mitochondrial structure and function and it makes them extensively swollen and distorted.[49,50] Mutants resistant to MGBG have been isolated from a number of different cell lines including CHO,[51] rat myoblast L6 line,[51] an adenovirus-transformed rat cell line (F4),[51] an SV40 transformed human cell line (Va₂),[52,53] and an adenosine-transformed rat cell line (F4).[54]

Mandel and Flintoff were the first to report isolation of stable, single-step mutants resistant to MGBG in CHO and rat myoblast L6 lines.[51] The spontaneous frequency of the mutants (which were about 1000-fold resistant to the drug) in CHO cells was about 0.2 to 0.5 × 10⁻⁶ and it was enhanced in a dose-dependent manner upon treatment with various known chemical and physical mutagens, e.g., EMS, 4-nitroquinoline oxide, β-propiolactone, methylmethane sulfonate, ultraviolet light, etc., which induce base substitution types of mutations.[55,56] The intracellular concentration of MGBG in the mutant cells was found to be greatly reduced, which seems to result from a marked deficiency in the cellular uptake of various naturally occurring polyamines (viz. spermine, spermidine, and putrescine).[51] None of these mutants showed any deficiency or alteration in the SAM-decarboxylase. The drug-resistance phenotype of these mutants behaved recessively in cell hybrids formed with the wild-type cells.[51] Wiseman et al.[52] have reported the selection of MGBG-resistant variants of the human cell line Va₂, which showed no significant differences in the drug uptake during short-term (2 to 60 min) incubation. The above results indicated that the drug-resistance in these mutants was due to an intracellular alteration in the binding sites. Subsequent studies by these authors indicate that a number of mitochondrial functions in the variant cells (viz. pyruvate oxidation, respiration) were more resistant to inhibition by MGBG as compared to the parental cells.[53] These results have led to the suggestion that a phenotypic alteration in mitochondria may be responsible for MGBG-resistance in these cells.[53]

An interesting observation regarding MGBG-resistant mutants has been made by Sircar et al.[54] These authors have isolated MGBG-resistant variants from an adenovirus-transformed rat cell line (F4). Similar to the mutants of CHO cells and rat L₆ myoblast, these mutants showed defective cellular uptake of MGBG. However, interestingly, these cells, while they continued to express adenovirus genes, showed reduced ability to grow on soft agar or in medium containing low serum or in nude mice. These results indicated that selection for

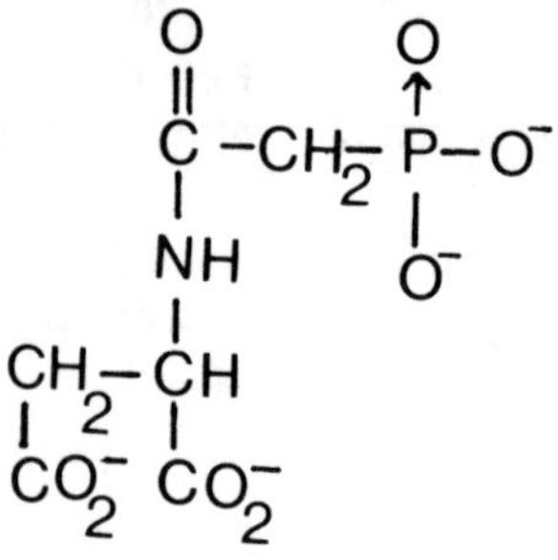

$$O \qquad\qquad O$$
$$\parallel \qquad\qquad \uparrow$$
$$C-CH_2-P-O^-$$
$$\vert \qquad\qquad \vert$$
$$NH \qquad\qquad O^-$$
$$\vert$$
$$CH_2-CH$$
$$\vert \qquad \vert$$
$$CO_2^- \quad CO_2^-$$

FIGURE 9. *N*-(Phosphonoacetyl)L-Aspartate.

MGBG-resistance may result in isolation of variants with phenotypic characteristics of normal cells and that such variants may be affected in a cellular function required for the maintenance of the transformed phenotype.[54]

## X. N-PHOSPHONOACETYL-L-ASPARTATE (PALA)

PALA (Figure 9) is a transition state analog inhibitor of the enzyme aspartate transcarbamylase (ATCase) which catalyzes the second-step in pyrimidine nucleotide biosynthesis. PALA is cytotoxic to mammalian cells because it blocks this essential pathway.[57] The first three enzymes of the pyrimidine biosynthesis, i.e., carbamyl-phosphate synthetase (CPSase), dihydroorotase (DHOase), and ATCase are found on single trifunctional protein referred to as CAD.[58] Kempe et al.[59] have reported isolation of stable, single-step mutants resistant to 0.1 m$M$ PALA from a number of different cell lines of Syrian hamster [viz., C13 (same as BHK21), C13/SV28, ST-1 and C13/SV28 II], mouse (SV40-Balb 3T3), and Chinese hamster (CHL) origins. The spontaneous frequency of PALA-resistant mutants in these cell lines was found to be in the range of $4.6 \times 10^{-5}$ to $2 \times 10^{-7}$. However, no resistant mutants were obtained from monkey MA-134 and human WI-38 cell lines (frequency $<4 \times 10^{-8}$). The rate of mutation to PALA-resistance in C13/SV28 (SV40 transformed BHK21 cells) line has been found to be about $2.0 \times 10^{-5}$ mutants/cell/generation.[59] Further serial selection in presence of increasing drug concentration with mutants of the C13/SV28 line has given rise to cell lines which are resistant up to 25 m$M$ PALA. Biochemical studies with these resistant lines have shown that they exhibit a parallel large increase in the amounts of the three enzymes (viz. ATCase, DHOase, and CPSase) which constitute the CAD complex. The observed relative increase in the activities of these enzymes showed a good correlation to the degree of resistance of the mutants to PALA.[59] Further, there were no changes either in the kinetic properties of the enzymes or in transport or degradation of PALA between normal and mutant cells.[59] Subsequent studies by Stark and co-workers have established that the observed increase in the enzymic activities is due to an increase in amount of the CAD protein, which in turn results from an amplification of the CAD gene complex in the mutant cells.[60-62] The amplified genes in PALA resistant mutants have been localized on the short arm of chromosome 9.[63] Thus cellular resistance to PALA develops from an increase in the intracellular target site for this drug.

## XI. PHOSPHONOFORMIC ACID

Phosphonoformic acid (PFA; Figure 10) is an antiviral agent which is a good inhibitor of viral DNA polymerase[64,65] but its effect on mammalian DNA polymerase is less pronounced.[65] Single-step mutants resistant to PFA have been isolated from S49 lymphoma cells after mutagenization with *N*-methyl-*N*'-nitro-*N*-nitrosoguanidine.[66] Biochemical studies

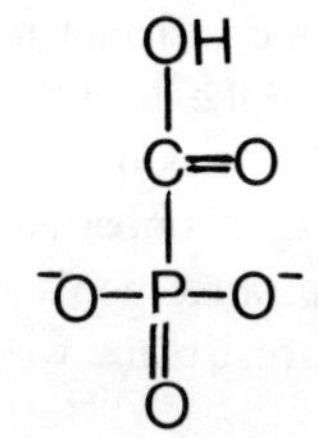

FIGURE 10.   Phosphonoformic acid.

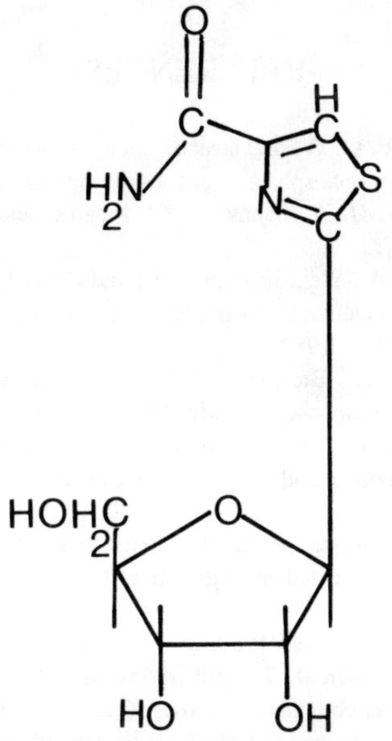

FIGURE 11.   Tiazofurin.

with these mutants have revealed that there was no defect in DNA polymerase activity. However, the activity of ribonucleotide reductase (as assayed by CDP reduction) was increased in the resistant cells. Treatment of normal or mutant cells with PFA inhibited ribonucleotide reductase, arrested cells in S phase of the cell cycle and decreased all deoxyribonucleotide pools, especially the dCTP pools. These results demonstrated that PFA can directly inhibit ribonucleotide reductase and in resistant cells, there is a mutation in this enzyme resulting in a large dCTP pool.[66]

## XII. TIAZOFURIN

Tiazofurin (2-β-D-ribofuranosylthiazole-4-carboxamide; Figure 11) is a c-nucleoside which exhibits antitumor activity against the L1210 and P388 leukemias. Studies on the mechanism of action of tiazofurin (TR) indicate that in vivo it is anabolized to a dinucleotide compound in which the nicotinamide of NAD is replaced by thiazole-4-carboxamide.[67,68] This anabolite has been referred to as TAD and it has been shown to be a potent inhibitor of IMP dehydrogenase resulting in depression in the concentration of all guanine nucleotides.[67,68] Mutants of CHO cells resistant to purine nucleoside analogs, which are either deficient in or affected in adenosine kinase do not show any increased resistance to tiazofurin, indicating that unlike other structurally related nucleoside analogs (viz., pyrazofurin), its phosphorylation does not occur via adenosine kinase.[69,70]

P388 leukemia cells that have become resistant to TR have been selected in culture by stepwise increases in the concentration of the drug.[68] The normal and TR-resistant cells were implanted in mice and formation of TAD was monitored. It was observed that resistance to TR in this murine cell line was because of impaired formation of TAD so that IMP dehydrogenase was not inhibited and triphosphate pools were not disturbed to a large extent as in sensitive cells.[68] A similar mode of resistance was also observed in CHO cells resistant to TR.[71]

# REFERENCES

1. **Graff, J. C. and Plagemann, P. G. W.**, Alanosine toxicity in Novikoff rat hepatoma cells due to inhibition of the conversion of inosine monophosphate to adenosine monophosphate, *Cancer Res.*, 36, 1428, 1976.
2. **Jayaram, H. N. and Cooney, D. A.**, Analogs of L-aspartic acid in chemotherapy for cancer, *Cancer Treat. Rep.*, 63, 1095, 1979.
3. **Tyagi, A. K. and Cooney, D. A.**, Identification of the antimetabolite of L-alanosine, L-alanosyl-5-amino-4-imidazolecarboxylic acid ribonucleotide in tumors and assessment of its inhibition of adenylosuccinate synthetase, *Cancer Res.*, 40, 4390, 1980.
4. **Tyagi, A. K. and Cooney, D. A.**, Biochemical pharmacology, metabolism and mechanism of action of L-alanosine, a novel natural antitumor agent, *Adv. Pharmacol. Chemother.*, 20, 69, 1984.
5. **Gupta, R. S.**, A novel synergistic effect of alanosine and guanine on adenine nucleotide synthesis in mammalian cells. Alanosine as a useful probe for investigating purine nucleotide metabolism, *J. Cell. Physiol.*, 104, 241, 1980.
6. **Tyagi, A. K., Cooney, D. A., Jayaram, H. M., Swiniarski, J. K., and Johnson, R. K.**, Studies on the mechanism of resistance of selected murine tumors to L-alanosine, *Biochem. Pharmacol.*, 30, 915, 1981.
7. **Gupta, R. S.**, unpublished observations, 1987.
8. **Sutton, B. M., McGusty, E., Wab, D. T., and Di Martino, M. T.**, Oral gold antiarthritic properties of alkylphosphine gold coordination complexes, *J. Med. Chem.*, 15, 1095, 1972.
9. **Sutton, B. M.**, in *Platinum, Gold and Other Chemotherapeutic Agents*, Lippard, S. J., Ed., American Chemical Society, Washington, D. C., 1983, 356.
10. **Snyder, R. M., Mirabelli, C. K., and Crooke, S. T.**, Cellular association, intracellular distribution and efflux of auranofin via sequential ligand exchange reactions, *Biochem. Pharmacol.*, 35, 923, 1986.
11. **Monia, B. P., Butt, T. R., Mirabelli, C. K., Ecker, D. J., Steinberg, E., and Crooke, S. T.**, Induction of metallothionein is correlated with resistance to auranofin, a gold compound, in Chinese hamster ovary cells, *Mol. Pharmacol.*, 31, 21, 1987.
12. **Bosch, L., Harbers, E., and Heidelberger, C.**, Studies on fluorinated pyrimidines. V. Effects on nucleic acid metabolism *in vitro*, *Cancer Res.*, 18, 335, 1958.
13. **Pasternak, C. A., Fischer, G. A., and Handschumacher, R. E.**, Alterations in pyrimidine metabolism in L5178Y leukemia cells resistant to 6-azauridine, *Cancer Res.*, 21, 110, 1961.
14. **Hashmi, S., May, S. R., Krooth, R. S., and Miller, O. J.**, Concurrent development of resistance to 6-azauridine and adenosine in a mouse cell line, *J. Cell. Physiol.*, 86, 191, 1975.
15. **May, S. R., Hashmi, S., Miller, O. J., and Krooth, R. S.**, Increased intracellular phosphoribosylpyrophosphate and accelerated orotic acid decarboxylation in a mouse cell line resistant to purine and pyrimidine ribonucleosides, *Somat. Cell Genet.*, 3, 263, 1977.
16. **Suttle, D. P. and Stark, G. R.**, Coordinate overproduction of orotate phosphoribosyltransferase and orotidine-5'-phosphate decarboxylase in hamster cells resistant to pyrazofurin and 6-azauridine, *J. Biol. Chem.*, 254, 4602, 1979.
17. **Jones, M. E.**, Pyrimidine nucleotide biosynthesis in animals: Genes, enzymes, and regulation of UMP biosynthesis, *Annu. Rev. Biochem.*, 49, 253, 19080.
18. **Newbold, R. F., Amos, J., and Connell, J. R.**, The cytotoxic mutgenic and clastogenic effects of chromium-containing compounds on mammalian cells in culture, *Mutat. Res.*, 67, 55, 1979.
19. **Douglas, G. R., Bell, R. D. L., Grant, C. E., Wytsma, J. M., and Bora, K. C.**, Effect of lead chromate on chromosome aberration, sister chromatid exchange and DNA damage in mammalian cells *in vitro*, *Mutat. Res.*, 77, 157, 1980.
20. **Campbell, C. E., Gravel, R. A., and Worton, R. G.**, Isolation and characterization of Chinese hamster cell mutants resistant to the cytotoxic effects of chromate, *Somat. Cell Genet.*, 7, 535, 1981.

21. **Campbell, C. E. and Worton, R. G.,** Linkage of genetic markers *emt* and *chr* in Chinese hamster cells, *Somat. Cell Genet.* 6, 215, 1980.
22. **Pittillo, R. F. and Hunt, D. E.,** Azaserine and 6-diazo-5-oxo-L-norleucine (DON), in *Antibiotics,* Vol. I, Gottlieb, D. and Shaw, P. D., Eds., Springer-Verlag, Berlin, 1967, 481.
23. **Lowy, B. and Williams, M. K.,** The presence of a limited portion of the pathway de novo of purine nucleotide biosynthesis in the rabbit erythrocyte *in vitro, J. Biol. Chem.,* 235, 2924, 1960.
24. **Kaufman, E. R.,** Isolation and characterization of a mutant Chinese hamster cell line resistant to the glutamine analog 6-diazo-5-oxo-1-norleucine, *Somat. Cell Molec. Genet.,* 11, 1, 1985.
25. **Yamamoto, K. R., Gehring, U., Stampfer, M. R., and Sibley, C. H.,** Genetic approaches to steroid hormone action, in *Recent Progress in Hormone Research,* Vol. 32, Greep, R. O., Ed., Academic Press, New York, 1976, 3.
26. **Sibley, C. H. and Yamamoto, K. R.,** Mouse lymphoma cells: mechanisms of resistance to glucocorticoids, in *Glucocorticoid hormone action,* Baxter, J. D. and Rousseau, G. G., Eds., Springer-Verlag, Berlin, 1979, 357.
27. **Huet-Minkowski, M., Gasson, J. C., and Bourgeois, S.,** Glucocorticoid resistance in lymphoid cell lines, in *Drug and hormone resistance in neoplasia,* Vol. 1, Bruchovsky, N. and Goldie, J. H., Eds., CRC Press, Boca Raton, Florida, 1982, 79.
28. **Ip, M. M.,** Steroids, in *Handbook of Experimental Pharmacology,* Fox, B. W. and Fox, M., Eds., Vol. 72, 1984, 633.
29. **Sibley, C. H. and Tomkins, G. M.,** Mechanisms of steroid resistance. *Cell* 2, 221, 1974.
30. **Pfahl, M., Sandros, T., and Bourgeois, S.,** Interaction of glucocorticoid receptors from lymphoid cell lines with their nuclear acceptor sites, *Mol. Cell. Endocrinol.,* 10, 175, 1978.
31. **Gehring, V. and Tomkins, G. M.,** A new mechanism for steroid unresponsiveness: Loss of nuclear binding activity of a steroid hormone receptor, *Cell* 3, 301, 1974.
32. **Yamamoto, K. R., Stampfer, M. R., and Tomkins, G. M.,** Receptors from glucocorticoid-sensitive lymphoma cells and two classes of insensitive clones: Physical and DNA binding properties, *Proc. Natl. Acad. Sci. U.S.A.,* 71, 3901, 1974.
33. **Bourgeois, S. and Newby, R. F.,** Diploid and haploid states of the glucocorticoid receptor gene of mouse lymphoid cell lines, *Cell* 11, 423, 1977.
34. **Bourgeois, S., Newby, F. R., and Huet, M.,** Glucocorticoid-resistance in murine lymphoma and thymoma lines, *Cancer Res.,* 38, 4279, 1978.
35. **Harmon, J. M. and Thompson, E. B.,** Isolation and characterization of dexamethasone-resistant mutants from human lymphoid cell line CEM-C7, *Mol. Cell. Biol.,* 1, 512, 1981.
36. **Pfahl, M. and Bourgeois, S.,** Analysis of steroid resistance in lymphoid cell hybrids, *Somat. Cell Genet.* 6, 63, 1980.
37. **Miesfeld, R., Okret, S., Wikstrom, A.-C., Wrange, O., Gustafsson, J. A., and Yamamoto, K.,** Characterization of a steroid hormone receptor gene and mRNA in wild-type and mutant cells, *Nature,* 312, 779, 1984.
38. **Johnson, D. M., Newby, R. F., and Bourgeois, S.,** Membrane permeability as a determinant of dexamethasone resistance in murine thymoma cells, *Cancer Res.,* 44, 2435, 1984.
39. **Kandutsch, A. A. and Chen, H. W.,** Inhibition of sterol synthesis in cultured mouse cells by cholesterol derivatives oxygenated in the side chain, *J. Biol. Chem.,* 249, 6057, 1974.
40. **Sinensky, M.,** Isolation of a mammalian cell mutant resistant to 25-hydroxy cholesterol, *Biochem. Biophys. Res. Commun.,* 78, 863, 1977.
41. **Sinensky, M., Armagast, S., Mueller, G., and Target, R.,** Somatic cell genetic analysis of regulation of expression of 3-hydroxy-3-methylglutaryl-coenzyme A reductase, *Proc. Natl. Acad. Sci. U.S.A.,* 77, 6621, 1980.
42. **Cavenee, W. K. and Baker, R. M.,** Characterization of dominant hamster cell mutants resistant to oxygenated sterols, *Somat. Cell Genet.,* 8, 557, 1982.
43. **Sinensky, M.,** Defective regulation of cholesterol biosynthesis and plasma membrane fluidity in a Chinese hamster ovary cell mutant, *Proc. Natl. Acad. Sci. U.S.A.,* 75, 1247, 1978.
44. **Sinensky, M., Duwe, G., and Pinkerton, F.,** Defective regulation of 3-hydroxy-3-methylglutaryl coenzyme A reductase in a somatic cell mutant, *J. Biol. Chem.,* 254, 4482, 1979.
45. **Cozarelli, N. R. and Low, R. L.,** Mutational alteration of *Bacillus subtilis* DNA polymerase III to hydroxy phenyl azopryrimidine resistance: Polymerase III is necessary for DNA replication, *Biochem. Biophys. Res. Commun.,* 51, 151, 1973.
46. **Arpaia, E., Ray, P. N., and Siminovitch, L.,** Isolation of mutants of CHO cells resistant to 6(p-hydroxyphenylazo)-uracil. I. A novel BrdU cross resistant phenotype, *Somat. Cell Genet.,* 9, 269, 1983.
47. **Arpaia, E., Ray, P. N., and Siminovitch, L.,** Isolation of mutants of CHO cells resistant to 6(p-hydroxyphenylazo)-uracil. II. Mutants auxotropic for deoxypyrimidines. *Somat. Cell Genet.,* 9, 287, 1983.
48. **Williams-Ashman, H. G. and Schenone, A.,** Methyl glyoxal bis(guanylhydrazone) as a potent inhibitor of mammalian and yeast S-adenosylmethionine decarboxylase, *Biochem. Biophys. Res. Commun.,* 46, 288, 1972.

49. **Mikeles-Robertson, F., Feuerstein, B., Dave, C., and Porter, C. W.,** The generality of methyl glyoxal bis(guanylhydrazone)-induced mitochondrial damage and the dependence of the effect on cell proliferation, *Cancer Res.,* 39, 1919, 1979.

50. **Porter, C. W., Mikeles-Robertson, F., Kramer, D., and Dave, C.,** Correlation of ultrastructural and functional damage to mitochondria of ascites L1210 cells treated in vitro with methylglyoxal bis(guanylhydrazone) or ethidium bromide, *Cancer Res.,* 39, 2414, 1979.

51. **Mandel, J. L. and Flintoff, W. F.,** Isolation of mutant mammalian cells altered in polyamine transport, *J. Cell. Physiol.,* 97, 335, 1978.

52. **Wiseman, A., Kramer, D. L., and Porter, C. W.,** Isolation and uptake characteristics of human cell variants resistant to the antiproliferative effects of methylglyoxal bis(guanylhydrazone), *Cancer Res.,* 43, 5937, 1983.

53. **Kramer, D. L., Zychlinski, L., Wiseman, A., and Porter, C. W.,** Biochemical and ultrastructural characterization of human cell variants resistant to the antiproliferative effects of methylglyoxal bis(guanylhydrazone), *Cancer Res.,* 43, 5943, 1983.

54. **Sircar, S., Palkonyay, L., Rodrigues, M., Allaire, S., Horvath, J., Thirion, J.-P., and Weber, J.,** Isolation of variants resistant to methylglyoxal bis(guanylhydrazone) from adenovirus-transformed rat cells, *Cancer Res.,* 47, 1339, 1987.

55. **Gupta, R. S. and Singh, B.,** Mutagenic response of five independent genetic loci in CHO cells to a variety of mutagens: Development and characteristics of a mutagen screening system based on selection for multiple drug resistant markers, *Mutat. Res.,* 94, 449, 1982.

56. **Gupta, R. S.,** in *Handbook of Mutagenicity Test Procedures,* 1984.

57. **Swyryd, E. A., Seaver, S. S., and Stark, G. R.,** N-(phosphonacetyl)-L-asparate, a potent transition state analog inhibitor of aspartate transcarbamyolase blocks proliferation of mammalian cells in culture, *J. Biol. Chem.,* 249, 6945, 1974.

58. **Mally, M. I., Grayson, D. R., and Evans, D. R.,** Controlled proteolysis of the multifunctional protein that initiates pyrimidine biosynthesis in mammalian cells: Evidence for discrete functional domains, *Proc. Natl. Acad. Sci. U.S.A.,* 78, 6647, 1981.

59. **Kempe, T. D., Swyryd, E. A., Bruist, M., and Stark, G. R.,** Stable mutants of mammalian cells that overproduce the first three enzymes of pyrimidine nucleotide biosynthesis, *Cell,* 9, 541, 1976.

60. **Padgett, R. A., Wahl, G. M., Coleman, P. F., and Stark, G. R.,** N-(phosphonacetyl)-L-aspartate-resistant hamster cells overaccumulate a single mRNA coding for the multifunctional protein that catalyzes the first steps of UMP synthesis, *J. Biol. Chem.,* 254, 974, 1979.

61. **Wahl, G. M., Vitto, L., Padgett, R. A., and Stark, G. R.,** Single copy and amplified CAD genes on Syrian hamster chromosomes localized by a highly sensitive method for in situ hybridization, *Mol. Cell. Biol.,* 2, 308, 1982.

62. **Ardeshir, F., Giulotto, E., Zieg, J., Brison, O., Liao, W., and Stark, G. R.,** Structure of amplified DNA in different Syrian hamster lines resistant to N-(phosphonoacetyl)-L-aspartate, *Mol. Cell. Biol.,* 3, 2076, 1983.

63. **Zieg, J., Clayton, C. E., Ardeshir, F., Giulotto, E., Swyryd, E. A., and Stark, G. R.,** Properties of single step mutants of Syrian hamster cell lines resistant to N-(phosphonoacetyl)-L-aspartate, *Mol. Cell. Biol.,* 3, 2089, 1983.

64. **Derse, D., Bastow, K. F., and Cheng, Y.,** Characterization of the DNA polymerases induced by a group of herpes simplex virus type I variants selected for growth in the presence of phosphonoformic acid, *J. Biol. Chem.,* 257, 10251, 1982.

65. **Shin, S., Donovan, J., and Nonoyama, M.,** Phosphonoacetic acid resistant RNA of Epstein-Barr virus in productively infected cells, *Virology,* 124, 196, 1983.

66. **Albert, D. A. and Gudas, L. J.,** Selection and characterization of mutant S49 T-lymphoma cell lines resistant to phosphonoformic acid: Evidence for inhibition of ribonucleotide reductase, *J. Cell. Physiol.,* 127, 281, 1986.

67. **Jayaram, H. N., Dion, R. L., Glazier, R. I., Johnson, D. G., Robins, R. K., Srivastava, P. C., and Cooney, D. A.,** Initial studies on the mechanism of action of a new oncolytic thiazole nucleoside, 2-β-D-ribofuranosylthiazole-4-carboxamide (NSC 286193), *Biochem. Pharmacol.,* 31, 2371, 1982.

68. **Jayaram, H. N., Cooney, D. A., Glazer, R. I., Dion, R. L., and Johns, D. G.,** Mechanism of resistance to the oncolytic C-nucleoside 2-β-D-ribofuranosylthiazole-4-carboxamide (NSC 286193), *Biochem. Pharmacol.,* 31, 2557, 1982.

69. **Mehta, K. D. and Gupta, R. S.,** Novel mutants of CHO cells resistant to adenosine analogs and containing biochemically altered form of adenosine kinase in cell extracts, *Somat. Cell Molec. Genet.,* 12, 1986.

70. **Gupta, R. S.,** Cellular resistance to purine nucleoside analogs involving deficiency or structural alterations in adenosine kinase, in *Drug Resistance in Mammalian Cells,* Gupta, R. S., Ed., CRC Press, Boca Raton, FL. 1989.

71. **Kuttan, R., Lai, M. M., and Saunders, P. P.,** Possible mechanism of action of 2-β-D-ribofuranosyl-thiazole-4-carboxamide in Chinese hamster ovary cells, *Proc. Am. Assoc. Cancer Res.,* 23, 218, 1982.

# INDEX

## A

AA, see 8-Azaadenine
AAU medium, 104, 178
N-Acetoxy N-acetylaminofluorene, 8, 38
ACTH, see Corticotropin
Actinomycin D, 147, 225, 227
ADA, see Adenosine deaminase
Adenine, 66, 80, 115—118
Adenine aminohydrolase, 112
Adenine analogs, 111—121
   collateral sensitivity of, 119—120
   mechanisms of action of, 114—119
   metabolism of, 112—113
   mutants resistant to, 120
   toxicity of, 113—114
Adenine-arabinoside (AraAde), 175—176
Adenine phosphoribosyltransferase, 114—115, 238, 248
Adenosine (Ado)
   7-deazaderivatives of, 90
   excess, 178
   inborn errors of purine metabolism and, 70—72
   medium containing, 104
   metabolism of, 72—73, 179
   mutants resistant to, 76—80
   structure of, 71
   supersensitivity to, 79—80
   transport of, 129
   toxicity of, 74—75
[$^3$H]Adenosine, 99, 103
Adenosine deaminase (ADA)
   araA as substrate for, 130—131
   deamination of APP by, 118
   deamination of DAP by, 118
   deamination of deoxyAMP by, 73
   deficiency in, 70, 72
   detoxification function of, 78, 85
   effect of aminopurine on, 119
   effect of Cof on, 114, 177—180
   effect of dCof on, 177—180
   gene for, 78—79
   impairment of activity of, 71, 74
   inhibition of, 126, 134, 136, 180
   overproduction of, 135, 179
   in wild type cells, 80
Adenosine-EHNA, 79—80
Adenosine kinase (AK)
   alteration in activity of, 134
   deficiency in, 179
   deficiency in activity of, 78, 100, 119
   effect of Ado on, 178
   effect of alanosine on, 248
   effect on araA, 130, 137
   mutants affected in, 94—100, 102
   phosphorylation by, 90, 93
   polypeptides of, 135

substrate for, 72—73, 81
Adenosine 3′,5′-monophosphate (cAMP, cyclic AMP)
   CHO cells and, 198—200
   formycin A in, 92
   increased production of, 74
   intracellular levels of, 72
   metabolism and action of, 187—189
   other mutant cell lines and, 200—201
   S49 cells and, 194—197
   as second messenger, 186—187
   Y1 cells and, 189—194
Adenosine phosphorylase, 248
S-Adenosylhomocysteine (SAH), 79—80
S-Adenosylhomocysteine hydrolase
   effect of ADA on, 72
   increased expression of, 80
   inhibition of, 75, 133—134
   mutations in, 85
   in SAH formation, 79
S-Adenosylmethionine (SAM), 55, 79—80, 222
S-Adenosylmethionine decarboxylase, 194, 196, 253
Adenylate (AMP)
   conversion of Ado to, 72, 112
   conversion of IMP to, 60, 70, 104
   deamination to IMP, 80
   effect of alanosine on, 178
   effect on PPRP levels, 113
   substitution for, 90
Adenylate cyclase, 187—192, 196—198, 200—202
Adenylate deaminase, 114, 180
Adenylic nucleosides, 178
Adenylic purines, 178
Adenylosuccinate (AMPS), 60
Adenylsuccinate synthetase, 248
Ado, see Adenosine
dAdo, see Deoxyadenosine
ADP
   assay with, 83
   phosphorylation of AMP to, 72
   reduction to dADP, 16
   regulation of, 175
   substitution for, 90
   as substrate, 76
dADP, 16, 73
β-Adrenergic agonists, 196—197, 200
AE$_1$ cells, 77
AG, see 8-Azaguanine
AH, see 8-Azahypoxanthine
β-AHA, 213
β-AHA$^r$ mutant, 213—216
AI, see Azainosine
AK, see Adenosine kinase
AK cells, 104—105, 118
AKR4 cells, 79
Alanine, 224—225
Alanosine, 104, 112, 178, 248—249

L-Alanosyl-AlCOR, 248
Alb, see Albizzin
Alb$^R$ mutant, 213—218, 228
Albizzin (Alb), 213—214, 217—218, 228
Aldehyde oxidase, 92
Alkaline phosphatase, 149
Amethopterin, 60, 66, 70, 146, 176
Amino acid analogs, 211—228
  amino acid transport mutants, 224—228
  aminoacyl-tRNA synthetase, 223—224
  asparagine synthetase, 212—216
  canavanine-resistant lines, 218—220
  glutamine synthetase, 216—218
  methionine adenosyl transferase, 222
  pyrroline-5-caraboxylate synthetase, 220—222
Amino acid transport, 198, 224—228
Aminoacyl-tRNA synthetase, 223—224
Amino alcohols, 223—224
Aminoimidazole carboxamide, 117
5-Amino-2-pentanone, 48
Aminopterin, 2—5, 7, 112, 146
2-Aminopurine, 115—119, 147
4-Amino-pyrazolo(3,4-d)pyrimidine, see Pyrazoloadenine
AMP, see Adenylate
cAMP see Adenosine 3′,5′-monophosphate
AMP deaminase, 72, 79—80, 180
cAMP phosphodiesterases, 187, 198—199
AMPS, see Adenylosuccinate
AMPS lyase, 61
AMPS synthetase, 61
Antifolate compounds, 2—4
Aphidicolin
  chemical structure of, 31
  effects and mechanism of action of, 30—32
  for isolating drug resistant cells, 18, 32—36
  resistance to, 20, 136, 175—176
  for solving basic biological problems, 36—38
APP, see Pyrazoloadenine
APP-ribonucleoside, 100
APRT, 112—114, 117—121
APRT$^+$ cells, 104
AraA, see 9-β-D-Arabinofuranosyladenine
AraAde, see Adenine-arabinoside
AraADP, 130
AraAMP, see 9-β-D-Arabinofuranosyladenine 5′-
  monophosphate
2-F-AraAMP, see 9-β-D-Arabinofuranosyl-2-
  fluoroadenine 5′monophosphate
AraATP, 131—136
9-β-D-Arabinofuranosyladenine (araA), 125—137
  cross resistance to, 35—36
  inhibition of DNA polymerase, 18
  pharmacology of, 127—134
    incorporation in nucleic acids, 133
    inhibition of DNA synthesis, 131—132
    inhibition of SAH hydrolase, 133—134
    metabolism, 130—131
    transport, 129—130
  resistance to, 134—136

structure of, 126—127
1-β-D-Arabinofuranosylcytosine, see Cytosine-
  arabinoside
9-β-D-Arabinofuranosyl-2-fluoroadenine (2F-araA),
  125—137
  pharmacology of, 127—134
    incorporation in nucleic acids, 133
    inhibition of DNA synthesis, 131—132
    inhibition of SAH hydrolase, 133—134
    metabolism, 130—131
    transport, 129—130
  resistance to, 134—136
9-β-D-Arabinofuranosylhypoxanthine (araH), 126
Arabinofuranosyl nucleoside analogs, 18
Arabinosides, 80
Arabinosyladenine, 79—80, 95, 102
Arabinosylcytosine, 76, 82
Arabinosyl 2,6-diaminopurine, 79
Arabinosylguanine, 79
AraC, see Cytosine arabinoside
AraCMP, 172
AraCTP, 166, 172, 176
AraCyt, see Cytosine arabinoside
AraH, see 9-β-D-Arabinofuranosylhypoxanthine
Arginine, 46, 212, 218—220
Argininosuccinate, 218
Argininosuccinate lyase (AS lyase), 218—219
Argininosuccinate synthetase (AS), 218—220, 228
Arginyl-tRNA synthetase, 218
AS, see Argininosuccinate synthetase
AS lyase, see Argininosuccinate lyase
ASC system, 213, 226, 228
AsnSyn, see Asparagine synthetase
L-Asparaginase, 212
Asparagine, 212
Asparagine synthetase (AsnSyn), 212—216, 228
Aspartate, 218
Aspartate transcarbamylase, 253—254
Aspartic acid, 212—214, 248
β-Aspartyl hydroxamate, 214
"A" system mutants, 224—226
"A" system transport, 213, 225—226
ATP
  cAMP synthesis from, 187
  binding of, 17
  conversion to IMP, 60
  enzyme activated by, 16
  formation of SAM from, 222
  in phosphorylation of serine, 189
  substitution for, 90
  varied concentration of, 99
dATP
  binding of, 17
  effect on CDP reductase, 174
  Km for, 32
  increased, 35
  inhibition by, 16, 132, 136
  pools of, 175
  sensitivity to, 176
ATP-dependent reactions, 75

Auranofin, 248—249
8-Azaadenine (AA)
  as APRT substrate, 150
  cross-resistance to, 103
  cytotoxicity of, 151
  inhibition by, 113—114
  phosphorylation by, 101
  resistance to, 117—118, 120
  structure of, 116
8-Azaadenosine, 90, 96—98, 102, 151
8-Aza-9-deazaadenosine (see Formycin A)
8-Aza-9-deazainosine (see Formycin B)
8-Azaguanine (AG)
  cytotoxicity of, 151
  resistance to, 152, 154
  selective efficiency of, 150
  structure of, 147
  studies with, 146
8-Azahypoxanthine (AH), 146, 150—151, 154
Azainosine (AI), 146, 150—151, 154
Azaserine, 70, 112, 179
6-Azauridine (6-AZU), 76, 248—250
6-Azauridine monophosphate (6-AZUMP), 248—250
Azaxanthine, 149
AZCA, see L-Azetidine-2-carboxylic acid
L-Azetidine-2-carboxylic acid (AZCA), 220—222
6AZU, see 6-Azauridine
6AZUMP, see 6-Azauridine monophosphate

**B**

*Bacillus subtilis,* 30, 32—34, 166
Bacterial *Ecogpt* gene, 65—67
BALB/c mice, 21—22
B cells, 71—72, 82, 85
BHK cells, 135, 244—245
Bleomycin
  chemical structure of, 18
  collateral sensitivity of, 20
  effect of aphidicolin on, 37
  effect of α-polymerase on, 38
  interaction with protein M2, 17
  resistance to, 36
Borrelidin, 224
8BrcAMP, see 8-Bromoadenosine 3′,5′-mono-
    phosphate
BrdU, 32
BrdU-black light, 36
BrdUMP, 162
BrdUrd, see 5-Bromo-2′-deoxyuridine
BrdUTP, 162, 168
Bredinine, 90, 94—95, 102, 119
8-Bromoadenosine 3′,5′-monophosphate
    (8BrcAMP), 190—192, 198, 200
5-Bromo-2′-deoxyuridine (BrdUrd), 18, 76, 160—
    162, 168, 252
5-Bromouracil (BrUra), 160
BrUra, see 5-Bromouracil
BuPdGTP, 36

**C**

CAD gene, 254
Calcium, 187
Calmodulin, 187
Can, see Canavine
Can$^r$ cells, 219—220, 228
Canavine (Can), 213, 218—220
4-Carbamoylimazolium-5-olate, 117, 119—120
*N*-Carbamoyloxyurea, 17—19, 25
Carbamyl-phosphate synthetase, 254
Carbohydrate analogs, 233—245
  resistant to 2-deoxygalactose, 234—243
    Dga$^R$, 234—243, see also Dga$^R$ mutants
    galactokinase activities in, 239—240
    mutation rates for, 237—238
    selection of, 234—237
    structural mutations in, 240—241
  resistant to 2-deoxyglucose, 244—245
  resistant to 3-O-methyl-D-glucose, 243—244
CCL39 cells, 36, 172—175, 178—180
CCRF-CEM cells, 131, 134—136
CDP
  effect on ribonucleotide reductase, 83
  inhibition of, 132, 136
  reduction to dCDP, 16, 160—162, 168, 252
  as substrate for ribonucleotide reductase, 166
dCDP, 16, 160—162, 168, 252
CDP reductase, 20, 161, 174—175
[$^{14}$C]formate, 62
Chinese hamster lung (CHL) cells, 3—4, 220—222,
    254
Chinese hamster ovary (CHO) cells
  AA-resistant, 120
  ADA in, 135
  alanine-resistant, 225
  alanosine-resistant, 248
  APRT in, 118
  AsnSyn, 213—217
  borrelidin-resistant, 224
  chromate-resistant, 250
  cycloleucine-resistant, 222
  Cyd-deaminase deficient, 176
  Dga resistance in, 242—243
  DHFR changes in, 3
  drug resistant properties of, 18
  dThd auxotrophs of, 174—175
  effect of aphidicolin on, 35
  inhibition of DNA synthesis in, 131
  isolates from, 6, 36, 175—176
  -K1, 225—226, 252
  MGBG-resistant, 253
  MG-resistant, 243—244
  Mtx-resistant, 4—5, 7—8
  mutagenesis studies in, 104—105
  mutants of, 49, 54, 94, 98—100, 198—200
  mutator gene in, 101
  ODC in, 51
  purine auxotrophs in, 60
  sensitivity of, 48—49

TR-resistant, 255
-tsH1, 227
tumorigenicity of, 23
TyrOH$^R$-resistant, 223—224
CHL cells, see Chinese hamster lung cells
Chloramphenicol acetyltransferase, 220
p-Chloromercuriphenylsulfonate (pCMS), 4
CHO cells, see Chinese hamster ovary cells
Cholera toxin, 190, 194, 196—197, 200
Chromate, 250
Chromosomes, 8—10, 31—32
CHY-2 cells, 228
[$^{14}$C]hypoxanthine, 62
Citrulline, 218—220
Class A mutants, 98—100
Class B mutants, 98—100
Class C mutants, 100
dCMP deaminase, 36, 174, 177
pCMS, see p-Chloromercuriphenylsulfonate
C-nucleoside analogs, 92—94, 99
Cof, see Corformycin
dCof, see Deoxycoformycin
Coformycin (Cof)
    effect on adenine, 114
    effect on ADA, 126, 130
    cellular resistance to, 177—180
    structure of, 128
Colchicine, 194, 251
Cordycepin (3'-deoxyadenosine), 76, 135
Corticotropin (ACTH), 189—194
Covidarabin, see Deoxycoformycin
Creatine phosphokinase, 21
CRM, see Cross reacting material
Cross reacting material (CRM), 100—101, 240—241
CTP, 63, 74, 165—166
dCTP
    competition with araCTP, 172
    effect of aphidicolin on, 30—32
    effect of araCTP on, 176
    effect of BrdUTP on, 162
    increased levels of, 166, 168
    inhibition of deoxynucleotidyltransferase by, 132
    Km for, 32
    pools of, 20, 34—36, 63, 172—175
    synthesis of, 177
CTPS, see CTP synthetase
CTP synthetase (CTPS), 36, 161, 166—168, 174—177
Cyc cells, 197
Cycloheximide, 31, 50, 225, 227
Cycloleucine, 213, 217, 222
Cyd, see Cytidine
dCyd, see Deoxycytidine
dCyd-AraCyt kinase, 173, 176—177
Cytarabine, see Cytosine arabinoside
Cytidine (Cyd), 36, 167
Cytidine-deaminase, 172, 176
Cytosine arabinoside (araC, AraCyt, cytarabine)
    effect of histidinol on, 223
    effect on DNA, 31, 172
    in isolating drug-resistant lines, 18
    metabolism of, 173
    resistance to
        of aphidicolin-resistant mutants, 32—34, 175—176
        of cells with biochemical defects, 176
        of cells with expanded dCTP pools, 172—175
        of dCyd kinase-deficient cells, 172
        in human tumor cells, 176—177
        of L1210 cells, 130
    toxic effects of, 165
Cytosine arabinoside kinase, 176

**D**

DAP, see 2,6-Diaminopurine
Daunomycin, 251
DDMP, see Metroprine
ddTTP, 37, 167
Deazaadenosine, 79, 93, 96, 102
3-Deazaaristeromycin, 79
7-Deazainosine, 102
7-Deazapurine, 92
7-Deazapurine nucleosides, 103
Deoxyadenosine (dAdo)
    cross resistance to, 35, 175
    effect of ADA on, 78
    effect on protein M1, 17
    inborn errors of purine metabolism and, 70—72
    for isolating resistant mutants, 18
    metabolism of, 73, 178
    mutants resistant to, 80—83
    phosphorylation deficiency in, 81—82
    phosphorylation of, 85
    as purine source, 179
    structure of, 71
    toxicity of, 75
3'-Deoxyadenosine, see Cordycepin
Deoxyadenosine-EHNA, 75—76, 79
DeoxyAMP, 73
DeoxyATP, 36, 71—72, 75, 80—82
Deoxycoformycin (covidarabin, dCof)
    cellular resistance to, 177—180
    effect on ADA, 74, 78, 130—131, 134
    effect on adenine, 114
    effect on DNA, 32
    effect on SAM, 79
    exclusion of IdUrd from, 168
    for leukemia or lymphoma, 71
    structure of, 126, 128
DeoxyCTP, 76, 84
Deoxycytidine (dCyd), 75—76, 131, 167, 179
Deoxycytidine kinase
    araA as substrate for, 130
    deficiency in, 81—84, 172
    deoxyadenosine as substrate for, 73
    effect on araA nucleotides, 135, 137
    reduced activity of, 176
Deoxycytidylate, 75
2-Deoxygalactose (Dga)
    mutants resistant to, 234—245
        Dga$^R$ mutants, 234—243, see also Dga$^R$ mutants

galactokinase activities in, 239—240
  mutation rates for, 237—238
  selection of, 234—237
  structural mutations in, 240—241
  structure of, 235
2-Deoxyglucose (Dgu), 234—235, 244—245
DeoxyGMP, 73
DeoxyGTP, 72, 76, 82, 84
Deoxyguanosine
  conversion to guanine, 62
  effect on protein M1, 17
  inborn errors of purine metabolism and, 70—72
  for isolating resistant mutants, 18
  metabolism of, 73—74
  mutants resistant to, 76, 83—84
  structure of, 71
  toxicity of, 75—76
Deoxyguanosine kinase, 73
Deoxyguanylates, 73
Deoxyinosine, 62, 70—73, 78
Deoxynucleotidyltransferase, 132
Deoxyribonucleoside kinase, 135
Deoxyribonucleosides, 75—76, 80—84
Deoxyribonucleoside triphosphates, 16, 83
Deoxyribonucleotide (dNDP)
  accumulation of, 71
  pools of, 20—22, 136
  reduction of rNDP to, 17
  sensitivity to, 72
  supply of, 175
Deoxyribonucleotide triphosphates, 137, 176
Deoxyribose-l-phosphate, 71
Deoxythymidine, 17—18, 35
Deoxyuridine, 167
Dexamethasone, 250—252
αDFMO, see α-Difluoromethylornithine
2dG$^R$ cells, 244—245
Dga, see 2-Deoxygalactose
Dga$^R$ mutants
  application to inactivation and expression, 242—243
  complementation analysis of, 241—242
  fluctuation test for, 234, 237
  mapping of, 242
  mutation rate for, 238
  null-allele, 240—241
  physiological characterization of, 239
  recessivity of, 241, 245
Dgu, see 2-Deoxyglucose
DHF, see Dihydrofolate
DHFR, see Dihydrofolate reductase
DHFR protein, 10
DHL-9 cells, 83
Diacylglycerol, 187
Diamine, 49
2,6-Diaminopurine (DAP), 113—118, 120
Diaminopyrimidines, 4
2,4-Diaminoquinazolines, 4
3,5-Diamino-l,2,4-triazole, see Guanazole
Diazoles, 17
6-Diazo-5-oxo-L-norleucine (DON), 250

Dibutyryl cAMP, 195, 199—201
Dichloro-Mtx, 5
α-Difluoromethylornithine (αDFMO), 47—56
  analogs of, 50
  clinical uses of, 55
  covalent binding of, 50
  effect on plating efficiency, 51
  high concentrations of, 56
  inhibition of ODC by, 47—49
  resistance to, 52—53
Dihydrofolate (DHF), 2
Dihydrofolate reductase (DHFR), 2—4, 6—9, 66
2,3-Dihydro-l-H-pyrazole 2,3-A imidazole (IMPY), 17
2,8-Dihydroxyadenine, 112
N$^2$-Dimethylguanine, 80
DMs, see Double minutes
DNA
  amplified, 6, 220
  BrdUrd in, 161
  cloned segments of, 154
  copy number of, 216
  exogenous, 66
  formycin A derivatives in, 92
  from *B. subtilis,* 166—167
  genomic, 199
  hmdUrd in, 164—167
  IdUrd in, 162
  levels of, 53
  M1 and M2, 24
  methylation of, 80
  in overproducing cells, 217
  phage, 215
  purines in, 146
  replication of, 154
  sangivamycin in, 91
cDNA, 53, 78, 215—219, 251
DNA glycosylase, 163
DNA polymerase
  altered, 32—35, 136, 176
  in DNA repair, 37—38
  effect of aphidicolin on, 30—31
  effect of araA on, 132—133
  elevated level of, 35
  functional roles of, 36—37
  inhibition of, 18, 254
  level of, 172
DNA reductase, 18
DNA repair, 75
DNA synthesis
  effect of aminopurine on, 119
  effect of aphidicolin on, 30—32
  effect of araA on, 126, 131—137
  effect of araC on, 172
  effect of BrdUrd on, 160
  effect of Can on, 218
  effect of dCTP on, 162
  effect of GMP on, 63
  effect of hydroxyurea on, 20, 25
  effect of Mtx on, 2
  effect of mycophenolic acid on, 62, 66

inhibition of, 75, 147, 165, 248
in mouse cells, 61
by γ-polymerase, 37
reversible inhibition of, 8, 16
DNA transfer, 180
DON, see 6-Diazo-5-oxo-L-norleucine
Double minutes (DMs), 8—10
DR2 mutants, 234, 236—240
Drug resistant cells, 16—24
bleomycin and ribonucleotide reductase, 20
gene amplification in, 23—24
hydroxyurea resistance and cross resistance, 18—23
modifications in cell proliferation, 20—23
ribonucleotide reductase inhibitors, 16—18
dTTP, see TTP

**E**

*Ecogpt* gene, 65—67
EHNA, see Erythro-9-(2-hydroxy-3-nonyl)-adenine
EMS, see Ethylmethanesulfonate
Epinephrine, 187
Erythro-9(2-hydroxy-3-nonyl)adenine (EHNA), 74, 78, 126—131, 177
*Escherichia coli,* 62, 114, 117—118, 126
*N*-Ethylmaleimide, 36—37
Ethylmethanesulfonate (EMS), 104—105, 192, 225, 228, 236
6-Ethylthiopurine ribonucleoside, 150

**F**

2F-araA, see 9-β-D-Arabinofuranosyl-2-fluoroadenine
2-F-araAMP, see 9-β-D-Arabinofuranosyl-2-fluoroadenine 5′monophosphate
2-F-araAMP monophosphate, 126—131
FdUMP, 165—166
FdUrd, see 5-Fluorodeoxyuridine
2-Fluoroadenine, 100—103, 117—118, 131
2-Fluoroadenosine, 90, 94—95, 103, 118
5-Fluorodeoxyuridine (FdUrd), 76, 101—103, 165, 173
Fluoropyrimidines, 165
5-Fluorouracil (FUra), 165—168, 174
5-Fluorouridine (FUrd), 76, 103, 165
FM3A cells, 35—36, 119, 136, 175
Folate analogs, 4—5
Folate utilizing enzymes, 6
Folic acid, 2—3
Follicle stimulating hormone, 198
Folyl glutamate snythetase, 6—7
Fom^R mutants, 98—99
Formamidoxime, 18
[^14C]Formate, 62
Formycin A (8-aza-9-deazaadenosine), 90—96, 98—99, 102, 105
Formycin B (8-aza-9-deazainosine), 90—96, 98—99, 102, 105, 129
10-Formyltetrahydrofolate synthetase, 6

Forskolin, 191—192, 196—197
Fumarate, 218
FUra, see 5-Fluorouracil
FUrd, see 5-Fluorouridine
FUTP, 166

**G**

Galactokinase, 234, 239—245
Galactosamine, 234—235
Galactose, 234, 239—243
GalK mutants, 240—245
GDP, 16
dGDP, 16
GDP pools, 63
Gene
for ADA, 78—79
for AK, 101
amplification of, 23—24, 53—54
CAD, 254
*Ecogpt,* 65—67
HPRT, 151—152, 154
inactivation and expression of, 242—243
mutation of, 31—34
mutator, 101
ODC, 56
variation in, 150—152
Glucagon, 187, 201
Glucocorticoids, 194, 250—252
Glucose, 198, 239, 241—244
D-Glucose, 234, 244
Glutamic acid, 220—222
Glutamine, 212—214, 217
Glutamine synthetase (GS), 213, 216—218, 228
Glycine, 224
GMP, see Guanylate
cGMP, 187
GMPP(NH)P, 196—197
GMP synthetase, 61, 63, 65
Gossypol, 18—20
Gramacidin, 251
GS, see Glutamine synthetase
GTP, 60, 63, 65, 70
dGTP, 16—17, 132, 175
dGTP pools, 63
Guanazole (3,5-diamino-1,2,4-triazole), 17—20, 25
Guanine
analogs of, 145—155
biochemical basis of resistance of, 147—150
cytotoxicity of, 146—147, 151
molecular mechanism of genetic variation in, 150—152
mutagenesis studies with, 152—154
effect on mycophenolic acid, 61—63
phosphoribosylation of, 66
phosphorylation of, 73
structure of, 147
toxicity of, 76
Guanine deaminase, 149—150
Guanine nucleotides, 114
Guanosine, 61—63, 71, 76

Guanylate (GMP), 60—65, 70, 113, 119—120, 180
Guanylate nucleotides, 63—65, 70, 80—83, 187
Guanylate ribonucleotides, 76
Guanylate synthetase, 250
Guanyl nucleotide, 189, 197, 202
dGuo-200-1 cells, 82—83

## H

HAT, see Hypoxanthine-amethopterin-thymidine
$^3$H-dUMP, 9
HeLa cells
   class A mutants of, 101
   DNA replication in, 30, 37, 167
   effect of mutagens on, 105
   hmdUrd-resistant, 163, 165
   hmUra generation in, 164
   human, 98, 132, 149
   inhibition of, 118
   mutants of, 104
HEp-2 cells, 132
Hepatoma variant HMO$_A$, 49—51
Herpes simplex, 30, 33—35, 126, 133—136
Hexose, 243—244
HGPRTase, see Hypoxanthine-guanine-phosphori-
      bosyltransferase
HisOH$^R$ lines, 223—224, 228
HisRS, 223
Histidinol, 213, 223
Histidyl-tRNA synthetase, 213, 228
HL60 cells, 176
hmdUMP, 168
hmdUrd see 5-Hydroxymethyl-2'-deoxyuridine
hmdUTP, 164—165, 167
HMG-CoA, see 3-Hydroxy-3-methyl-glutaryl-
      coenzyme A
HMO$_A$ cells, see Hepatoma variant HMO$_A$
hmUra, see 5-Hydroxymethyuracil
L-Homocysteine, 75, 79
Homogeneously staining regions (HSRs), 8—10,
      212, 216
HPRT, see Hypoxanthine-guanine-phosphori-
      bosyltransferase
HPRT gene, 151—154
HPUra, see 6-(p-Hydroxyphenylazo)uracil
HSRs, see Homogeneously staining regions
HTC cells, 49—50
[$^3$H]Tubercidin, 99, 103
Human chorionic gonadotropin, 198
9-(Hydroxyalkyl)adenines, 177
25-Hydroxy-cholesterol, 252
8-Hydroxy-2,6-diaminopurine, 118
6-N-Hydroxylaminopurine, 119
5-Hydroxymethyl-2'-deoxyuridine (hmdUrd), 161,
      163—168
Hydroxymethyldeoxyuridylase phosphorylase, 167—
      168
3-Hydroxy-3-methyl-glutaryl-coenzyme A (HMG-
      CoA) reductase, 252
5-Hydroxymethyuracil (hmUra), 163—168
6-(p-Hydroxyphenylazo)uracil (HPUra), 252

Hydroxyurea
   DNA synthesis inhibition by, 8
   excess, 136
   related compounds and, 15—25
      bleomycin, 15
      cellular properties of drug resistant cells, 16—23
         bleomycin collateral sensitivity, 20
         resistance and cross resistance, 18—20
         resistance and modifications in cell prolifera-
            tion, 20—23
         ribonucleotide reductase hypersensitivity, 20
         ribonucleotide reductase inhibitors, 16—18
         ribonucleotide reductase, 16, 23—24
      resistance to, 35—36, 160—161
      structure of, 19
Hydroxyurethane, 18
Hypoxanthine
   analogs of, 145—155
      biochemical basis of resistance of, 147—150
      mechanism of cytotoxicity of, 146—147
      molecular mechanism of genetic variation in,
         150—152
      mutagenesis studies with, 152—154
   effect of adenine aminohydrolase on, 112
   effect of PNP on, 72
   effect on adenine, 80
   effect on DNA synthesis, 61
   effect on IMP, 180
   phosphoribosylation of, 66
   phosphorylation of, 62
   rate of formation of, 117
   structure of, 147
Hypoxanthine-amethopterin-thymidine (HAT)
      medium
   basis for, 60, 146
   growth in, 152, 155, 160, 162
   hmdUrd-resistant cells in, 163
   reversion rate measurement with, 153
   revertant isolation in, 154
   selection for HGPRT cells, 104
   sensitivity to, 150
   variation of, 120
Hypoxanthine-guanine-phosphoribosyltransferase
      (HGPRTase, HPRT)
   in Ado metabolism, 72
   decreased activity of, 147, 149
   deficiencies in, 83—84, 119, 176
   in deoxyguanosine metabolism, 76
   loci of, 104, 112, 150, 153
   loss of, 153, 155
   phosphoribosylation by, 66
   in purine nucleotide synthesis, 61
Hypoxanthine phosphoribosyltransferase, 248

## I

IdUMP, 162, 168
IdUrd, see 5-Iodo-2-deoxyuridine
IdUTP, 162
IMP, see Inosine 5'-monophosphate
IMP dehydrogenase, 61—65, 119—120, 255

IMPY, see 2,3-Dihydro-l-H-pyrazole 2,3-A
    imidazole
Inosine (Inox)
  in AE₁ cells, 77
  conversion of adenosine to, 70, 78, 135
  conversion of hypoxanthine to, 72
  conversion to guanine, 62
  effect of mycophenolic acid on, 65
  oxidized, 18
  structure of, 71
Inosine 5'-monophosphate (IMP)
  anabolism of, 147
  conversion of ATP to, 60
  conversion to GMP, 62—63
  conversion to AMP, 104
  deamination of AMP to, 80
  starvation of, 180
  synthesis of, 70
Inosine phosphorylase, 248
5'-Inosinic acid (PI-IMP), 18
Inosinic purines, 178
Inox, see Inosine
Interferon, 200—201
5-Iodo-2-deoxyuridine (IdUrd), 161—165, 168
5-Iodotubercidin, 93
3-Isobutyl-1-methylxanthine, 187
S-Isobutylthioadenosine, 79
Isoleucine, 226—227
Isoproterenol, 194, 196


**J**

J774.2 mutants, 200—201


**K**

Ka mutants, 195
KB/AraC cells, 176—177
Kinetin riboside (KR), 94—95, 102
Kin mutants, 192—196
KR, see Kinetin riboside


**L**

L1210 cells
  AG in, 147
  alanosine-resistant, 248
  cultured, 133
  effect of AG on, 146
  effect of Can on, 218
  effect of tiazofurin on, 255
  2-F-araA transport in, 129—132
  GTP levels in, 62—63
  isolates from, 5
  leukemic, 133—135
  melphalan-resistant, 228
  mRNA in, 91
L5178Y cells, 153, 248
LDL, see Low-density-lipoprotein
*Leishmania,* 92, 93
Lesch-Nyhan syndrome, 150, 152, 154

Leucine, 226—228
Leucyl-tRNA synthetase, 227
LHF cells, 23
Low-density-lipoprotein (LDL), 38
"L" system mutants, 226—228
"L" system transport, 213, 228


**M**

MAIQ, see 4-Methyl-5-amino-1-formylisoquinoline
    thiosemicarbazone
MAT, see Methionine adenosyltransferase
MDCK cell, 201
MeAIB, see 2-Methylaminoisobutyric acid
MeAPR, see 6-Methyl aminopurine riboside
Melphalan, 228
MeMPR, see 6-Methylmercaptopurine riboside
6-Mercaptoguanosine, 76
6-Mercaptopurine (MP)
  cross resistance to, 102, 119
  cytotoxicity of, 151
  mode of action of, 154
  phosphorylation by, 101
  structure of, 147
  studies with, 146
  toxic effects of, 149
Methasquin, 4
Methionine, 217
Methionine adenosyltransferase (MAT), 79, 213, 222
Methionine sulfoximine (Msx), 213, 216—217
Methotrexate (Mtx), 1—10
  alterations in transport of, 4—6
  cytotoxicity of, 2—3
  DHFR and, 3—7
  genetics of resistance of, 7—9
  polyglutamation defects in, 7
  purine synthesis blocking by, 60
  structural features of, 2
4-Methyl-5-amino-1-formylisoquinoline thiosemicar-
    bazone (MAIQ), 17, 20
2-Methylaminoisobutyric acid (MeAIB), 221, 225—
    226
6-Methyl aminopurine riboside (MeAPR), 90, 98
5-Methylcytosine, 80
3-O-Methyl-D-glucose (MG), 234—235, 243—245
5,10-Methylene THF synthetase, 6
Methylglyoxal bis(guanylhydrazone) (MGBG), 253
7-Methylguanine, 80
Methylmercaptopurine ribonucleoside (MMPR), 135
6-Methylmercaptopurine riboside (MeMPR), 90—
    92, 94—98, 100, 102
N-Methyl-N'-nitro-N-nitrosoguanidine (MNNG),
    32—33, 192, 227, 254
Methyl-N-nitroso guanidine, 244
α-Methylornithine (αMO), 47—50
6-Methylpurine, 119
5-Methyltetrahydrofolate, 36
5-Methyl THF, 5
Methylthioadenosine, 80, 112—113
6-Methylthiopurine ribonucleoside, 150
5-Methyluracil, 80

Metroprine (DDMP), 5, 7
αMFMO, see α-Monofluoromethylornithine
MG, see 3-O-Methyl-D-glucose
MgATP, 188—189
MGBG, see Methylglyoxal bis(guanylhydrazone)
MMPR, see Methylmercaptopurine ribonucleoside
MNNG, see *N*-Methyl-*N*′-nitro-*N*-nitrosoguanidine
αMO, see α-Methylornithine
α-Monofluoromethylornithine (αMFMO), 47
Mouse neuroblastoma cells, 65
MP, see 6-Mercaptopurine
Msx, see Methionine sulfoximine
Msx$^R$, 228
Mtx, see Methotrexate
Mtx-resistant cells, 3
Mutagenesis studies, 152—154
Mutants
    aphidicolin-resistant, 32—36
    CHO, 198—200, see also Chinese hamster ovary
        cells
    cross-resistance studies with, 101
    Dga-resistant, 234—237
    galactokinase activities in, 239—241
    immunological studies with, 100—101
    mycophenolic acid-resistant, 63—65
    S49, 194-197, see also S49 cells
    toyocamycin-resistant, 101—104
    variants of, 200—201
    Y1, 189—194
Myco-0 cells, 65
Myco-lA cells, 64—65
Mycophenolic acid, 59—67
    bacterial *Ecogpt* gene and, 65—67
    cellular effects of, 60—63
    mutant cell lines resistant to, 63—67
    structure of, 61
Myoblast cell lines, 21—22

**N**

NAD$^+$, 63, 92
NADH, 63
NBMPR, see Nitrobenzylthioinosine
dNDP, see Deoxyribonucleotides
rNDP, see Ribonucleotides
Nitrobenzylthioinosine (NBMPR), 77
NPS-ACTH, 193
NSU1 cells, 84
dNTPs, 30—32, 35, 37
Nucleic acid, 62—63, 133
Nucleoside-resistant mutants, 76—84
    of adenosine, 76—80
    of deoxyadenosine, 80—83
    of deoxyguanosine, 83—84
Nucleosides
    adenylic, 178
    analogs of, 90—94
    cross resistance to, 175—176
    metabolism of, 72—74
    toxicity of, 74—76
    transport of, 76—78, 80—81, 83

Nucleoside triphosphate, 168
Nucleotidase, 85, 149
Nucleotide pools, 35, 62—63, 201

**O**

ODC, see Ornithine decarboxylase
ODC cDNA, 53
ODC mRNA, 46, 50—54
OMP, see Orotidine-5′-monophosphate
Ornithine, 220—222
Ornithine analogs, 45—56
    chemical structures of, 41
    clinical uses of, 55
    effects on cells in culture, 48—49
    inhibition of, 196
    mammalian cells resistant to, 49—54
    mechanism of action of, 48
    regulation of ODC activity in, 54—55
    role of ODC, 46—47
Ornithine decarboxylase (ODC)
    activity of, 52—55
    in cancer therapy, 55
    inhibition of, 48—49, 55, 248, 250
    in Kin mutants, 193
    levels of, 51
    overproduction of, 53—54
    regulation of, 50
    role of, 46—47
    stimulation of, 198—199
    synthesis of, 53, 194
Orotate, 167
Orotate phosphoribosyltransferase, 165, 250
Orotidine decarboxylase, 93, 248
Orotidine-5′-monophosphate (OMP), 248—249
OS3 cells, 190—191

**P**

P388 cells, 146, 248, 255
P815 cells, 179
PAA, see Phosphonoacetic acid
PALA, see Phosphonoacetyl-L-aspartate
Papaverine, 188
Parasitic infections, 55
P5C, see Pyrroline-5-carboxylate synthetase
*Penicillium stoloniferum*, 60
PF, see Pyrazofurin
PFA, see Phosphonoformic acid
Phagocytosis, 200—201
Phenothiazines, 187
Phenotypes, 7, 9, 33—34
Phenylalanine, 226—227
Phosphodiesterase, 201
Phosphonoacetic acid (PAA), 34, 136
Phosphonoacetyl-L-aspartate (PALA), 253—254
Phosphonoformic acid (PFA), 254—255
Phosphoribosyl formylglycinamide, 118
Phosphoribosyl formylglycinamide synthetase, 250
Phosphoribosylpyrophosphate (PRPP)
    adenine sites of action and, 117

depletion of, 76
effect of Ado on, 74
effect of DAP on, 118
elevated levels of, 249
in guanine phosphoribosylation, 83
in hypoxanthine coversion, 147
in purine metabolism, 148
in purine nucleotide synthesis, 61
salvage synthesis of, 112
synthesis of, 113, 178
PI-IMP, see 5′-Inosinic acid
cis-Platinum, 176
*Pneumocystis carinii pneumonia,* 55
PNP, see Purine nucleotide phosphorylase
Polyamines, 46—49
Polyamine synthesis, 55, 91
Polyglutamation, 3, 7
Polymerase, 37—38
Probenecid, 188
Proline, 212, 220—222, 224—226
Prostaglandin E$_1$, 196—198, 200—201
Protein elevations, 23—24
Protein kinase, 186—202
  activated, 188
  cAMP-dependent, 186, 189—190, 197—202
  mutants of, 192—196, 201
Protein M1
  altered, 35
  analysis of, 24
  binding to, 16—17
  elevation of, 18
  regulation of, 23
  sensitivity of, 82
  as target for gossypol, 18
Protein M2
  analysis of, 24
  dimer formation by, 17
  elevation of, 18
  inactivation of, 18, 20
  overproduction of, 35
  regulation of, 16, 23
Protein overproduction
  by amino acid transport mutants, 224—228
  by aminoacyl-tRNA synthetase, 223—224
  by asparagine synthetase, 212—216
  by canavanine-resistant lines, 218—220
  by glutamine synthetase, 216—218
  by methionine adenosyl transferase, 222
  by pyrroline-5-caraboxylate synthetase, 220—222
Protein phosphotransferases, 188
PRPP, see Phosphoribosylpyrophosphate
PRPP aminotransferase, 60, 117
PRPP glutamine amidotransferase, 70
PRPP synthetase, 60, 63, 70, 113
Purine
  Ado as source for, 179
  analogs of, 114—115, 150
  auxotrophs of, 60
  biosynthesis of, 180
  cross resistance to, 119
  effect on mycophenolic acid, 61—62

inosinic, 178
  metabolism of, 70—72, 148
  as substrate for nucleoside transport, 76
Purine deoxyribonucleoside kinase, 130
Purine nucleoside analogs, 89—105
  AK$^-$ mutant selection, 104—105
  biochemical effects of, 90—94
  cellular resistance to, 94—104
    cross-resistance studies, 101
    immunological studies, 100—101
    mutants affected in adenosine kinase, 94—100
    mutants resistant to toyocamycin, 101—104
Purine nucleoside phosphorylate, 92
Purine nucleosides, 76—77, 83—84
Purine nucleotide formation, 117
Purine nucleotide phosphorylase (PNP), 70—73, 76, 84
Purine nucleotide synthesis, 62—65, 70, 250
Purine ribonucleoside, 102
Puromycin, 252
Putrescine, 46—50, 53—54
Pyrazofurin (PF), 90, 93—96, 98—102
Pyrazoloadenine (APP), 100, 102, 116—119
Pyrazolopyrimidine nucleosides, 90
Pyrazolopyrimidine ribosides, 105
Pyridoxal phosphate, 46
Pyridoxamine phosphate, 48
Pyrimethamine, 5, 7, 9
Pyrimidine deoxyribonucleotides, 75—76
Pyrimidine nucleosides, 76—77, 102—103
Pyrimidine phosphoribosyltransferase, 168
Pyrimidine ribonucleosides, 76
Pyrimidine ribonucleoside triphosphate, 63
Pyrimidines
  biosynthesis of, 74—75, 78
  derivatives of, 101
  halogenated and other 5-position, 159—169
    5-bromo-2′-deoxyuridine, 160—162
    5-fluorouracil, 165—166
    5-hyroxymethyl-2′-deoxyuridine, 166—168
    5-iodo-2′-deoxyuridine, 162—165
  metabolism of, 173
Pyrroline-5-carboxylate (P5C) synthetase, 213, 220—222
Pyrrolopyrimidine nucleosides, 90, 105

**R**

Ribavirin (virazole), 64—65, 94—95, 102
Ribonucleotide reductase
  affinity for araATP, 136
  allosteric effectors of, 17
  altered, 23—24, 82—84, 134, 136
  effect of araATP on, 132
  effect of deoxyGTP on, 76
  effect of PFA on, 254
  effect on deoxynucleotide supply, 174
  hypersensitivity of, 20
  increased activity of, 21
  increased level of, 35
  inhibitors of

dATP as, 178
  cellular properties of, 16—18
  BrdUrd as, 160—162, 168
  chemical structure of, 19
  deoxyadenosine toxicity and, 75
  DNA synthesis and, 137
  gossypol as, 20
  hydroxyurea as, 160—161
  introduction to, 16
  mutations of, 80
  reduction by, 17, 166
  role in nucleoside resistance, 175—176
  as site of action for hydroxyurea, 22
  subunits of, 25
Ribonucleotides (rNDP), 17, 65
Ribose-1-phosphate, 71, 135
Ribose-5-phosphate, 60, 70
RNA
  AG in, 147
  effect of nucleoside analogs on, 90—94
  2-F-araA in, 133
  FUra in, 166, 168
  methylation of, 91
  polyadenylated, 92
  production of, 216
  purines in, 146
  synthesis of, 2, 218
mRNA
  ADA deaminase, 135
  AS, 219—220
  effect of ADA on, 78
  from mutant cells, 192
  for HPRT, 152
  increase in, 215
  in L1210 cells, 91—92
  levels of, 53, 223
  M1 and M2, 24—25
  ODC, 46, 50—54
  α subunit of, 197
  transcription of, 225, 251
rRNA, 90
tRNA, 80, 91, 227

**S**

S49 cells
  AMP deaminase-deficient, 79
  cAMP-resistant, 186
  araA accumulation in, 129
  deoxyadenosine phosphorylation in, 81—82
  deoxycytidine kinase-deficient, 84
  dexamethasone-resistant, 250—251
  GMP levels in, 63
  GTP levels in, 62—63
  mutants of, 64—65, 77, 194—199
  nucleoside transport-deficient clones in, 80
  ODC activity of, 52
*Saccharomyces cerevisae,* 114
SAH, see S-Adenosylhomocysteine
SAH hydrolase, see S-Adenosylhomocysteine
  hydrolase

SAICAR synthetase, 248
SAM, see S-Adenosylmethionine
SAM decarboxylase, 46, 50
SAM synthetase, 85
Sangivamycin, 90—91, 102—105
SC2 mouse cells, 20, 23
SCID, see Severe combined immunodeficiency
  disease
Serine, 226
Serine hydroxymethyl transferase, 6
Severe combined immunodeficiency disease (SCID),
  70—71
Sodium butyrate, 199—200
Sodium fluoride, 197, 200
Somatic cell hybrid analysis, 9
Spermidine, 46—50, 54—55, 253
Spermidine synthetase, 55
Spermine, 46—49, 253
Spermine synthetase, 55
Steroidogenesis, 194
*Streptomyces,* 90
Sulfate transport, 250
Sutherland's Second Messenger Hypothesis, 186

**T**

T cells, 71, 76, 81—85
TCN, see Tricyclic nucleoside
12-O-Tetradecanoylphorbol-13-acetate (TPA), 193—
  196, 199
Tetrahydrofolate (THF), 2, 66
TG, see 6-Thioguanine
dThd, see Thymidine
Theophylline, 187—188
THF, see Tetrahydrofolate
6-Thioguanine (TG)
  AK mutants and, 103
  cytotoxicity of, 151
  effect on cloning ability, 149
  phosphorylation of, 101
  resistance to, 120, 151—154
  selectivity efficiency of, 150
  structure of, 147
  studies with, 146
  toxic effects of, 149
6-Thioguanosine, 76, 103, 151
Thiopurines, 147
Thiosemicarbazones, 17
Threonine, 224
Threonyl-rRNA synthetase (ThRS), 224
ThRS, see Threonyl-rRNA synthetase
Thymidine (dThd)
  cross resistance to, 172—175
  deprivation of, 177
  effect on dCyd-AraCyt kinase deficient cells, 176
  effect on IMP, 66
  excess, 35—36, 136
  sensitivity to, 79
  suppression of toxicity by, 167
Thymidine kinase, 160, 162—163, 165, 196
Thymidine phosphorylase, 168

Thymidine synthetase, 6—7
Thymidylate, 2
Thymidylate kinase, 162, 168
Thymidylate synthetase, 3, 35—36, 165—168
Tiazofurin, 96, 255
dTMP, 162, 168
TMQ, see Trimetrexate
Toyocamycin, 90—91, 94—98, 100—105
Toy$^r$ cells, 101—104
TPA, see 12-O-Tetradecanoylphorbol-13-acetate
Transglutaminase, 198—199
Triamcinolone, 252
Triazinate, 7
Triazines, 4
Tricyclic nucleoside (TCN), 90—91, 94—95, 102—103
Trifluoperazine, 187
Trimetrexate (TMQ), 5, 7
Trypanosomiasis, 55
TTP, 63, 84
dTTP
    accumulation of, 162
    as araATP substrate, 132
    binding of, 17
    endogenous production of, 174
    excess, 173
    Km for, 34
    pools of, 175
    reduction of GDP and ADP by, 16
ddTTP, 37, 167
Tubercidin (7-deazaadenosine)
    cross resistance to, 96, 102—103, 135
    dose response curves of, 97—98
    resistance to, 76, 94—95, 100, 105
    structure of, 91
[$^3$H]Tubercidin, 99, 103
Tubercidin nucleotides, 90
TyrOH$^R$ cells, 223—224
Tyrosine aminotransferase, 50
Tyrosinol, 223—224
TyrRS, 223—224

**U**

UDP, 16, 36, 166, 174, 252
dUDP, 16, 252
UDP-Gal, 234
Ultraviolet light (UV), 8, 32—33, 36—38, 104—105
UMP, see Uridine monophosphate
dUMP, 166, 167
hmdUMP, 168
Uracil-DNA glycosylase, 165
hmUra, see 5-Hydroxymethyuracil
Urd, see Uridine
hmdUrd see 5-Hydroxymethyl-2'-deoxyuridine

Uridine (Urd), 77—78, 104, 167, 178
Uridine kinase, 165—166, 248
Uridine monophosphate (UMP), 248
UTP, 63, 74, 165, 174
hmdUTP, 164—165, 167
UV, see Ultraviolet light

**V**

Vaccinia, 33—34
Valine, 226—227
V79 cells
    AK$^+$, 105
    aphidicolin-resistant, 136
    aphidicolin-sensitive, 33
    aphidicolin-treated, 30
    BrUTP in, 162
    chromate-resistant, 250
    CTP levels in, 165
    CTPS mutants of, 36
    effect of thymidine on, 166
    galactokinase activity in, 241
    galK in, 245
    hmdUrd-resistant, 163, 165, 167
    hmUra generation in, 164
    mutants of, 98
    mutation rate for, 238—239
    mycophenolic acid-resistant, 64
    wild-type, 236—237
V$_{max}$ mutants, 195, 226, 238
Vinblastine, 194, 251
Vincristine, 176
Virazole, see Ribavarin

**W**

WI-L2 cells, 81, 133
WT cells, 99—100

**X**

Xanthine, 61—62, 66, 147
Xanthine-guanine-phosphoribosyltransferase, 61—62, 65—66
Xanthine oxidase, 72, 112, 118
Xanthosine, 62
Xanthosine 5'-monophosphate (XMP), 60, 63, 66
XMP, see Xanthosine 5'-monophosphate
X-rays, 37, 153

**Y**

Y1 cells, 186, 189—194, 199
Y6 cells, 190—191